MYXOMATOSIS

MYXOMATOSIS

A History of Pest Control and the Rabbit

PETER W. J. BARTRIP

Tauris Academic Studies
LONDON • NEW YORK

Published in 2008 by Tauris Academic Studies,
an imprint of I.B.Tauris & Co Ltd
6 Salem Road, London W2 4BU
175 Fifth Avenue, New York NY 10010
www.ibtauris.com

In the United States of America and Canada distributed by
Palgrave Macmillan, a division of St. Martin's Press
175 Fifth Avenue, New York NY 10010

ISBN: 978 1 84511 572 2

A full CIP record for this book is available from the British Library
A full CIP record for this book is available from the Library of Congress

Library of Congress catalog card: available

Printed and bound in Great Britain by CPI Antony Rowe, Chippenham
from camera-ready copy edited and supplied by
Oxford Publishing Services, Oxford

Contents

List of Tables
and Illustrations

List of Abbreviations

ACRC	advisory committee on rabbit clearance
ACROLP	Advisory Committee on Rabbits and other Land Pests
AEC	Agricultural Executive Committee
AI	Avian Influenza
AHT	Animal Health Trust
ARC	Agricultural Research Council
BAF	Board of Agriculture and Fisheries
BAP	Bureau of Animal Population
BBC	British Broadcasting Corporation
BFAWS	British Federation of Animal Welfare Societies
BSc	Bachelor of Science
BSE	Bovine Spongiform Encephalopathy
BTO	British Trust for Ornithology
BVA	British Veterinary Association
CAEC	County Agricultural Executive Committee
CJD	Creutzfeldt-Jakob Disease
CLA	Country Landowners' Association
CSIR	Council for Scientific and Industrial Research (till 1949)
CSIRO	Commonwealth Scientific and Industrial Research Organization (from 1949)
CSVO	Chief Superintending Veterinary Officer
CVO	Chief Veterinary Officer
DAS	Department of Agriculture Scotland
DCVO	Deputy Chief Veterinary Officer
DORA	Defence of the Realm Act
DSc	Doctor of Science

DVO	Divisional Veterinary Officer
DVSM	Diploma in Veterinary State Medicine
FMD	foot and mouth disease
FRCP	Fellow of the Royal College of Physicians
FRS	Fellow of the Royal Society
FRSE	Fellow of the Royal Society of Edinburgh
HO	Home Office
ICD	Infestation Control Division
ICI	Imperial Chemical Industries
LPAC	Land Pests Advisory Committee
MA	Master of Arts
MAC	Myxomatosis Advisory Committee
MAF	Ministry of Agriculture and Fisheries (till October 1954)
MAFF	Ministry of Agriculture, Fisheries and Food (from October 1954)
MC	Military Cross
MD	Doctor of Medicine
MIRD	myxomatosis-induced rabbit depopulation
MRC	Medical Research Council
MRCVS	Member of the Royal College of Veterinary Surgeons
MSBI	Mammal Society of the British Isles
NA	National Archives
NAS	National Archives of Scotland
NATO	North Atlantic Treaty Organization
NC	Nature Conservancy
NFU	National Farmers' Union
NFUS	National Farmers' Union Scotland
NSW	New South Wales
NUAW	National Union of Agricultural Workers
PHLS	Public Health Laboratory Service
PP	*Parliamentary Papers*
PREM	Premier

P&J	*Press and Journal*
QC	Queen's Counsel
QJF	*Quarterly Journal of Forestry*
RCA	Rabbit Clearance Areas
RCC	Rabbit Clearance Committee
RCS	Rabbit Clearance Society
RCVS	Royal College of Veterinary Surgeons
RPO	regional pest officer
RSPCA	Royal Society for the Prevention of Cruelty to Animals
ScD	Doctor of Science
SHAC	Stop Huntingdon Animal Cruelty
SLF	Scottish Landowners' Federation
SPCA	Society for the Prevention of Cruelty to Animals
SR&O	Statutory Rules & Orders
SSSI	Site(s) of Special Scientific Interest
SVO	Superintending Veterinary Officer
SWN	*Southern Weekly News*
TGWU	Transport and General Workers' Union
TUC	Trades Union Congress
UFAW	Universities Federation for Animal Welfare
ULAWS	University of London Animal Welfare Society
VO	Veterinary Officer
WAEC	War Agricultural Executive Committee

Acknowledgements

I am delighted to acknowledge the financial support of the Wellcome Trust (History of Medicine Section) in the form of generous Research Expenses and Research Leave Awards covering the period 2003–2006. Without these awards this book would not have been written. I acknowledge also a period of research leave granted by the University of Northampton which helped me to get my project up and running. The following people graciously granted me interviews and permission to quote their words: Lord Carrington, Mrs Georgina Coleby (née Ottaway), Cyril Skinner and Stuart Wicks. I much appreciate their assistance. I am grateful to the curators, archivists, librarians and other staff of the Bodleian Library (especially the Radcliffe Science Library), BBC Research Central, BBC Written Archives Centre, British Library National Sound Archives, British Newspaper Library, National Archives, National Archives of Scotland, Museum of English Rural Life (particularly Caroline Benson for her help with illustrations), Christopher Reed of the RSPCA Archives, Jane Thornton Higgs, curator of the Eden Valley Museum and Tony Mutimer-Still. The editors of the *Edenbridge Chronicle* and the *Kent and Sussex Courier* kindly printed appeals for information from people who remembered or were involved in the first myxomatosis outbreak. John Sheail generously allowed me a pre-publication view of his paper 'Wartime rodent-control in England and Wales' in B. Short et al. (eds), *The Frontline of Freedom: British Agriculture in the Second World War* (*Agricultural History Review* supplement 4: BAHS, 2007). Steve King and John Stewart were good enough to read my manuscript – for which, many thanks. I am grateful too to Denis Galligan, Director of the Centre for Socio-Legal Studies, the University of Oxford, for according me associate research fellow status and providing me with office space. 'Myxomatosis' by Philip Larkin is reprinted from *The Less Deceived* by kind permission of The Marvell Press, England and Australia. For permission to reproduce illustrations I am grateful to the British Library, the Museum of English Rural Life, Newsquest and the *Press and Journal* (Aberdeen).

Peter Bartrip
March 2007

Chapter 1

Before Bough Beech

A New Disease?

In September 1953 a number of dead rabbits were found on Major Williams's Bough Beech estate near Edenbridge in Kent. Early indications suggested syphilis. A month later, on 13 October, it was confirmed that further rabbit deaths on the estate had actually been caused by myxomatosis.[1] A disease hitherto unknown in England, except in the context of scientific investigation, had reached the United Kingdom. Soon myxomatosis was breaking out elsewhere, initially in Kent and Sussex, but before long in other counties. Within a short time, but also *for* a short time, myxomatosis virtually eliminated the wild rabbit from Great Britain.

When myxomatosis was discovered at Bough Beech it was not a new disease; in fact, by October 1953 it had been rampaging through France for over a year and across other parts of continental Europe for a somewhat shorter period. Since 1950 it had been present among the wild rabbit population of Australia – to devastating effect from 1951. It had first been reported among laboratory animals in Uruguay as long ago as the 1890s. In October 1953 myxomatosis was not even new to Britain, for experiments with it as a potential means of rabbit control date back to the early 1930s. Furthermore, beginning in June 1952, staff at the North of Scotland College of Agriculture tried to exterminate rabbits on the Heisker (Monach) Islands in the Hebrides using myxomatosis virus.[2] Neither was the appearance of the disease in England in October 1953 altogether unexpected. In view of its presence in northern France many observers, whether they welcomed or dreaded the prospect, considered that its arrival in Britain was 'inevitable'.

So what is myxomatosis and what was its history before it was spotted at Bough Beech? Myxomatosis is a highly infectious, sub-cutaneous, viral pox disease. It was actually the second animal virus known to science, the first being foot and mouth.[3] For years myxomatosis was thought to spread mainly by contact. Since the 1940s, however, it has been known that blood-sucking insects, principally mosquitoes and fleas, serve as vectors. The significance of transmission via these vectors was fully appreciated in the early 1950s. Although hares are very occasionally affected, the disease is virtually confined to rabbits. Rabbits native to the Americas can contract it, but they are only mildly affected and do not develop generalized myxomatosis. The European wild rabbit (*oryctolagus cuniculus*), on the other hand, is highly susceptible, as are their domesticated or laboratory counterparts, all of which belong to the *oryctolagus* genus.[4]

Once the virus has entered a rabbit's bloodstream, it multiplies and spreads rapidly. The incubation period is usually about five or six days. Symptoms include swellings, mainly on the head and around the genitals and anus; mucous discharge, especially from the eyes; and 'general dopeyness'. Facial swelling can be severe enough to distort features, cause blindness and create difficulty in feeding and drinking. If an infected wild rabbit does not die on the roads or in the jaws of a predator, it is likely to succumb to secondary lung infection about eight days after the incubation period or 10–14 days after initial infection. Infected domestic rabbits often survive for longer periods or have a better recovery rate as a result of the care given by owners. Where a virulent strain of the virus is present the mortality rate can exceed 99 per cent. Vaccination with Shope fibroma virus can provide temporary protection.[5]

Hilda Kean states that myxomatosis was 'developed by scientists during the [Second World] war as a way of "containing" the wild rabbit population.' She goes on to say that parliament discussed the prospect of introducing it in Britain in 1951 but was 'forced to reject this option in the face of public outrage'.[6] None of this is true. The disease was not developed by scientists either in the war or at any other time. It was a naturally-occurring virus against which the European wild rabbit had no resistance. It was first described by Guiseppe Sanarelli (1864–1940), who coined the name *myxomatosis cuniculi*. He encountered the disease when it broke out with devastating effect, though 'without obvious reason', among laboratory rabbits in the Institute of Hygiene, Montevideo in 1896. Every infected rabbit died of the disease within a few days of showing any symptoms and Sanarelli reported his findings in 'Das Myxomatogene Virus' (*Zentralblatt für Bakteriologie und Parasitenkunde*, 23 (1898) 865).[7]

Sanarelli was born in Monte San Savino, Italy, in April 1864. He graduated in medicine and surgery from the University of Siena in 1889 before continuing his studies at the Pasteur Institute in Paris. In 1893 he became professor of hygiene at his Alma Mater. After two years he accepted an invitation from the Uruguayan government to establish an institute of experimental hygiene at the University of Montevideo, where he remained until 1898. He then returned to Italy, occupying chairs in hygiene first at the University of Bologna, then the University of Rome, where he remained until 1935. Sanarelli published important work on various diseases, including cholera, tuberculosis, typhoid and yellow fever, registering 'firsts' in several fields. Surprisingly, *Morton's Medical Bibliography* does not mention his discovery of myxomatosis as a disease of rabbits, though it does refer to his claim for priority in observing Shwartzman phenomenon (a type of vasculitis or inflammation of a blood vessel).[8]

In the decade or so following Sanarelli's initial report, myxomatosis appeared among hutch rabbits in other South American cities, including Rio de Janeiro and São Paolo. At the end of the 1920s G. M. Findlay, of the Imperial Cancer Research Fund in London, noted that the disease was 'restricted to certain countries of South America – the Argentine, Brazil and Uruguay.'[9] Perhaps because it affected only laboratory rabbits at isolated locations on one continent, myxomatosis was little studied until the 1930s, by which time the first outbreaks outside South America, in 'rabbitries' in the Santa Barbara, Ventura and San Diego areas of California, had occurred.[10] As Thomas Rivers noted in 1930: 'Since Sanarelli's original communication only ten papers ... dealing with infectious myxoma of rabbits have appeared.'[11] Few of these were published in English language journals.[12] There was, furthermore, considerable disagreement between different authors about the nature of the virus and the disease, including, indeed, about whether there was more than one virus or different strains of the same virus.[13]

The Australian Connection

In 1919 the Brazilian researcher, Dr Henrique Beaurepaire Aragão, was the first person to suggest the potential of myxomatosis as a means of controlling rabbits in countries such as Australia where they had become serious agricultural pests.[14] The rabbit was not, of course, native to Australia. A few domesticated animals arrived with the first fleet in 1788, and further consignments soon followed. An attempt to establish a warren was made at Parramatta in 1806 and wild rabbits were introduced in Tasmania in the 1820s. Notwithstanding that they damaged vegetation, 24 more were introduced to Barwon Park near Geelong, Victoria, in 1859. Their progeny spread rapidly and before long the rabbit had taken 'possession of Australia as if he were the conqueror of the country'. It spoiled crops, consumed indigenous flora, and cost millions of pounds in lost agricultural output, soil erosion and pest control measures (including the notorious and ineffective rabbit-proof fence, which, from 1907, crossed the country from north to south).[15] By 1913 W. E. Abbott was writing about the rabbit plague that had 'cost our Governments many millions of pounds and our Pastoralists and Farmers so much that the sum is incalculable'.[16] By the 1930s David Stead, sometime 'Special Rabbit Menace Commissioner' to the government of New South Wales (NSW), could write of a pest that had prospered to such a degree that it threatened 'literally to engulf the nation's most vital national industries' and doom the entire countryside to a disaster of 'gigantic proportions'.[17]

As early as the 1880s the NSW government offered financial incentives to anyone who could rid the colony of the invaders' unwelcome presence. Pasteur's attention was attracted but proposals to experiment with chicken cholera came to nothing because the Australian authorities refused to allow the great man's nephew to import the bacillus.[18] When, nearly 40 years later Aragão made his suggestion, he went so far as to send a sample of the virus. Aragão's proposal, though given serious scientific consideration, was not adopted. Agriculturalists were keen; elsewhere, however, there were misgivings that the disease might not cause a large and protracted epidemic leading to the wholesale destruction of rabbits. Some doubted whether public opinion would countenance the extermination of rabbits by biological means. Others questioned the wisdom of elimination given the value of rabbits as food.[19] In the 1920s Aragão sent further virus samples, this time to the NSW Department of Agriculture for trial and in 1927 experiments on transmissibility and specificity were carried out at the department's veterinary research station in Glenfield. H. C. White reported the results in his 'Observations on rabbit myxoma' in the 1927–28 annual report of NSW's director of veterinary research. The station's director, H. R. Seddon, doubted whether the disease would either eliminate an entire colony or spread from one colony to another. He also stressed the need for reassurance that myxomatosis would not spread to other species.[20]

Then, in 1933, at the request of Australia's Council for Scientific and Industrial Research (CSIR, and from 1949 the Commonwealth Scientific and Industrial Research Organization, CSIRO), the physiologist and pathologist Sir Charles Martin began to investigate the potential of myxomatosis as a biological weapon against rabbits. The inception of this project owed much to the inspiration, enthusiasm and drive of Dr Jean Macnamara, an Australian paediatrician with a special interest in poliomyelitis. In 1933, while holding a Rockefeller Foundation travel scholarship in the United States, she met Dr Richard Shope of Princeton University, New Jersey. Following the myxomatosis outbreaks among domesticated rabbits in California, Shope was working on the development of a vaccine and Macnamara saw diseased rabbits in his laboratory. She had no previous knowledge of myxomatosis and was unaware of the attention her compatriots had already devoted to it. She was, however, quick to recognize that the disease might provide a solution to Australia's rabbit problem. She used her extensive and high-level network of personal and professional contacts to press for an investigation. At the request of the Australian high commissioner in London, she drew up a memorandum that led to Martin's enquiry. She even travelled to Cambridge at her own expense to discuss the project with Martin.[21]

London-born Charles James Martin (1866–1955) took up a post in

Australia as demonstrator in physiology at the University of Sydney in 1891, soon after he qualified in medicine. Following a spell as lecturer, then professor, of physiology at Melbourne University he returned to Britain, first as director of the Lister Institute of Preventative Medicine, later as professor of experimental pathology at London University. He served as a pathologist with Australian forces on the Greek island of Limnos during the First World War and received a knighthood in 1927. After retiring from his London chair, in 1930, Martin returned to Australia, at the invitation of the CSIR, to direct its nutrition division at the University of Adelaide, where he was appointed professor of biochemistry and general physiology. Following his relocation to the UK in 1933, he carried out research on myxomatosis at Cambridge University's Institute of Animal Pathology. By conducting his work in Britain Martin avoided Australia's strict quarantine regulations. He reported his findings in the institute's fourth annual report (1934–35) and, in more or less the same form, in a CSIR bulletin.[22]

Martin considered that if a pathogenic microbe was to be used as a biological control it had to possess certain characteristics 'to the highest degree'. First, it would have to produce a disease sufficiently infectious to spread through an entire population. Second, the virulence of the disease would have to be such that few animals would survive as the basis of a resistant population. Third, those animals that recovered from the disease should be incapable of conferring disease-resistance on their progeny. Fourth, the disease would have to be specific to the animal for which it was intended. Fifth, the microbe would have to be easy to store, propagate and apply.[23]

Martin tested the virus on tame and wild rabbits housed in cages and compounds. He knew that most reports on myxomatosis referred to the disease's 'extreme infectiousness'. Thus, he cited Findlay's observation that 'even in a large airy room it is difficult to avoid infecting other rabbits'.[24] Martin's conclusions were slightly different, however. He found it difficult to transmit the disease except when the animals were in close contact. He could not demonstrate that flies spread it and generally had little to say about the role of other insects as possible vectors. He did find myxomatosis 'an unusually fatal disease', indeed, one with 'an extraordinarily high fatality for a naturally-contracted infection'. However, an entire population was 'seldom' wiped out and those few rabbits that did survive acquired a 'solid' degree of immunity from further attack. Gradually, therefore, a population capable of resisting the disease came into existence. More positively, in terms of rabbit control, this population appeared incapable of conferring sufficient immunity to their offspring 'to militate against the effectiveness of myxomatosis as an agent for the destruction of rabbits'.[25] Also positive was the 'highly specific' nature of myxomatosis. Not only was it confined to rabbits, but also the European wild rabbit (the species present in Australasia) and its domesticated relatives in Europe, North America and elsewhere, appeared to be uniquely susceptible.[26]

From his researches Martin concluded that the myxomatosis virus possessed in abundance the characteristics necessary to exterminate 'rabbits in a circumscribed area'. Beyond this the possibilities were less certain: 'the readiness with which the infection will spread to colonies in the neighbourhood depends not on the virus but upon the amount of intercourse between the animals of … separated colonies.'[27] In his CSIR paper he recommended 'field experiments on an insulated area in Australia'. If these succeeded he felt it would then be necessary to develop 'an appropriate scientific organization, such as was found to be necessary for the control of the prickly-pear'.[28]

Meanwhile, Martin sought an isolated location in the UK where he could conduct a large-scale field experiment. In 1936 he asked the naturalist and farmer, Ronald Lockley, for permission to introduce myxomatosis to the island of Skokholm, Pembrokeshire. Lockley, who for years had been attempting to clear the 240-acre island of its thousands of rabbits in order to preserve the pasture for his sheep, consented. In September he and Martin marked and then released 83 infected rabbits at locations across the island. Although 12 of the animals were found dead soon afterwards, no other impact was observed by the time the island had to be evacuated for the winter a few weeks later. When 'the island was visited in the following spring, there was no trace of the disease in a population that seemed as numerous as ever'. The following summer, 55 infected rabbits were released. On this occasion fatalities occurred among introduced and native animals but by September the disease appeared to have died out 'with no obvious effect on the numbers of rabbits'. A third attempt, in spring 1938, involving the inoculation with myxomatosis of seven rabbits in one warren, also petered out following some deaths but without exterminating the warren. Lockley speculated that the tendency of sick rabbits to isolate themselves in the open during the contagious period was responsible for the failure of the disease to take hold. In fact, as was subsequently discovered, the experiment failed because of Skokholm's lack of suitable insect vectors. Broadly similar experiments in Denmark in the 1930s produced similarly disappointing results, with the disease dying out in fairly short order.[29] In 1936 a former diplomat who appeared as a witness before a British select committee on agriculture (rabbit damage) referred to these Danish experiments but hesitated to recommend myxomatosis as a means of rabbit control in Britain. He thought the disease sounded 'very unpleasant' and considered that rabbits already had more inhumanity practised on them than 'any other animal in the country'.[30]

Martin was apparently so disappointed by the failure of the Skokholm experiments that he 'more or less retired from this field of research soon after'.[31] His work was taken forward in Australia by Dr L. B. Bull, deputy chief of the animal health division at CSIR. Once the chief quarantine officer had granted permission to import the virus he tested the susceptibility to myxomatosis of various domesticated, laboratory and native animals in strictly enclosed conditions. The main objective was to establish whether the disease was specific to rabbits, though Bull's research was also important in demonstrating the importance of blood-sucking insects as disease vectors. The strain of virus used was of South American origin, though obtained from the Rockefeller Institute for Medical Research in the USA. Animals tested included sheep, pigs, dogs, cats, guinea pigs, ferrets, wallabies, wombats, cockatoos and bats. In no instance did a tested animal contract the disease.[32] As Fenner and Fantini point out, since little was then known about the mutability of viruses, the possibility that the myxomatosis virus could mutate and then affect supposedly insusceptible animals, perhaps even humans, apparently received no consideration.[33] As it was, the way appeared clear for field trials.

The trials took place at a number of remote locations, the first being Wardang Island, in the Spencer Gulf, South Australia, in late 1937. Although 238 rabbits died, approximately half of those on the island when the disease was introduced, the outbreak petered out after a few months. Follow-up trials in 1938–39 produced more deaths but, because of the rabbit's tremendous reproductive capacity, little or no net reduction in the total population. Overall, the experiments 'failed to show that extermination by means of this epizootic was possible'.[34] In 1941, far better results were achieved at Point Pearce, on the Yorke Peninsula of the South Australia mainland, where most of the rabbits were infested either naturally or artificially with native stick flea. Over a 60-day period all but 17 of 500 rabbits in 13 warrens died. This outcome suggested to Bull that in some locations myxomatosis might be useful in rabbit control provided insect vectors were available. Further trials at Mount Victor, Koonamore and Melton took place in 1942. Some successes were achieved but overall the results were not especially encouraging, the main problems being the tendency for the disease to run its course and die out and the capacity of the rabbit rapidly to repopulate.[35] Bull and his co-author wrote in 1944:

> The general results of the study, and especially those of the field experiments and field trials, show that myxomatosis cannot be used to control rabbit populations under the most natural conditions in Australia with any promise of success. Nevertheless, it seems possible that in some parts of Australia under special conditions, including the presence of insect vectors in abundance and the absence of predatory animals, the disease could be used with some promise of temporary control of a rabbit population.[36]

Fenner and Fantini have observed that 'Bull's extreme pessimism is difficult to understand' given his knowledge that insect vectors were capable of spreading myxomatosis and that under suitable conditions mosquitoes could transmit it from one colony to another.[37] Nevertheless, this pessimism, which influenced some of Bull's colleagues such as Francis Ratcliffe, the officer-in-charge of CSIRO's newly-established wildlife survey section, probably inhibited further experimentation. Other factors also played their part. Among these, 'wartime and immediately postwar conditions' and 'the rather illogical aversion of health authorities to allow field studies of the virus in any but sparsely populated areas' loomed large. With traditional control measures neglected during the war years, rabbits prospered mightily. In the early 1950s one observer estimated that Australia held up to three billion of them.[38]

Further field trials commenced only after Dame (as she now was) Jean Macnamara ruffled CSIRO feathers by suggesting that previous experiments had been 'pathetically limited', not least because the virus had never been tested in a fertile region. Although these accusations stung CSIRO personnel, and precipitated acrimonious correspondence in the Australian press, they also prompted reflection, reassessment and recognition that the virus should be tested in 'good country'.[39] In January 1950 new trials commenced, this time in higher rainfall and relatively prosperous though remote agricultural land on the borders of NSW and Victoria. The familiar pattern was observed. A few local outbreaks of the disease occurred, but by the end of November, when the field workers returned to Canberra, results were 'thoroughly disappointing in that the infection failed to spread effectively even within the warren colonies into which it was introduced'.[40]

Within a few weeks, however, reports began to reach Canberra that hundreds of rabbits were dying in the locality of the experiments. This development, as the eminent virologist Macfarlane Burnet later wrote, made 'front page news for Australia and everyone in the country was on the lookout for sick rabbits'. The disease spread rapidly northwards across NSW and northwest towards the arid interior; the coastal fringes of the southeast were, however, little affected. By the end of summer, that is early in 1951, it had reached southern Queensland. Yet even within affected areas its spread was patchy. Along watercourses and in the vicinity of lakes and temporary pools rabbits died in large numbers; elsewhere they continued to prosper. Various theories about mode of transmission were put forward. Mostly these pointed to the involvement of two species of mosquito; their significance as vectors explained the clustering of the disease in areas where surface water was present.[41]

With the arrival of winter the occurrence of the disease subsided, though without disappearing altogether. With the coming of spring arrangements were made to spread the disease artificially. Burnet later recalled his experience:

> In October [1951] I spent a night in a country hotel in Northern Victoria and was intrigued to read a notice: 'An officer of the Lands Department will attend at the stock-yards on Tuesday next to inoculate rabbits with myxomatosis. Landowners should bring 10–20 live rabbits.' That sort of thing went on over most of Southeastern Australia. In retrospect it is hard to be sure that the inoculations made any significant difference in the result.[42]

In fact, as early as February 1951 CSIRO was disseminating detailed instructions on 'How to Spread Myxomatosis'.[43] In the course of the year serious outbreaks recurred, including in arid areas. In a lecture delivered in October 1952 Burnet stated that it was 'impossible to say how many rabbits were killed'. With the mortality rate as high as 99.5 per cent in some localities, he estimated that between 25 and 50 per cent of Australia's rabbit population, 'perhaps three or four hundred million rabbits' had been killed.[44] As Fenner and Fantini point out, '33 years after Aragão had first made the suggestion that myxomatosis should be used to control rabbits in Australia, myxomatosis had been demonstrated to be a highly effective means of biological control.'[45]

The subsequent history of myxomatosis in Australia is covered at length elsewhere, most recently and comprehensively by Fenner and Fantini. Since this history is beyond the scope of the present study it will not be considered further here. Instead, the focus will switch to the arrival and pre-Bough Beech history of myxomatosis in Europe. Before leaving Australia, however, it is well to note that until 1951 and the myxomatosis epizootic, the moral dimension was largely absent from discussions about the potential of myxomatosis as a biological control. Such considerations did not arise until serious outbreaks of the disease occurred. Earlier reluctance to introduce myxomatosis centred on concerns about the wisdom of importing and liberating a virulent micro-organism hitherto absent from Australia (except under conditions of strict quarantine), the specificity of the disease, and its potential to solve the rabbit problem either in the short or long terms. Once the disease was epizootic, questions about cruelty did arise and it was suggested that the RSPCA was considering legal action against CSIRO. In the event no prosecutions occurred and ethical objections never loomed large. As Fenner and Fantini point out, 'the economic and ecological cost of rabbit infestations in Australia outweighed ethical sensitivities'. There was more concern about the public health and water pollution threats posed by millions of dead and decomposing rabbits. In addition, an outbreak of human encephalitis in the Murray Valley created public and press fears about a link with myxomatosis. In an effort to allay such worries three leading Australian scientists volunteered to be inoculated with the myxomatosis virus in order to demonstrate human immunity to the disease.[46]

It should also be noted that Australian agriculture, at least in the short term, flourished in the virtual absence of the rabbit. In 1953 *The Times* reported Australia's minister for external affairs' statement about 'a remarkable increase in the carrying capacity of ... pastures. ... If the gains made in the past three years were maintained, Australia's stock-carrying capacity would be increased by tens of millions and the value of the wool clip by many millions of pounds.' Quantification of economic gains attributable to myxomatosis is problematic, not least because of the difficulty of distinguishing between the influence of the epizootic and that of the weather (conditions in 1952–53 were generally favourable to farming). Furthermore, different sources provide different figures and different comparisons. Lockley states: 'It is estimated that the increase of agricultural production since the success of myxomatosis in the southeastern States of Australia, has been worth some £50,000,000 annually.' Rolls notes that 'Australia's annual wool clip increased suddenly by 70,000,000 lbs.' Both these figures were regularly cited in the press. For its part, Australia's Bureau of Agricultural Economics assessed the value of increased sheep production in 1952–53 alone to be £34 million, excluding savings made

on rabbit control.[47] Whatever the exact amount, myxomatosis produced significant financial benefits for Australian agriculture. British
farmers and others took note.[48]

One question remains: did the Australian authorities deliberately
deploy myxomatosis in the hope of eliminating or controlling the
country's rabbits? The issue is important in relation to the present
study where a central question concerns the involvement of the British government or private individuals in bringing the disease to the
UK. CSIR and other agencies, including state governments, were
interested in the possible use of the disease as early as the 1920s but
also in the 1930s and 1940s. However, the authorities had profound
misgivings about introducing the virus even under strictly controlled
conditions – hence, the location of Martin's research in Britain. The
apparent confirmation, in the 1940s, that myxomatosis affected
rabbits alone allayed some of these fears. Even so, Australia's early field
trials took place in remote, semi-arid locations. In 1950, however, the
disease was introduced into a fertile farming area that contained people
along with domesticated and wild animals and, importantly, blood-
sucking insects. It was understood well before this time that mosquitoes
and fleas could spread myxomatosis. As Ratcliffe et al. acknowledged
in 1952, citing papers by Aragão in 1920 and Bull and Mules in 1944,
'when we started our field experiments with myxomatosis [in the
Murray Valley in May 1950] it was known that two species of fleas and
about half a dozen species of mosquitoes could transmit the infection.'[49]
To be sure, Bull and Mules had concluded in 1944 that myxomatosis
'can be readily transmitted … by species of mosquitoes'.[50] So the
question arises: was CSIRO intent on creating an epizootic in 1950?

In relation to this question, the terminology employed in most
accounts is confusing. The 1950 introductions are frequently referred
to as 'trials' or 'experiments', but words like 'release' and 'liberation'
are also used. Thus, Fenner and Ratcliffe write of the 'field trials of
1950' but also about the 'first experimental liberation of the virus …
on an irrigated dairy farm at Gunbower, in Victoria, some 150 miles
downstream from Albury'.[51] Similarly, Ratcliffe et al. use the term
'field trials', but also discuss the 'seven liberations of the virus … on
five sites in the Murray Valley'.[52] Ken Myers, who joined CSIRO's

Wildlife Survey Section in 1950, wrote in 1954 about 'the "escape" of the virus from the experimental sites in 1950'.[53] In Britain an official publication referred to 'liberations of the myxoma virus ... between May and November, 1950'.[54] For their part, Fenner and Fantini devote one section of their chapter on 'the introduction of myxomatosis into Australia' to 'Field Trials by the Wildlife Survey Section, 1950' and another to 'The Escape: Spread through South-Eastern Australia, 1951.'[55] The word 'escape', which is clearly incompatible with the notion of 'liberation', implies previous confinement; conduct of a scientific trial suggests an experiment under carefully controlled conditions. However, a report in *The Times* states that early 'in 1951 [*sic*], in order to deal with the rabbit menace, a disease known as myxomatosis was deliberately spread among rabbits in some districts in Victoria and New South Wales.'[56]

Myxomatosis was introduced into the Murray Valley in 1950 without control or confinement. Indeed, the expectation appears to have been that conditions suited the takeoff of the disease.

> As Aragão (1943) had shown that myxomatosis in South America was probably maintained among the local wild rabbits (*Sylvilagus braziliensis, syn. Minensis*) by mosquito bites, and Bull & Mules (1944) had demonstrated that several Australian species of mosquitoes could transmit the disease, a series of field trials was undertaken between January and November 1950, on six sites in the well-watered Murray Valley.[57]

So, notwithstanding Myers's use in this passage of the term 'field trials' and his use of related terms such as 'field experiments' elsewhere in the paper, it is hard to avoid the conclusion that 1950 saw a deliberate attempt to introduce myxomatosis. The rate of spread and the extent, of the (generally welcome) epizootic that ensued might have taken most observers by surprise; its occurrence should not have.[58]

The French Connection
Australia's myxomatosis outbreak received media coverage in Britain and continental Europe.[59] In January 1952 the Pasteur Institute in

Paris informed Francis Ratcliffe of its interest in the disease as a possible solution to France's rabbit problem. It requested and received offprints of articles and a sample of the virus. The Australians also provided details of how to prepare the virus in bulk. Fenner and Fantini have been unable to locate information about the use made of the information and materials sent from Australia.[60] Nevertheless, the first outbreak of epizootic myxomatosis among rabbits in Europe occurred in France in 1952.

In Australia the rabbit was regarded more or less universally as an unmitigated menace. In France, however, largely because of the importance of wild rabbits to huntsmen and of domestic rabbits in the rural economy, attitudes were more ambivalent. Although the wild rabbit was officially regarded as an agricultural pest that should be destroyed, powerful forces favoured its preservation for sporting purposes. As Lockley wrote:

> The rabbit occupies a unique position in France as the main game of the average sportsman. Probably 80 per cent of those holding permits to shoot do so primarily for killing rabbits. That is to say, about 80 per cent of the cartridges fired by 1,850,000 *chasseurs* are aimed at rabbits. About 70 per cent of wild rabbits killed are shot. Probably three cartridges are fired for each rabbit killed with a gun.[61]

All this meant considerable revenue for the French treasury, the Conseil Supérior de la Chasse, local communes and businesses involved in the manufacture of guns, cartridges and other shooting equipment. Accordingly, French law conferred the protection of a closed season on the rabbit. Ambivalence about the value of rabbits existed even within the Ministry of Agriculture, where the rabbit was entirely a matter for the *service de la chasse* rather than the pest control division. Tenant farmers could reclaim from the holder of the shooting rights on their land the cost of the agricultural damage caused by rabbits. Since the amount of compensation so obtained could exceed the rent payable on a holding, a large rabbit population could be profitable.

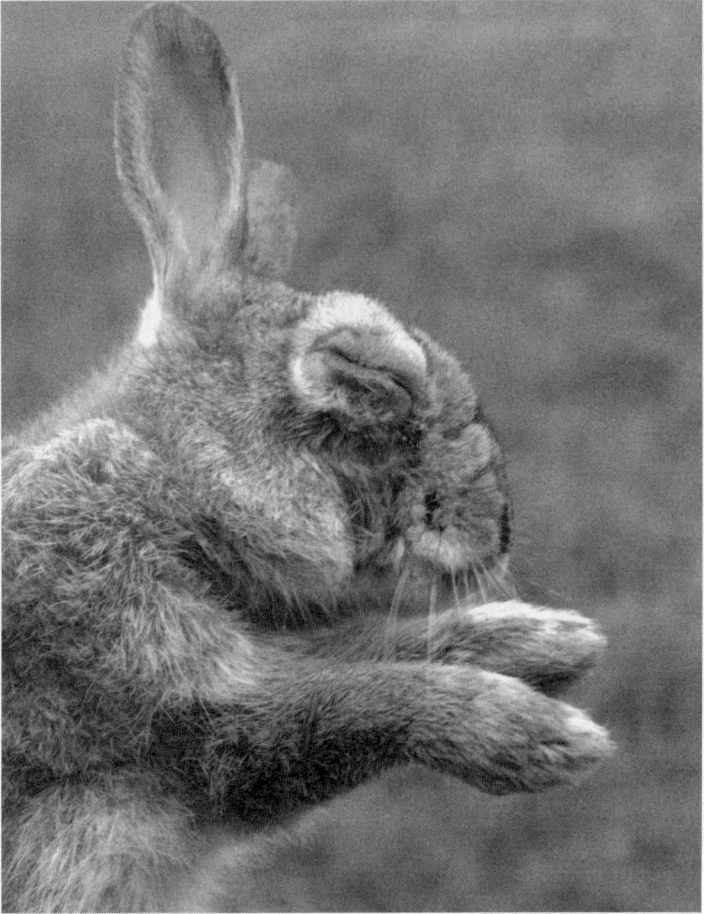

1. Rabbit with myxomatosis.

Indeed, some farmers supposedly sowed crops with a view to attracting rabbits and submitting a compensation claim. And landowners did not necessarily object to paying substantial sums of compensation, for heavy rabbit infestation could greatly increase the value of shooting rights. Rabbit rearing for meat and fur, involving up to 100 million animals at any one time, was also an important domestic industry that provided an income for numerous people, many of whom were supplementing retirement pensions.[62]

Dr Paul Armand Delille initiated France's myxomatosis outbreak in June 1952. As a member of the French Académie de Médicine and commander of the Légion d'honneur, Delille had pursued a distinguished career as a physician and bacteriologist. By 1952, at which point he was in his late seventies, he had retired to his 300-hectare country estate (Chateau Maillebois) near Dreux in the department of Eure-et-Loir to the west of Paris. The estate, farmed by his son Lionel, was infested with rabbits and Delille conceived the idea of controlling them by means of myxomatosis, which he knew to be highly contagious. Accordingly, he obtained a small amount of virus from his friend Professor Hauduroy, of the Laboratoire de Bacteriologie in Lausanne, Switzerland, and used it to inoculate two wild rabbits, which he then released on his property. Delille maintained that he never intended to cause anything other than the destruction of the rabbits on his walled estate (though he subsequently went on to recommend myxomatosis for rabbit control). As an amateur entomologist he believed that northern France carried no insects that could serve as vectors and carry the disease beyond his grounds. However, rabbits soon began to die both on his property and on surrounding land. In July 70 domestic rabbits died in a village eight kilometres from Maillebois. By August the disease was present in a village 45 kilometres away. It then 'raced across the interior of France' before entering Belgium and Holland, killing rabbits by the hundreds of thousand, if not millions, as it progressed. In October the disease gained official recognition.[63]

The escape of sick rabbits and insect vectors that were, in fact, present probably caused the spread of the disease beyond Delille's estate. The deliberate removal of dead and dying animals by those who wished to spread the disease may also have been a factor. The spread of myxomatosis to locations far from the estate probably owed much to human agency, witting or unwitting, including the transfer of infected but still symptomless animals either for food or to restock hunting grounds or rabbit farms. Ultimately, of course, Delille was responsible. He became the subject of severe criticism from hunters who, by the autumn of 1953, had 'little but sparrows on which to loose their cartridges', and rabbit breeders who feared for their livelihoods.[64] He later faced legal proceedings. Two actions against him failed but on appeal he was held liable in one instance. Because the plaintiff's agricultural gains were held to compensate for his sporting losses, Delille was required to pay only 5000 francs (about £5) as opposed to the one million francs (£1000) sought. To most farmers, foresters, nurserymen and horticulturalists Delille was a benefactor. In the summer of 1956 he was awarded a gold medal in recognition of his services.[65]

When, in September 1953, weeks before the disease reached Britain, Dr J. W. Evans of Britain's Ministry of Agriculture visited France to investigate the country's myxomatosis outbreak, he found that the disease had spread unevenly. In heavily infested areas, which he defined as land holding 400 rabbits per hectare, 99 per cent had been destroyed. He reported their elimination from the low-lying coastal country of southern France. There were, however, survivors on high country inland. He also found that 30–40 per cent of domestic rabbits had died. According to Lockley, the Pasteur Institute estimated that around 35 per cent of domestic and 45 per cent of wild rabbits in France had died of myxomatosis by the end of 1953.[66] It was still too soon to gauge the impact of the disease on agriculture and forestry, but anecdotal evidence indicated higher production for farmers and successful tree planting in areas where this had previously been impossible. There were, however, downsides; in fields where rabbits had died in large numbers, pheasants and cattle had died of septicaemia. Furthermore, in the absence of rabbits on which to prey, foxes were said to be invading farms and taking poultry. Even so, Evans reported that 'those who have the benefit of agriculture and forestry at heart are delighted'. Others were less enthusiastic, whether on humanitarian grounds or, in the case of hunters, because of lost sport. There were also unwelcome economic outcomes. Evans quoted a daily newspaper that predicted serious consequences for gunsmiths, manufacturers of cartridges and other shooting goods, furriers, dealers in game, hoteliers and the tourist industry more generally, and even the French state because revenues from the sale of hunting permits plummeted.[67]

Faced with the decimation and possible demise of the rabbit, the French authorities took various steps, some of which sought to con-

trol the disease and protect the rabbit. The deliberate spread of myxomatosis was made a punishable offence with a maximum penalty of
five years' imprisonment; then the National Assembly moved to prohibit the importation of viruses. Myxomatosis became a notifiable
disease. Areas in which it was present had to be identified by means of
signs bearing the words: '*Myxomatose, maladie contagieuse du lapin*'. All
rabbits inside such areas were to be destroyed. Regulations were
enacted for the disinfection and isolation of domestic rabbits and the
safe disposal of corpses. Rabbit farmers were required to provide
regular reports about the sanitary status of their holdings. A mass
inoculation programme was introduced and by the time Evans prepared
his report as many as 3.5 million animals had been inoculated. In some
of the worst affected areas restocking began, with or without official
sanction. Some reports suggested that immune American cottontail
rabbits were being imported either surreptitiously, with US airmen
based in France playing a part, or even with official sanction. Evans
could not authenticate these reports but considered that if such practices
were taking place it amounted to a 'calamity' because the incomers,
larger than their European counterparts, threatened to be more
destructive of trees and crops than the rabbits they were replacing.[68]

Finally, Thompson and Worden suggest that French public
opinion, which was greatly exercised by myxomatosis in 1953, had by
1955 ceased to care much. Rather, the disease had come to be
accepted 'with a Gallic shrug'.[69] This is an unconvincing judgement.
The enactment of substantial government regulation, the civil liti-
gation against Delille (ongoing at the end of 1955), the dramatically
differing esteem in which the originator of France's myxomatosis outbreak was held by different sectors of French society and the high value
French shooters continued to place on rabbit hunting, all suggest that
the disease remained a controversial issue years after its introduction.[70]

Chapter 2
The War on the Rabbit

Expensive Guests

It is generally agreed that European wild rabbits are not native to the British Isles, but originated on the Iberian Peninsula, or the western Mediterranean basin more generally.[1] There is less agreement about the manner in which they reached Britain from continental Europe. Since the end of the nineteenth century most authorities, including Ronald Lockley and John Sheail, have accepted that the Normans introduced them, possibly in the twelfth century.[2] Earlier writers often considered the Romans responsible.[3] A middle position is that both the Normans and the Romans brought them, the Roman colonies possibly having died out by the eleventh century.[4]

John Marchington, who carefully reviews the evidence for Norman and Roman involvement, concludes that there is 'virtually no evidence' for a Roman introduction and a 'very strong' case for Norman responsibility. However, on a basis of 'logic' rather than hard evidence, he maintains that the Romans probably did bring rabbits to Britain, though whether they then became at all widespread in the wild is another matter. Marchington also speculates that rabbits may have arrived, with or without human assistance, by land before rising sea levels at the end of the ice age created the English Channel and separated the British Isles from the continental land mass. This theory accords with other suggestions that the British rabbit dates from the Neolithic period.[5] However they arrived, there is no disputing that rabbits have been present in Britain for some 900 years and possibly for far longer.

Although attitudes varied from place to place, time to time, interest group to interest group and person to person, rabbits were long considered a welcome presence in the British Isles. Whether farmed in warrens or living wild in the countryside they were a useful source of fur for clothing and meat. Rabbit flesh is said to have been a luxury food in the Middle Ages. Lorwin states that 'few wild' but a 'great number of domesticated rabbits' were consumed in Elizabethan England. For her part, Ayrton notes that rabbit meat was esteemed in the Elizabethan period 'and throughout the seventeenth and eighteenth centuries'. Thereafter, she maintains, it went out of favour, becoming 'positively disliked in the First World War and again in the Second, when meat was short'.[6] There is, however, little documentary support for a post-eighteenth-century collapse in the public's appetite for rabbit flesh.

At the end of the nineteenth century Simpson wrote that the meat:

> esteemed by all classes – is relished by the invalid as much as by persons in robust health, served by the expert cook in a dozen dainty ways, and regarded as almost a luxury by the poor, to whom the rabbit often affords a means of making a savoury dinner, with the aid of food scraps, such as could not be easily procured in any other way. In all towns and populous districts the demand is practically unlimited.[7]

Arscott, referring to the late nineteenth or early twentieth centuries, agrees. She sees rabbit as 'the most democratic of foods since it was eaten by every rank from farmhand to noble'. In 1898 Alexander Shand took a slightly different line; he saw the rabbit as 'a most useful and respectable animal' whose culinary 'merits have been unfairly ignored, simply because he is cheap and common'. He detected a growing popularity and predicted that it would 'cut a more conspicuous figure in the future than in the past'. Meanwhile, it was principally 'a favourite food of the poorer classes', even though they had little idea about how to prepare it. Of one thing he was certain, rabbits would always be present 'not only in sufficiency but in a superabundance, and out of sheer charity to the farmers we are bound to consume him'.[8]

That rabbit was consumed by the less affluent in the 1930s is indicated by its prominence in Norah Fletcher's *500 Sixpenny Recipes*, a book that shunned game and all high priced meat cuts in favour of 'less expensive raw materials'.[9] Forty years later, in *English Food*, Jane Grigson considered the animal 'the staple protein of poor country families' until myxomatosis transformed it into a luxury food. Before this happened the only meat a newly-married and poverty-stricken friend ate in the first years of her marriage were the rabbits her husband was able to shoot in the fields around her village.[10]

Rabbit recipes can be traced through half a millennium. Maxine McKendry reproduces a fifteenth-century recipe for 'spicy creamed rabbit'. In the mid-eighteenth century Hannah Glass described six rabbit dishes.[11] Some 130 years later *Mrs Beeton's Book of Household Management* listed ten, including a boiled dish with the less than alluring ingredients of rabbit and water.[12] In the 1920s the same author's *All-About Cookery* included 23 recipes ranging from rabbit boiled, casseroled, creamed, curried, fricasseed, fried with tartare sauce, jugged, marbled and stewed, to rabbit broth, darioles, patties, pie, pilau, pudding, ragout and soup. In addition, the animal could be prepared larded and braised or as a dish for invalids. The book also supplied information about trussing and carving.[13] Fletcher's *500 Sixpenny Recipes* (1934) listed 15 rabbit dishes including rabbit surprise, braised rabbit with lettuce and jugged rabbit with chestnuts.[14] The 1950 edition of *Mrs Beeton's Book of Household Management* carried as many as 33 rabbit recipes across 16 pages of text. Additions to the 1923 repertoire included rabbit *à la minute*, American style, barbecued, and roast with a sauce *espagnole*.[15]

It is difficult to draw conclusions from any of this about the extent to which rabbit actually featured in the British diet either by choice or necessity, or the degree to which it was eaten by urban dwellers as opposed to their rural counterparts, or by members of different social classes. Histories of food, diet and nutrition in the United Kingdom are notably silent about the rabbit's place in the British kitchen.[16] It is likely, however, that rabbit meat was an important raw material in British cuisine, especially among less affluent country dwellers.

Because rabbits provided the hunter with sport, they received protection under game and other laws as early as 1389. As 'gentlemen's game' they could be hunted only by those who possessed sufficient property. In the course of the seventeenth century rabbits (and deer) ceased to be viewed as wild, and hence owned by no one; instead, they were classed as 'enclosed' animals and thus the private property of landowners. An act of 1692 (3 & 4 William and Mary c.10) formalized the position and rabbits ceased to be protected under the game laws (which made hunting for hares, pheasants, partridges and moorland birds the exclusive privilege of the landed gentry). Accordingly, by the eighteenth century rabbits were 'game' only in the sense of being animals hunted for sport; in the eyes of the law they were private property. Those who took or killed them without permission were 'treated as thieves, which is to say very harshly indeed', the theft of an enclosed animal being punished far more severely than the poaching of game. The Game Reform Act, 1831 (1 & 2 Will. IV c.32) made all game the private property of landowners. Thereafter, the more draconian aspects of the criminal law having been repealed over the preceding decades, trespass in pursuit of rabbits in daytime was punishable by a fine of up to £2 (£5 if a group of five people or more were involved) plus costs, or up to two months' imprisonment.[17]

During the medieval and early modern periods, rabbits appear to have been relatively uncommon in the wild, except in the vicinity of warrens, and hence not serious agricultural pests. Sentiment swung against the animal only as its numbers increased significantly, beginning in the eighteenth century, with changes in field sport fashion and agricultural practice. Until this time:

> feral colonies stood little chance of survival because of the high density of natural predators in the countryside. Although these predators did not depend on rabbits for food, they killed large numbers of young which effectively stopped the small rabbit colonies from growing in size. The slaughter of predators from 1750 onwards by farmers and gamekeepers anxious to protect their stock gave rabbits a new lease of life and their population increased.[18]

This wholesale, ruthless and efficient destruction of predators was undertaken by landlords who had acquired the means to engage in field sports involving small game. Some wished to hunt rabbits; others wanted to encourage them because they attracted foxes, which could in turn be hunted – though the rabbit's habit of creating holes and undermining terrain through its burrowing was less welcome to horse riders. It was also thought that numerous rabbits would keep the fox away from domestic and game fowl. Landlords often had little desire to protect rabbits *per se*; they were more concerned to cull creatures such as hawks, polecats and weasels that killed the partridges, pheasants and hares they wanted to shoot. Rabbits were accidental beneficiaries. In addition, they benefited fortuitously from the creation of game preserves and the encouragement of undergrowth that could provide cover for foxes and more desirable small game.[19]

Changing agricultural practices also favoured the rabbit. In the first place, the enclosure of land, which involved planting miles of hedgerows, created a perfect habitat adjacent to field crops. In the second, the introduction of winter cropping boosted food availability at a time of year when dearth had hitherto led many rabbits to starve.[20] Seemingly, every change suited the rabbit. It is hard to be clear about numbers. A late seventeenth-century estimate of one million has been dismissed as no 'more than a guess'. It appears, however, that 'during the nineteenth century the rabbit population rose at a phenomenal rate'.[21] The creature became abundant even in Norfolk and Scotland where it had hitherto been localized or scarce.[22]

When did farmers begin to regard the presence of rabbits as inimical to good husbandry? It has been stated that 'old farming books gave no reference to rabbits as pests before 1849'.[23] In 1917 Pickworth Farrow maintained that rabbits had become a problem only 'during the last few decades or more recently still' as they benefited from the decline of their natural enemies.[24] A few years later Tansley and Adamson also traced the proliferation of rabbits to 'comparatively recent years' and their preservation for sporting purposes.[25] Some 80 years earlier, however, rabbit infestation of agricultural land was sufficiently serious for most of the witnesses who appeared before a select committee on the game laws to support the 'total' destruction of rabbits (and hares). Rabbits, the committee noted, were 'universally condemned as mischievous vermin'. This and other sources suggest there are good grounds for viewing the 1840s as the decade when rabbits came to be widely regarded as enemies of agriculture.[26]

In 1872 Alexander Taylor, a Kincardineshire farmer, told another select committee on the game laws that rabbits were 'pure vermin'; given the opportunity farmers would 'exterminate [them] completely'. Sir James Elphinstone MP agreed that their extermination was highly desirable.[27] Landowners, who were not farmers but who held shooting rights on tenants' farms that they could either let or enjoy themselves, did not necessarily agree. As for tenant farmers, whose crops were consumed and livelihoods threatened, until the passing of the Ground Game Act in 1880 they could exercise no control without the permission of the landowner. If a landlord reserved the rabbits on a tenant's farm either for his own use or for sale to a shooting tenant, a farming tenant who killed them committed a criminal offence.[28]

The 1872–73 select committee judged that some areas had recently seen 'a considerable diminution of both hares and rabbits on cultivated lands'.[29] Nevertheless:

> There can be no question that the existence of a large number of hares and rabbits upon an arable farm is most prejudicial to its profitable occupation, and your committee cannot too strongly reprobate the practice of some landlords and their shooting tenants of keeping up a large stock of those animals on cultivated lands to the injury of the crops of the farming tenants.[30]

The committee recommended that rabbits should be denied all legislative protection and that landowners should be liable to compensate their tenant farmers for rabbit damage.

In the short term nothing happened, but in 1880 parliamentary proponents of the Hares and Rabbits Bill (later the Ground Game Act, 1880) argued that tenant farmers should acquire the inalienable right to kill rabbits and hares on their land. Although some MPs agreed with the 1872–73 committee that ground game wrought less damage than in earlier years, others questioned such assessments. For example, James Howard, Liberal MP for Bedford and author of several books on agriculture, stated that in many districts ground game 'constituted a great and widespread evil'. Albert Pell, the Conservative MP for South Leicestershire, while allowing that rabbits had their uses, referred to 'the immense amount of mischief' they did 'upon the small class of farms'. The rabbit, he observed succinctly, 'was a most destructive little animal'.[31] Over the following decades such views were aired regularly. As A. D. Middleton of Oxford University's Bureau of Animal Population put it in 1940: 'We can assume without any misgivings that the rabbit is a pest. ... No one with the slightest practical knowledge of agriculture, forestry, or horticulture will have any hesitation in condemning the rabbit as a major pest on developed land.'[32]

Laws and Orders

Subject to certain restrictions relating to common and moor land, the Ground Game Act (1880) established the inalienable right of occupiers of land to kill and take the hares and rabbits on land they occupied. This right, shared with the landowner, could be extended in writing to one other authorized person but could not be renounced or withdrawn through any kind of agreement. If ground game were shot, occupiers needed to possess a gun licence under the terms of the Gun Licence Act, 1870. They did not, however, need a game licence.[33]

The Ground Game Act infringed the rights of property but such infringement was justified, in the act's preamble, in the interest of 'good husbandry' and, in particular, 'to enable ... occupiers to protect their crops from injury and loss'. In practice, the act satisfied few. Indeed, Harting observes that it 'caused more misunderstanding, ill-feeling and general dissatisfaction' than any other statute of 'modern times'.[34] As a rabbit control measure the act was seriously flawed. Landlords who wanted to preserve ground game could bribe or threaten (perhaps with eviction) tenants who exercised their newly-acquired right too enthusiastically. Landlords could also retain land where rabbits bred. Tenants had no entitlement to enter land adjacent to their holdings for the purpose of killing rabbits. Perhaps most importantly, notwithstanding the recommendation of the 1872–73 committee, the owners or occupiers of land overrun by rabbits had no obligation to compensate neighbours for damage done by straying animals.[35] On large holdings there was the additional problem that tenants could employ only one rabbit catcher, no matter how many acres they rented. For all these reasons it is highly unlikely that the act led to any reduction in Britain's rabbit population. No further steps to control rabbits were taken until the First World War when the state intervened to safeguard a country 'nearly starved out by the German submarine campaign'.[36]

An Order in Council issued in March 1917 under the Defence of the Realm Act, 1914, allowed the Board of Agriculture and Fisheries (BAF) to take or authorize such action as it deemed necessary to prevent or reduce damage to crops, trees or pasture by game birds, hares or rabbits.[37] The aim, of course, was to protect the nation's food supply during a national emergency. Under the terms of the order, War Agricultural Executive Committees (WAECs) could authorize entry onto any land for the purpose of killing rabbits.[38] The Corn Production Act, 1917, conferred similar powers on BAF, though under its terms the cost of any control measures was recoverable from neglectful occupiers of land.[39] Sheail describes these powers as 'quite unprecedented'. However, the absence of documentation makes it impossible to say how much use was made of them.[40] Probably there was limited recourse to dictatorial methods for 'the success of the food production campaign depended on the goodwill of farmers and landowners'.[41] In any case, with the manpower shortages of wartime, rabbit catchers were hard to find. As Lord Dunmore informed readers of *The Times* at the end of 1917, 'there are thousands of rabbits on my property in Scotland, but it is impossible to trap and market them owing to the fact that there are no trappers available.'[42]

With the end of the war, emergency regulations lapsed and repeal of the Corn Production Act 1917, in 1921, terminated the right of public bodies to control rabbits on private land.[43] Ostensibly, things were different in forestry, for the legislation that established the Forestry Commission, in 1919, empowered the commissioners, after giving a landowner or occupier due opportunity to comply, to arrange for the destruction of rabbits, hares or vermin such as squirrels and to recover the cost.[44] In practice, these powers were never exercised, even though the commission conservatively estimated that rabbit damage cost it around £30,000 per annum (mostly in fencing and wages for rabbit catchers).[45] Yet, in England, Wales and Scotland rabbit control was an important issue throughout the interwar period. As the Game and Heather-Burning (Scotland) Committee reported in 1921: 'It is generally agreed that with the possible exception of the rat, the rabbit is the most serious four-footed pest that farmers have to deal with. It is therefore desirable that it should be, as far as possible, destroyed.'[46]

As early as 1922 the Council of Agriculture recommended reinstating lapsed powers for controlling rabbits on agricultural land and a government bill came before the Commons.[47] The bill sought to empower county councils to take action against occupiers of land who failed to control rabbits with the result that neighbouring property was damaged. It was not enacted.[48] Rabbit (or rabbit and rook) bills came before parliament almost every year between 1922 and 1930, sometimes at a rate of more than one a year. Although the details varied from bill to bill, the main thrust was re-enactment of section ten of the Corn Production Act with county councils having powers of intervention to destroy rabbits wherever occupiers of land failed to exercise control. For various reasons, however, including pressure of parliamentary business, opposition from lobby groups (the Society for the Protection of Wild Birds opposed the Rabbits and Rooks Bill, 1925, while furriers objected to the Rabbits Bill 1928), or fear that 'county council officials will swarm over private property', no legislation was enacted.[49]

Although Lord Clinton observed in parliament that 'of all the curses with which agriculture is endowed the rabbit is absolutely the worst', the extent to which there was widespread demand for legislative controls is unclear.[50] The House of Lords select committee on the Rabbits and Rooks Bill, 1927, observed that, except for unionized farmers, there was not 'much proof of any general demand for the Bill or any desire to give evidence in its favour'. It accepted that rabbits, unlike rooks, which had 'redeeming qualities', were 'destructive animals' and 'unmitigated nuisances to the good farmer and forester', but considered the terms of the bill 'unworkable in practice'. It went no further than to voice the 'opinion that any owner or occupier suffering from damage to his crops by rabbits which come from places outside the land he occupies should be entitled to compensation and should be empowered to claim it in the County Courts.'[51]

The proposal came to nothing. A Rabbits Bill came before parliament twice in 1929–30. The government was sympathetic and the bill even passed in the Commons. Ultimately, however, it came to nothing.[52] In the absence of legislation, it remained for farmers, foresters and others to protect themselves as best they could against the incursions of rabbits from the land of neighbours who neglected to practise rabbit control either through bad husbandry or because they were game preservers.

In 1927 Lord Bledisloe, parliamentary secretary to the Ministry of Agriculture and Fisheries (MAF), explained the need to control rabbits in terms of their growing numbers and the changed social conditions of the postwar world that were resulting in a relaxation of traditional control measures:

> The widespread splitting up of estates has resulted to a large extent in the discontinuance of the organised destruction of both rabbits and rooks, and there is an increasing tendency to let the sporting rights on agricultural estates to shooting syndicates, many of which have far less sympathy with the difficulties of the farming community than the old-fashioned landowners, who formerly retained the shooting in their own hands. Evidence from all over the country goes to show that there is an increase in the number of rabbits destroying both crops and timber.[53]

When, in 1935, *The Times* tried to 'explain the palpable increase of rabbits during the past few years', it emphasized the 'succession of dry summers and mild winters'. Beyond this it pointed the finger at the 'well-intentioned' but flawed Ground Game Act, 1880, which in practice had often placed rabbit control entirely in the hands of farmers who lacked the time and expertise to practise it effectively. Meanwhile, the depressed state of agriculture in the interwar years meant neglect of hedgerows and the spread of briar and bramble among which rabbits could thrive and multiply.[54] As Sir Emrys Jones, Gloucestershire's wartime cultivation officer put it, the countryside of the 1930s was 'a wilderness in modern terms. The hedges were overgrown, the whole place ridden with millions of rabbits. It looked hardly possible to grow any sort of corn crop; if the rabbits didn't have it the mildew caught it'.[55]

In 1936 a Hampshire landowner, Sir Ronald Sperling, brought the rabbit issue back into the public domain with a letter to *The Times* in which he claimed that rabbits were increasing 'faster than ever', that they were costing the country £70 million a year and that something needed to be done.[56] A week later an editorial headed 'Too Many Rabbits' expressed agreement. Rabbits 'prolific and ubiquitous' as they were, 'are expensive guests, and where a landowner or a farmer fails to keep down their numbers there seems to be a strong case for the intervention of a public authority to mitigate the nuisance.'[57] Shortly afterwards Lord Merthyr moved the appointment of a select committee of the House of Lords to consider how to protect agriculture against 'the ravages of rabbits'.[58]

This inquiry was then and remains the only full-scale official investigation of the problem of rabbit damage in Britain. It sat for the best part of four months and took evidence from 38 witnesses. These witnesses included civil servants, farmers, landowners, land agents, and a professional rabbit trapper, manufacturers of traps and furs, plus representatives of the National Farmers' Union, animal welfare groups, forestry organizations, the British Field Sports Society and the County Councils' Association.

Many witnesses informed the committee (though the evidence was purely anecdotal) that the rabbit population was rising. For example, a Perthshire farmer observed that 'rabbits have multiplied amazingly and there is now hardly a place where they are not increasing'. The Scottish Land and Property Federation (supported by the Royal Scottish Forestry Society) considered it 'an undoubted fact that rabbits have been increasing enormously within recent years and have become a perfect plague in many places'. Suggested reasons for the increase included favourable summers, agricultural depression and the

collapse of the price of rabbit meat owing to cheap imports from Australia and elsewhere. At a time of growing international tension, food
production was again coming to be viewed as a branch of national
defence and some witnesses, such as Sir Roy Robinson, chairman of
the Forestry Commission, favoured a policy of extermination: 'the
destruction of the rabbits would do more than any other single
measure in this country to enhance production from the soil whether
it is timber or food or anything else.' Though this opinion was by no
means unanimous, most of the witnesses who appeared before the
select committee, even those representing animal protection bodies,
accepted the need for vigorous control measures.[59]

The committee's report considered the extermination of the rabbit
to be neither possible nor desirable (it was 'an important source of
cheap food'). If occupiers chose to let rabbits damage their property
and they alone suffered, the question of redress did not arise. However, occupiers of neighbouring land deserved protection. To this end
the committee recommended that following 'fair and impartial
enquiry' county councils should be empowered to order the destruction of rabbits, or the implementation of other precautions, wherever
rabbits caused damage on neighbouring property. In the event of non-
compliance, councils should also be empowered to institute legal proceedings and to supply trained personnel to undertake the destruction.
Occupiers of these neighbouring lands should also be able to claim
compensation from the offender.[60] In a letter to *The Times*, Sperling,
who gave evidence to the committee, described the report as 'very
lukewarm'.[61] Even so, the possibility of legislating to give effect to the
select committee's recommendations, was discussed on a number of
occasions in 1937–38, including in cabinet. Several bills were prepared.
Ultimately, however, for broadly the same reasons that all previous
interwar proposals had foundered, no legislation ensued.[62] Rabbits,
'horrid liver-fluked ravenous animals' that they were, remained 'an
absolute menace to British agriculture'.[63]

Little more than a month before the Second World War broke out
parliament finally passed the Prevention of Damage by Rabbits Act.
The act applied to England and Wales only (excluding greater London). Part I allowed local authorities who received a complaint from a

third party to require the control of rabbits within a reasonable period of time (not less than three weeks) whenever those rabbits were causing or likely to cause 'substantial damage' to the 'crops, trees, shrubs, pasturage, fences, banks or works on land in the occupation of any other person'. Failure to comply was punishable by fine of up to £25 plus a maximum of £5 per day for each succeeding day of non-compliance. Councils could kill the animals and then recover the costs from the occupier.[64]

Lord Sempill, who had introduced the bill in the House of Lords, noted that after repeated failures to introduce legislation against the rabbit, 'open war is now declared'.[65] For his part Sperling attributed the success of the bill in large part to 'the publicity given to the subject by *The Times*, and to ... the energy and perseverance of UFAW [which] was quick to recognize that excess of rabbits meant the perpetuation of gross cruelty by trappers, and threw the whole of its organization into the campaign.' At the same time, he recognized that it was 'not enough to get an Act passed'; it was up to county councils to enforce it.[66] Certainly, there was much to be done, for many authorities considered Britain's rabbit population, estimated at 50 million in the late 1930s, had increased to an 'extraordinary' extent in recent years. So much so that, 'in the early part of the war [the rabbit] was in sole possession of much valuable land'.[67]

Days before the outbreak of the Second World War, Defence (General) Regulations, which applied to the UK as a whole, empowered the agriculture and fisheries minister 'to authorize persons at any time to enter upon any land' to kill rabbits or various other pests.[68] A few weeks later the Rabbits Order allowed county WAECs in England and Wales to require the destruction of wild rabbits wherever they were satisfied that the animals were causing or likely to cause crop, pasture or tree damage. The order differed from the prewar act in that WAECs could take action without prior complaint from a third party, without issuing notice to the occupier and without first providing occupiers with the opportunity to deal with their rabbits. The Rabbits Order of 27 March 1940 amended and clarified the 1939 order.[69]

The extent to which WAECs made use of the powers conferred upon them by these orders is unknown. The Hampshire committee appears to have taken its responsibilities very seriously. Despite objections it destroyed the rabbits on a preserved (and fenced) warren on the Duke of Wellington's estate at Stratfield Saye and took a very robust line with Lieutenant-Colonel Cradock, an uncooperative landowner at Knighton Twyford near Winchester.[70] At the end of 1941 a leading article in *The Times* noted that:

> In the past two years many farmers and others have been warned by the War Agricultural Committees that they must kill off the rabbits on their land and, failing prompt compliance, the committees have put in their own rabbit catchers to do the work. In this way the drive against rabbits has been greatly intensified, and the general experience of the man who goes out with a gun now is that rabbits are nothing like as plentiful as they have been in years past.[71]

Another leader in the same newspaper in early 1943 referred to 'the intensive campaign for the destruction of rabbits which has been carried on for the past three winters'. As a result of these efforts 'there cannot be nearly so many rabbits in the country as there were. In some districts the rabbit is now a rare sight.'[72] At the end of the war an article on 'The Course of Nature' posed the question: 'What change in rural England strikes the exile most forcibly on his return from years of service overseas?' One man's answer was 'the almost complete absence of rabbits in the field'.[73]

The wartime rabbit regulations lapsed with the return of peace. Part I of the Prevention of Damage by Rabbits Act was repealed by the Agriculture Act, 1947. This act 'had two interrelated aims: the promotion of a "stable" agricultural sector to ensure fairer returns for farmers, farm workers and landlords; and an "efficient" system to increase food production and relieve the tightly rationed consumer'.[74] The second of these objectives called for pest and weed control. The act allowed the minister of agriculture, through CAECs and in the interest of 'preventing damage to crops, pasture, human or animal foodstuffs, livestock, trees, hedges, banks or any works on land', to order the destruction of a range of birds and mammals, including rabbits. The penalty for failing to comply was a fine of up to £25 and a maximum £5 for each subsequent day of non-compliance. Where necessary, the ministry could authorize a third party to do the work and recover the cost from the responsible person.[75] The Agriculture (Scotland) Act, 1948, included similar provisions.[76]

In 1948 the Committee on Industrial Productivity's import substitution panel 'drew attention to the fact that the existence in Great Britain of many millions of rabbits feeding on crops, grassland and young trees constituted a dollar liability'. It proposed an intensive campaign to eliminate the wild rabbit and the creation of a specialist rabbit section within MAF's Infestation Control Division (ICD). The government accepted these recommendations and set up a working party on the control of wild rabbits to prepare operational plans, create research and training programmes, and establish field trials. When it became clear, however, that further statutory powers were needed to implement the proposals, the idea was shelved.[77]

In February 1950 an article in *The Times* observed that the rabbit problem was worsening:

> From various parts of the country come reports of the rapid and, some say, alarming increase in the number of rabbits. The position in many areas is back to where it was at this time of the year in 1940, when the rabbits, already far too numerous, became during the winter far too bold. Many will remember the nibbled crocuses, or worse, the completely eaten wallflowers, of that rabbit-infested spring.

After several years of scarcity the rabbit was back in gardens from which it had been absent for ten years. The writer attributed its return mainly to the natural operation of the population cycle, caused by a run of mild winters that extended the breeding season and produced fewer hard-weather fatalities. A further factor was the collapse in the market price for rabbit meat caused by a glut of imports from Australia and New Zealand.[78]

Persuaded of the growing rabbit menace and the reluctance of many farmers to recognize it, in July 1950 MAF convened a conference to consider ways of addressing the problem through the voluntary cooperation of interested parties. Attended by representatives of the CLA, NFU, NUAW, TGWU, Nature Conservancy (NC) and Forestry Commission, the conference led to the establishment of voluntary rabbit clearance areas within which landowners and occupiers were expected to engage in a programme for the 'rapid and progressive reduction of the rabbit population'. For its part, the ministry undertook that CAECs would invoke s.98 of the Agriculture Act against those who were uncooperative.[79]

In 1951 the Committee on Cruelty to Wild Animals, which recommended the extermination of the wild rabbit on grounds of the cruelty involved in ongoing control measures and protection of the national economy, endorsed rigorous application of existing powers. It also thought that consideration should be given to tougher measures.[80] In practice, little was done; in 'few cases' were farmers compelled to destroy rabbits under the provisions of the 1947 Act.[81] Furthermore, as the writer and farmer Robert Henriques observed in his 'Farmers' Ordinary' column in the *Field*: 'Despite Section 98 of the Agriculture Act, 1947, empowering the Minister of Agriculture to go and kill the rabbits himself, he has scarcely attempted it.'[82] Lord Carrington attributed the act's weakness to administrative complexity and an individualistic approach:

> There is … a specific legal duty on a person to control rabbits on his land only if he has been served with a notice to remedy conditions found to exist at a particular time, and that duty is fulfilled when the requirements of the notice are satisfied. The procedure of individual inspection and the service of individual notices requires much time and effort, and as each notice must provide for a reasonable period for compliance it is impossible to arrange for collective action.[83]

The ICD regarded the 1950 conference as the 'the first serious attempt at large scale coordinated control'. By the end of 1953 over 350 voluntary rabbit clearance areas, covering more than 1.5 million acres of England and Wales had been established.[84] To this extent the ministry's efforts were successful. But efforts to organize voluntary clearance schemes in Scotland failed and rabbit control on land under the control of government departments such as the War Office could be worse than that exercised by farmers. The recalcitrant could be sanctioned only through the flawed procedures of the Agriculture Act, 1947 and its Scottish equivalent. As a Labour MP noted in 1954, the 1950 conference produced 'only a little progress … here and there' and 'the voluntary scheme has failed'.[85]

So far as can be determined, rabbit numbers continued to rise.[86] It has been repeatedly suggested that by the early 1950s Britain's rabbit population stood at between 60 and 100 million animals. Even if the lower figure is correct, this would still mean that for all the anti-rabbit measures taken during the war, the population had increased by ten million in little more than a decade. On the eve of the myxomatosis outbreak the rabbit problem may never have been worse.[87]

Gasses and Traps

How was rabbit control effected on the eve of the myxomatosis outbreak? Aside from natural methods involving disease and predators such as stoats, weasels, buzzards, cats and foxes, there were six ways of controlling rabbit numbers: shooting, ferreting, netting, snaring, gassing and trapping.[88] Of these, the most controversial was the gin or steel trap and the most innovative, gassing.

Hilda Kean states that 'once the effects of gas warfare in the trenches upon men was known, the practice of gassing wild rabbits in their warrens became subject to criticism.'[89] Far from this being the case, 'use of poison gases in war-time' prompted the Board of Agriculture and Fisheries, in conjunction with the War Office, to explore the potential of mustard and chlorine gas in rabbit control. These experiments took place at Methwold, Norfolk, in 1918.[90] There is no evidence that gas was used to kill rabbits before the war and none to support the contention that gassing rabbits was 'hindered by common antipathy engendered by the horrors of gas warfare in the trenches of the first world war'.[91] In reality, it was the 'very unsatisfactory' results of the early experiments that created doubts about the usefulness of gas.[92] The development of gas technology was also delayed by uncertainty, removed only in 1939 (in England and Wales), about whether legislation for the protection of animals permitted the gassing of wild rabbits.[93] Such uncertainty did not prevent experimentation with carbon monoxide (motorcar exhaust fumes), which was fed into burrows through garden hoses. Indeed, ULAWS regarded this as a quick and humane way of destroying even the largest rabbit colonies. But using motorcars to generate gas had obvious limitations in terms of vehicular access to burrows on remote or rough terrain.[94] So the lack of an easily portable alternative was another factor that delayed widespread use of gas.

In 1936 the House of Lords select committee heard that 'several cyanide products are now on the market'. One of these was produced by Imperial Chemical Industries (ICI) under the trade name, 'Cymag'. First introduced in 1933–34 (for the overseas market), Cymag was a pale fine powder consisting of sodium cyanide and magnesium sulphate. An American alternative, 'Cyanogas' had calcium cyanide as its main ingredient. Whatever type was employed, the method of application was the same. Powder was deposited in the mouth of a burrow or blown through it by means of a fan or pump. As the powder was exposed to moisture, either in the atmosphere or soil, it was converted into lethal hydrogen cyanide (prussic acid).[95]

Experiments on W. H. Buckley's Castell Gorfod estate in Carmarthenshire and on an island in Loch Lomond in the 1930s indicated that 'cyanide dust' could clear rabbit-infested land efficiently and cost-effectively without damaging potentially valuable meat or fur. ULAWS and the RSPCA approved it and manufacturers were inundated with orders.[96] In 1938–39 Ronald Lockley, encouraged by ULAWS and assisted by the British agents for Cyanogas, organized a gassing campaign that all but wiped out the 10,000 or so rabbits on the island of Skokholm.[97] However, effective though it could be, gas had its downsides. First, it was suitable only on relatively heavy soils where rabbits lived in burrows with openings that could be sealed. Second, since it was fatal to humans it needed to be handled by skilled operatives and deployed only on dry and calm days in areas removed from people or farm animals. Careful storage was also necessary. Third, although it was safe to eat the meat or utilize the pelts of gassed rabbits, the animals inevitably died underground and were in many cases irretrievable, at least without labour-intensive and hence expensive excavations. As a result, furriers were unenthusiastic about it. Fourth, in unscrupulous hands it could be misused, as it was in Scotland at least, by salmon poachers who tipped cans of cyanide powder into rivers.[98]

Doubt about the legality of gassing wild rabbits was resolved at the end of the 1930s. In 1937 the House of Lords select committee recommended that the practice 'should be legalized beyond doubt'.[99] Two years later the Prevention of Damage by Rabbits Act made it clear that gas could be used with no breach of animal protection legislation.[100] From 1941 landowners and farmers were able to purchase cyanide gas powder at subsidized rates and large quantities (over 79 tons in 1949) were used. In 1951 the Committee on Cruelty to Wild Animals reported that 'gassing with cyanide, where it is practicable, is an extremely effective and humane method of control and should be used in preference to any other method for destroying animals which live underground.'[101] This was not a universal view. The journalist, James Wentworth Day, claimed that 'a gassed rabbit suffers probably just as much as a myxomatous one. His eyes are blinded. His nostrils are choked. His throat is rasped and semi-throttled. His lungs are torn and bleeding. It is high time that the gassing of rabbits was also made illegal.'[102] During the 1950s and beyond, however, cyanide gas, which was readily available without licence from chemists and agricultural suppliers, remained 'a main method of attack' against the wild rabbit. MAF and the Department of Agriculture for Scotland (DAS) encouraged its use and early attempts to prevent the spread of myxomatosis relied heavily on gassing burrows in the affected areas.[103]

In this chapter the gin, or as it was sometimes called, the spring or steel trap has already been mentioned. The word 'gin' in the sense of a contrivance for catching game dates back at least as far as the thirteenth century. Designs varied but essentially a gin trap consisted of little more than a flat pan fitted with powerful spring-loaded metal jaws, which could be toothed or smooth. The apparatus was fixed to the ground, usually in the mouth of a burrow or on a known rabbit run, by means of a peg and chain, and covered with a thin layer of soil. When set, the jaws were held open by catches that were released when

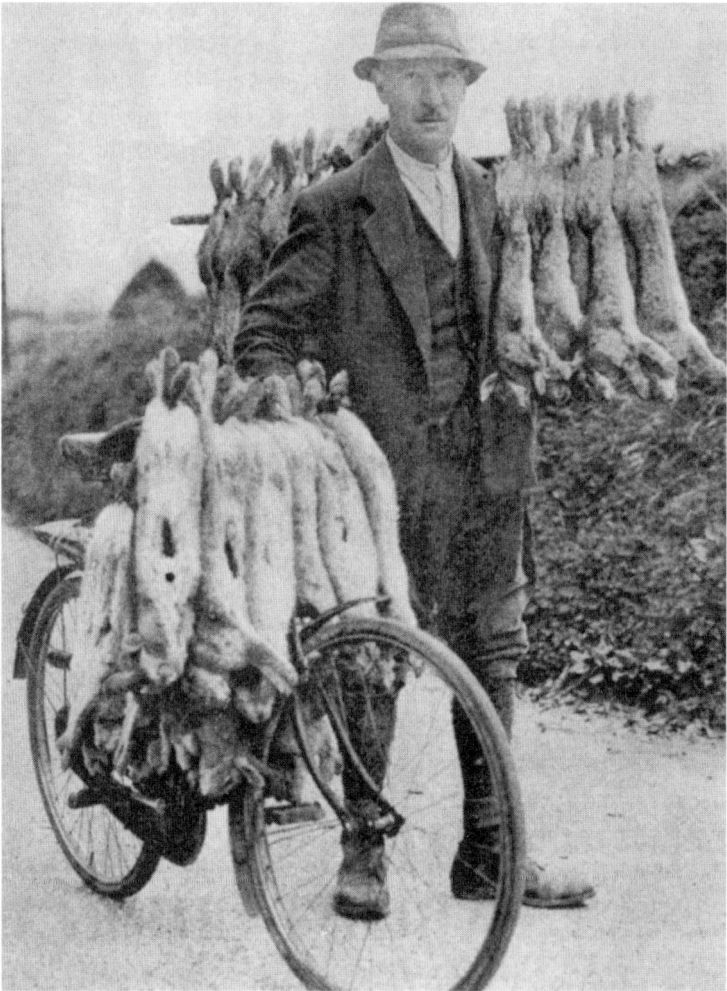

2. Before myxomatosis struck.

weight was placed on the pan. When the jaws snapped shut, they gripped the leg of the rabbit (or any other animal) that triggered the mechanism. There the creature usually remained, injured but alive, until the trapper returned or the animal escaped minus part of a limb or two.

Sheail states that after the passage of the Ground Game Act, and especially from 1900, the gin became the main means of catching rabbits. Kirkman observes that use of the gin received a substantial fillip during the First World War when the price of rabbit flesh shot up.[104] Certainly the gin trap possessed advantages over alternative control methods; it was inexpensive (only snaring was cheaper), readily available, easy to carry, speedily set, even by someone with little or no skill, and highly efficient in operation. Where rabbits were prolific, a gang of experienced trappers tending a large number of traps could clear out thousands of animals in a single night. With all these advantages, it is not surprising that by 'the 1930s the old fashioned rabbit catcher with his nets, ferrets and snares had given way to the commercial trapper'.[105] Even gas provided no real competition.[106]

Over the years, two criticisms were levelled against the gin trap. First, it did little or nothing to advance genuine rabbit control; indeed, it was often claimed it increased the population. Second, it was cruel. The idea that the gin trap was counter productive was argued by ULAWS/UFAW over a period of many years. The argument had several component parts, some of which were more persuasive than others. It was claimed that commercial trappers had no interest in exterminating rabbits, as against 'cropping' them. To eliminate them would be contrary to the trapper's interest because he would be compromising his future livelihood. Hence, 'trappers always stop work when the yield ceases to be profitable in consequence of rabbits having fled to neighbouring property, stayed in their burrows, or been caught.' It was also stated that traps accounted for many of the rabbit's natural enemies (for example stoats, weasels and cats). While both these claims are plausible, other arguments against traps, for example, that they caught few does, were less convincing. The House of Lords select committee was 'not impressed' by any of the arguments that trapping was counter productive. It suspected that 'the real foundation of the opposition to gin traps comes from those who object to their use on the ground of their cruelty' and it is hard to disagree with this conclusion.[107]

Although solicitude for animals in Western culture can be traced back through the centuries, if not millennia, so too can notions of man's dominion over animals and his right to treat them as he wished, even to the point of inhumanity. Keith Thomas has shown that some seventeenth century writers, thinkers and clerics believed that wanton cruelty and killing were wrong. However, it was only in the eighteenth century that concern for the feelings of animals became at all wide-spread.[108] The animal protection legislation of the early nineteenth century was concerned first with the abuse of domestic animals, then with the prohibition of baiting and fighting; from the 1870s, anti-cruelty organizations turned their attention to vivisection.[109] Concern about the cruelty of the hunting field, though not unknown even in the early nineteenth century, was unusual. Such prominent figures as Lord Llangattock, a staunch opponent of vivisection in the late nine-teenth century, and W. H. Buckley, for many years a leading light in ULAWS, were both hunt masters in Wales.[110] Even the Society for the Prevention of Cruelty to Animals (RSPCA from 1840) was reluctant to criticize hunting, certainly until well into the second half of the twentieth century. Nevertheless, the society did have concerns about rabbit traps and snares, and in the Victorian period offered prizes for the invention of more humane devices.[111]

The 1872–73 select committee on game laws, for all its focus on rabbits, ignored the issues of trapping or cruelty. Section six of the Ground Game Act, 1880 prohibited occupiers (but apparently not owners) from night shooting, using poisons and setting spring traps anywhere but in rabbit holes. However, this clause owed more to concern about maiming and killing animals other than rabbits than to a wish to avoid cruelty to rabbits *per se*.[112] Only with the enactment of the Protection of Animals Act, 1911 (s.10) did it become a legal requirement to inspect spring traps set for hares or rabbits at reason-able intervals and at least once every day between sunrise and sunset. The Committee on Cruelty to Wild Animals reported that trappers who sold rabbits for food (though perhaps not others) tended to inspect regularly because they did not want their catch to spoil or be stolen by a predator.[113] But enforcement of the requirement for regular inspection was virtually impossible.

From 1928 ULAWS campaigned vigorously against the gin trap, by convening meetings and conferences, lobbying MPs, giving evidence to official committees, contributing articles to journals and writing letters to the press. It also published a number of pamphlets to support its case. These included W. H. Buckley's, *The Rabbit Problem in Agriculture* (*circa* 1933), A. H. B Kirkman's, *Man versus Rabbit* (1934) and C. W. Hume's, *Instructions for Dealing with Rabbits* (1936). In 1935 a Gin Traps (Prohibition) Bill sought to ban the manufacture, sale, use and possession of traps.[114] Although it failed to become law, it did lead to the appointment of a House of Lords select committee that, among other things, considered the case for abolishing traps. The committee, though in no doubt that trapping was cruel, accepted that:

> if the rabbit has got to be killed, most methods of killing it are, unfortunately, cruel. It is impossible to tell if a rabbit suffers more by having its leg broken in a gin trap than when strangled by a snare, dying in a hole from the effects of a gun-shot wound or other injury or from gas.

It urged the ministry to investigate the potential of humane traps. Meanwhile, it agreed with those farmers and others who had testified that 'gin traps are probably an effective and economical method of killing rabbits'. It recommended that 'gin traps should in no circumstances be set in the open', but judged that complete abolition 'would undoubtedly tend to allow rabbits to increase'.[115] A few years later these conclusions were given force of law by the Prevention of Damage by Rabbits Act, 1939, which specified that spring traps were permissible, but only if set within rabbit holes.[116] From 1941, however, such was the priority given to rabbit destruction in the war years that open trapping was permitted at the discretion of WAECs to tackle the problem of surface-dwelling rabbits in woodland and on rocky ground.[117] Although the ban on trapping in the open was reinstated with the end of the war, the Committee on Cruelty to Wild Animals found that it was 'flagrantly and deliberately disregarded'.[118]

Public sentiment against the gin trap continued to run high in the 1950s. In 1954 the cook, Dorothy Hartley, cautioned against eating trapped rabbits 'broken-legged and killed in fever and slow misery. … They are definitely unhealthy food.'[119] The Committee on Cruelty to

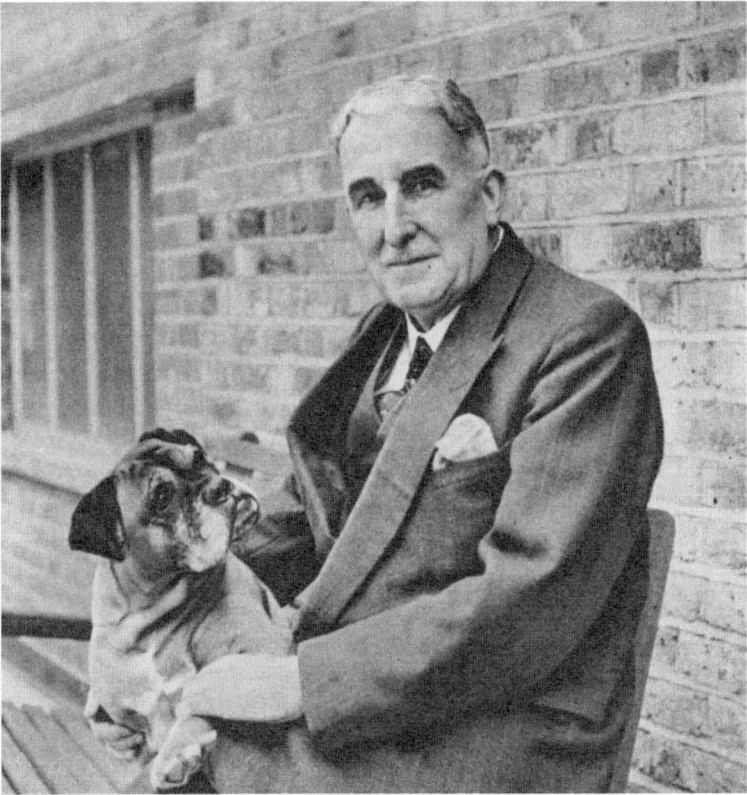

3. Major C. W. Hume.

Wild Animals received more representations from the public about
the cruelty of gins than it did about any other subjects it addressed.[120]

Its report described the trap as 'a diabolical instrument which
causes an incalculable amount of suffering'. Even so, it did not
recommend its immediate abolition: 'the rabbit is such a pest in this
country that it is impossible in present circumstances to control it
properly without some use of the gin or some other efficient trap.'[121]
Only in 1954, with effect from 1958, did attempts to ban the spring
trap finally succeed when the Pests Act, 1954 proscribed the sale,
ownership and use of spring traps that could catch anything other
than rats, mice or other small ground vermin.[122]

Chapter 3

Narrative of a Disease

Discovery

On 19 August 1953 a MAF official sent a 'very confidential' letter about myxomatosis to the country's four regional pest officers (RPOs). The letter noted that the disease had been recently introduced into France by a private individual with 'spectacular results' and went on:

> For various reasons which you will know and appreciate we feel it is very desirable to proceed cautiously before considering its introduction into this country. It is very doubtful, however, whether we could do anything to prevent its being introduced by some private individual. It seems probable that its use would not be illegal, and there is apparently nothing to prevent some enterprising but irresponsible person from getting hold of a supply of the virus.

MAF did not want to be caught unawares by an outbreak of the disease so it urged the RPOs to be alert to any reports of rabbit deaths from myxomatosis. At the same time it urged them to ensure that CAECs 'get no inkling of what we are about'.[1]

Less than a month later, on 15 September 1953, MAF's animal health division sent a circular to all its veterinary officers.[2] This referred to Australian efforts 'to get rid of rabbits by deliberate spreading of a virus disease known as Myxomatosis' and to recent developments in France where the disease was 'said to be spreading rapidly and to be causing some alarm'. The disease was not thought to be present in the United Kingdom but officers, though instructed not to make any 'special inquiries or investigations', were asked to inform head office if any suspected cases came to their attention.[3] Within a month a British outbreak had been confirmed. It is likely that the disease had already struck when the ministry issued its 15 September circular. It may even have been present in mid-August.[4]

The first development in Britain's myxomatosis outbreak involved the discovery of some dead rabbits on Major Sidney Williams's 2000-acre Bough Beech estate near Edenbridge in Kent. As Geoff Wicks, the tenant of Syliards Farm where the rabbits were first found, told the BBC: 'We began to see rabbits lying about all over the place, helpless, heads swollen up. Like raw meat their heads were with large blisters.'[5]

MAF files provide somewhat conflicting accounts of the circumstances of this discovery. It appears that around mid-September 1953, Wicks informed A. V. Neal, the Tonbridge-based assistant pest officer for Kent, that he had found dead rabbits on his land. Neal did not know what to make of the specimen Wicks showed him but he took it away to show the county pest officer, Mr Gregory. Gregory diagnosed syphilis and took no further action.[6] Because dead and dying rabbits continued to be found, Williams's gamekeeper, Frederick Feeke, notified Leslie Thompson, head of the syndicate that rented the shooting on the affected land. He, in turn, contacted MAF's divisional veterinary office and E. P. Thorne, a superintending veterinary officer, diagnosed myxomatosis. For further confirmation, two carcasses were sent for diagnosis to the Veterinary Investigation Office at Wye College in Kent. Postmortem examination 'revealed all the signs of myxomatosis'.[7]

Neal has left a slightly different account. In a letter dated 24 October 1953, he claimed that on 28 September Feeke, the gamekeeper 'casually mentioned seeing one or two dead rabbits'. Neither man attached any importance to the sighting because 'its [sic] not uncommon to find a dead rabbit occasionally'. Neal wrote nothing about a diagnosis of syphilis or any further developments until Friday 9 October when Gregory told him that Wicks 'had complained of seeing several dead rabbits', one of which was in his possession. Neal was instructed to collect the animal and report to his boss. That afternoon Feeke told him that Thompson had sent two corpses to Wye on the previous evening.[8]

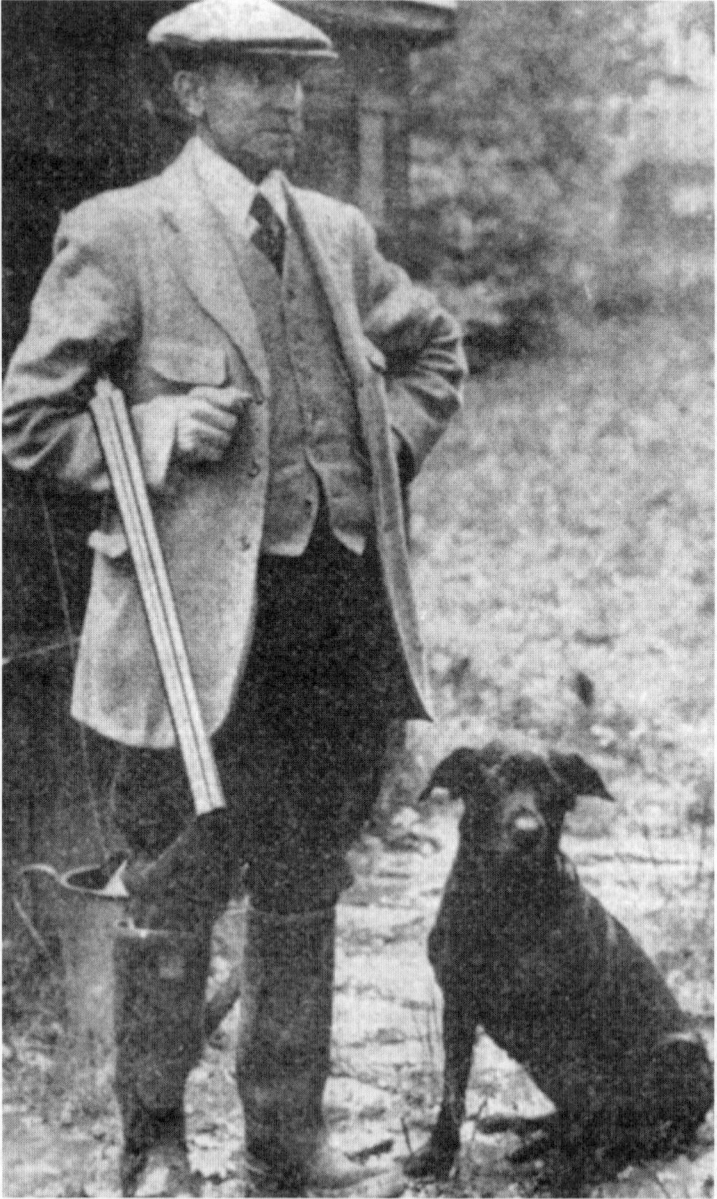

4. Frederick Feeke, Major Williams's gamekeeper.

At this remove it is difficult to say who found the
and when. Neither is it clear whether an early misdi
ensuing delay allowed the disease to gain a foothold.
ponse might have given the containment measures late᷅   _ a
better chance of success.

Whatever the precise circumstances surrounding the discovery of
myxomatosis at Bough Beech, from 9 October onwards events moved
quickly. Late that afternoon the veterinary investigation officer at Wye
informed MAF of his diagnosis. When the lesions were described to
the ministry's deputy chief veterinary officer he agreed that the rabbits
had 'almost certainly died from myxomatosis'. MAF's animal health
division then took a number of steps. First, it arranged for Thorne to
visit Bough Beech as soon as possible. Second, it confidentially
warned the estate's owner, Major Williams, that myxomatosis was
'strongly suspected' and advised against further shooting in the woodland where the diseased rabbits had been located (Williams raised no
objection). Third, it made arrangements to inject laboratory rabbits
with matter from the diseased animals.[9]

Thorne set off for Edenbridge early on Saturday 10 October in an
effort to 'secure full details of the case' and to catch some live rabbits
for testing. Accompanied by Neal he toured the Bough Beech estate,
which comprised five tenanted farms, and came across about a dozen
dead and six live but very sick rabbits, all with the same lesions as the
animals found previously. The two men also discovered that the
disease 'was rather more widespread than ... first thought'. It was
affecting several parts of the estate, including three different farms.
Altogether, several hundred acres appeared to be affected. Also on 10
October J. R. Hudson, B.Sc. MRCVS, a senior research officer at
MAF's veterinary laboratory in Weybridge, Surrey, went to Wye to
give his opinion about the disease affecting the Bough Beech rabbits.
He examined some of the ailing animals and agreed they were suffering from myxomatosis. On the basis of this opinion and other information, a MAF official noted that 'it may safely be presumed that the
disease is in fact myxomatosis'. Hudson had already made his way to
Paris to discuss the outbreak at the Pasteur Institute and try to obtain
some vaccine for laboratory rabbits. Though he rated prospects for

securing a supply of vaccine from the French 'poor', he was more hopeful of obtaining some 'precise information' about manufacture. In fact, the institute did make some vaccine available and MAF subsequently manufactured it at its Weybridge laboratory.[10]

On Sunday 11 October one of MAF's four regional pest officers, W. D. Baylis, accompanied by Thorne, Neal, Feeke and Surrey's pest officer, made a thorough inspection of the Bough Beech estate to assess whether the outbreak could be prevented from spreading by isolating the infected area and killing all the rabbits within it.

> After many enquiries it appeared to me [Baylis] that no rabbits with the disease had been seen outside a comparatively small area, so I decided there might be a hope of containing the area by wiring as soon as possible, because the disease might not spread other than by contact at this time of the year. I also decided that the area could not be cleared of rabbits for some time because of the large amount of undergrowth. But could in my opinion be cleared say by March 1954 by all acceptable methods, primarily gassing, all methods [sic], driving and shooting with nets.[11]

Two days later, on 13 October, a myxomatosis outbreak was officially confirmed and the minister of agriculture and fisheries, Sir Thomas Dugdale, met officials to discuss the appropriate response. They decided to fence 200 acres of the Bough Beech estate and kill all rabbits in the enclosed area. Neither the farmers nor the landowner raised any objection. Indeed, Major Williams agreed that the ministry could take any steps it deemed fit provided Feeke was kept informed. Wicks, of Syliards Farm, cooperated by ploughing a furrow into which the base of the fence could be set to make it rabbit proof. Sir William Slater, secretary of the ARC, though not consulted, was from the first sceptical about the chances of eradicating the disease, as was the government's chief veterinary officer. Nevertheless, under Baylis's supervision, Forestry Commission workers and pest officers moved in to erect 5000 yards of rabbit-proof netting, 10,000 yards of support wire and 1000 timber posts. About 40 operatives, including 'selected' London rat catchers and men provided by Surrey AEC, completed the

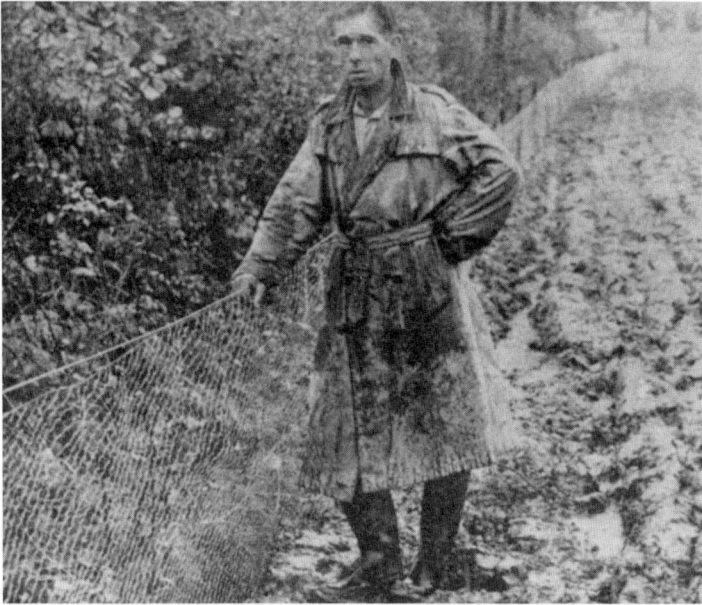

5. Mr Wicks of Syliards Farm.

exercise in about 48 hours between 16 and 18 October. As L. R. Sankey of MAF's Infestation Control Division (ICD) noted, this represented a 'remarkable achievement' on the part of Baylis and his men. The fence was then patrolled while rabbits were gassed and shot.[12]

Notwithstanding the extent of scrub and woodland in the enclosed area the extermination programme proceeded faster than anyone expected. In fact, pest officers from Kent, Surrey, East Sussex and Hertfordshire, armed with spades, slashers, flame-throwers and even a bulldozer, completed the work in only 11 days, killing over 400 rabbits.[13] As the exercise proceeded Major C. J. Armour, an ICD research officer, sprayed larvicide onto pools within and beyond the enclosure to control the mosquitoes thought to be the main vectors of myxomatosis. With October drawing to an end and winter approaching, it appeared that the goal of containment might have been achieved.[14]

On 19 October MAF and the DAS issued a joint press release to announce the discovery of myxomatosis (origin unknown) near Edenbridge. Information was given about the steps being taken to contain the disease and the appointment of a myxomatosis advisory committee chaired by Lord Carrington. The release noted that the disease was confined to a small area and that there was 'little likelihood' that it would spread, at least not before spring 1954 when conditions would be more favourable. The public was assured not only that the rabbit was a pest rather than a commercial asset, but also that myxomatosis would not necessarily result in its extermination. Neither should there be any 'immediate cause for concern' beyond the need to vaccinate domestic rabbits, which the government, already in touch with the Pasteur Institute in France, had well in hand. Overall, the release sought to reassure the public and emphasize that the authorities, after close study of the Australian and French outbreaks, were fully in control.[15]

In reality, limited attention had been paid to these overseas epizootics. A scientific civil servant (Dr J. W. Evans) spent a few days in France and submitted a report, but his visit (in late September 1953) did not take place until myxomatosis had reached the Channel coast.[16]

A week after the press release it emerged that a second outbreak of myxomatosis had occurred at Park Farm, Salehurst, near Robertsbridge in East Sussex, about 25 miles from Bough Beech. The affected farm was a 653-acre holding that comprised 200 acres of woodland and 100 acres of grassland (which supported a beef herd of Sussex cattle); the rest of the farm produced hops and fruit. Around mid-October the farm manager, Mr Mills, began noticing a few dead rabbits on open land surrounding an area of woodland. As the number of deaths increased, the matter came to the attention of the police at Hurst Green. On 26 October they reported to MAF's divisional veterinary office the presence of dead and dying rabbits showing signs of swollen eyes and mucous emissions. By the next day 40 rabbits had been affected and Major A. Franklin, one of the MAF's divisional veterinary officers, met J. D. Paterson of the Veterinary Investigation Service at Wye. Paterson confirmed myxomatosis in one dead and one sick rabbit.[17]

This second outbreak raised questions about the value of MAF's containment policy. It appeared, however, that the policy remained

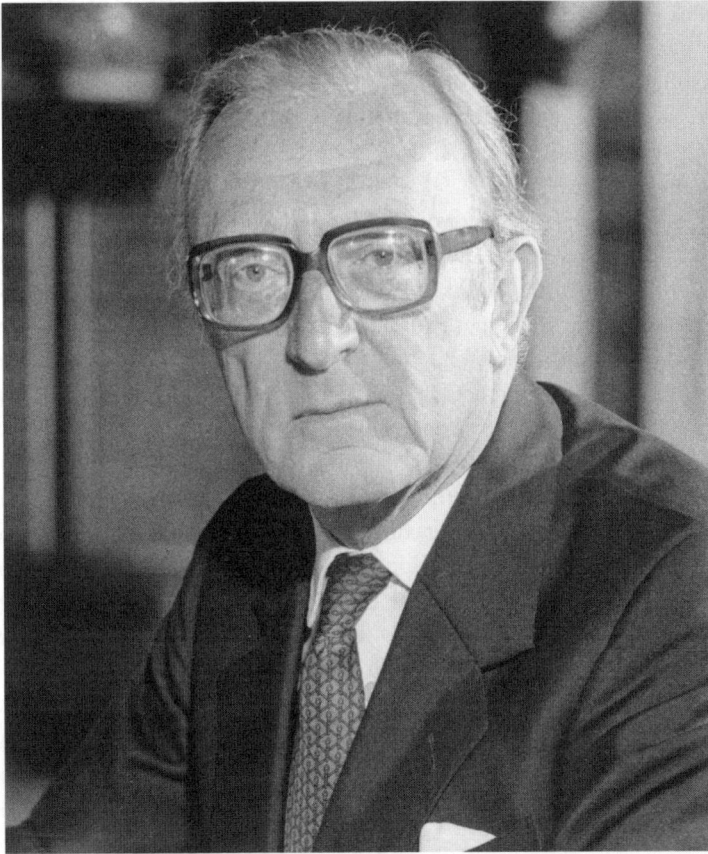

6. Lord Carrington.

feasible because the diseased rabbits at Salehurst, though found on open ground, appeared to have come from a comparatively small patch of woodland around which a fence could be erected. Accordingly, J. N. Ritchie, MAF's chief veterinary officer, advised that the policy of containment and extermination applied at Bough Beech could and should be extended to the new outbreak. He cautioned, however, that the occurrence of any further outbreaks would render the policy impractical.[18] Hugh Gardner, senior under secretary in MAF, agreed; he thought it was appropriate to keep the disease in check pending the deliberations of the MAC and the imminent arrival of winter frosts, which might mean no further outbreaks.[19] Lord Carrington accepted this advice: 'I think that it is just defensible to try and stop a second outbreak ... but if there are further outbreaks I suggest we should consider very seriously whether we can continue the present line.'[20]

It soon emerged that diseased rabbits were also present in an adjoining plantation (Maynard's Wood) at Salehurst. This would require fencing around 100 acres of woodland. The farmers concerned expressed their willingness to assist in the work by lending tractors and trailers, supplying stakes free of charge, and ploughing a furrow around the circumference of the woods so that the bottom of the fence could be buried. Even with these offers of help, the policy of containment and extermination promised to be difficult and expensive. As at Bough Beech, the two woodlands contained dense undergrowth that would make it difficult to use gas. Baylis questioned whether extermination were possible in such conditions. However, Sankey, second in command at the ICD, dismissed such misgivings and suggested that the woods could be bulldozed if necessary. Accordingly, on 29 October, with the support of men loaned by the Ministry of Works and Forestry Commission, fencing operations began. Again, progress was quick; two days later Sankey reported that the woods had been fenced.[21] There remained the problem of mosquito infestation. Sewage beds and pools of water formed by recent heavy rainfall provided ideal conditions for the insects, even in late October. It was therefore necessary, as at Edenbridge, to embark on a larvicide spraying programme. Meanwhile, police in Kent, Sussex and Surrey were requested to report any cases of dead or dying rabbits; but neither round Edenbridge nor Robertsbridge were diseased animals discovered outside the enclosed areas.[22]

At the end of October the ministry heard that a case of myxomatosis had been discovered near Faversham.[23] The report proved false, but on 1 November police notified the discovery of dead rabbits at another location, this time on two farms in the parishes of West Firle and Alciston to the east of Lewes, East Sussex. Myxomatosis was confirmed on the following day. Again rabbit deaths had been first spotted by local people about a fortnight earlier. In fact, Baylis judged that the disease had been present in the area for at least a month. The new outbreak, about 20 miles from Robertsbridge and 25 from Edenbridge, was located on 'open farms adjoining heavily [rabbit] infested downland'. Far from being concentrated in one small and relatively remote spot, sick and dead rabbits were found three-quarters of a mile or more apart. With the main Lewes to Eastbourne road running through the affected land, it was quickly apparent that there was 'no practicable possibility of fencing the area in and exterminating the rabbits'.[24] Even so, Baylis suggested that it might be possible to restrict the spread of infection by driving the rabbits into a wood at the centre of the outbreak and destroying them there by gassing and other means and also by gassing burrows in neighbouring hedgerows.[25]

Perhaps surprisingly, this operation proceeded smoothly as did the containment exercise at Salehurst. On 7 December Sankey noted that no diseased rabbits had been found beyond the fenced area at Salehurst and few at the unfenced site near Lewes. Neither were there signs that the Lewes outbreak was spreading. Throughout the greater part of November no rabbits were found beyond the three areas already known to be infected. Suspected outbreaks at Llandenny in Monmouthshire, Handy Cross near High Wycombe in Buckinghamshire, Smarden in Kent, Lindfield in Sussex, Lee Bay near Ilfracombe in Devon, and as far north as Staffordshire all proved to be false alarms. The news from the Edenbridge area, however, was less good. Diseased rabbits had been found outside the enclosed area, including on the Hever Castle estate. The estate refused MAF permission to gas burrows and, though it promised it would take the necessary action, MAF doubted whether the work would be done thoroughly. Then infected rabbits were found elsewhere, most significantly at two locations remote from Kent and East Sussex: at St Osyth (27 November) and Holland-on-Sea (5 December), both near Clacton, Essex, and at Southwold, East Suffolk (2 December).[26]

The disease was quiescent over the rest of the winter. Some predicted that cold weather would end the outbreak.[27] By mid-March 1954 the position was little changed. Some new cases had recently come to light near Bough Beech and a fresh outbreak had been discovered near Thorpe le Soken, a short distance from the first Essex cases at St Osyth.

There were still only 12 centres of infection in four counties: six in Kent, the rest in East Sussex, Essex and Suffolk. But with winter coming to an end and myxomatosis apparently 'smouldering' in all these locations, it was clear that frost and snow had not done for the disease.[28] Spring and summer saw it take off with a vengeance. It was confirmed in Wales (Radnorshire) on 8 May and in Scotland (Kincardine) on 13 July. By the end of July 137 outbreaks had been recorded in 28 English and Welsh and 2 Scottish counties. By the end of October every county in England and Wales, plus 28 of the 33 Scottish counties, had experienced outbreaks (Table 3.1). By the fourth week of November only Selkirk, of all the counties in Great Britain, remained free of the disease. By the end of 1954 Scotland had experienced 127 separate outbreaks with Aberdeenshire and Perthshire the most affected counties, each with 15 outbreaks.[29]

Ireland's minister for agriculture, James Dillon, informed the Dail that he 'refused to have anything to do with the introduction of myxomatosis to eradicate rabbits' even though they had become a 'serious menace' to agriculture. Dillon was determined to resist pressure from farmers and politicians on the grounds that the risk of introducing a new animal disease was 'out of all proportion to the likely benefits'. In July 1954, however, the disease was confirmed in the counties of Carlow, Kildare and Wicklow. Deputy Joseph Hughes accused farmers of spreading it.[30]

Robin Page, a boy in 1954, has written of the arrival of myxomatosis in his corner of Cambridgeshire:

> We read of the disease's progress in the paper, but it seemed a long time reaching us and perhaps, we thought, it would miss us completely; then one day, Jim [a farmworker] found a rabbit, helpless, with swollen discharging red eyes, blind and emaciated. Myxomatosis had arrived and it swept through the parish like a plague. Soon all the rabbit warrens were deserted, except for corpses, and rabbit pie became a thing of the past.[31]

Table 3.1. County-by-County Spread of Myxomatosis (England and Wales) October 1953–October 1954

Date	County
October 1953	East Sussex, Kent
November	Essex
December	East Suffolk
March 1954	Isle of Wight
May	Bedfordshire, Cornwall, Gloucestershire, Norfolk, Radnorshire, West Suffolk, West Sussex
June	Anglesey, Berkshire, Buckinghamshire, Cardiganshire, Devon, Oxfordshire, Pembrokeshire, Surrey
July	Brecknockshire, Caernarvonshire, Cambridgeshire, Carmarthenshire, Denbighshire, Dorset, Flintshire, Hampshire, Herefordshire, Hertfordshire, Lincolnshire (Kesteven), Lincolnshire (Lindsey), Merionethshire, Northamptonshire, Nottinghamshire, Shropshire, Somerset, Warwickshire, Wiltshire, Worcestershire
August	Cheshire, Cumberland, Durham, Glamorgan, Leicestershire, Lincolnshire (Holland), Monmouthshire, Montgomeryshire, Staffordshire, Yorkshire (ER), Northumberland
September	Huntingdonshire and Soke of Peterborough, Lancashire, Yorkshire (NR), Yorkshire (WR)
October	Derbyshire, Isle of Ely, Middlesex, Rutland, Westmorland

Source: NA MAF 131/115.

Young Page's belief that the disease might bypass his area was well founded, for its pattern of spread was erratic. Radnorshire in mid-Wales was affected at a very early stage. Its first outbreak preceded Surrey's, even though the Surrey border was close to Edenbridge, and occurred several months before that of Middlesex. Equally oddly,

Anglesey's outbreak predated Hampshire's, notwithstanding its remoteness from Bough Beech. Cornwall's first cases were discovered in May 1954 whereas Devon's occurred in June and Somerset's in July. Further north, the disease reached Scotland at a time when a score of English counties remained untouched. Indeed, 16 outbreaks across nine Scottish counties had occurred before a clutch of English counties, including Middlesex and Derbyshire had been affected. Once the disease had reached Scotland the rate of spread across the country was even more dramatic than in England (see Tables 3.1 and 3.2). All this was indicative of human, as well as insect, transmission for 'the natural spread is extremely slow, probably on an average less than a radius of one mile per month outward from each centre of infection' (see Chapter 4).[32]

Table 3.2. County-by-County Spread of Myxomatosis (Scotland), July 1954–May 1955

Date	County
July 1954	Kincardine, Sutherland
August	Aberdeen, Angus, Dumfriesshire, Fife, Orkney, Perthshire, Stirlingshire
September	Ayrshire, Banffshire, Clackmannan, Lanarkshire, Moray, Nairn, Peeblesshire, Ross and Cromarty, Zetland
October	Argyll, Berwickshire, Bute, Caithness, East Lothian, Inverness, Kinross, Kirkcudbright, Midlothian, Renfrew, West Lothian, Wigtown
November	Dumbarton, Roxburgh
May 1955	Selkirk

Source: NAS AF74/177.

Another peculiarity of the spread of myxomatosis was that some counties were affected worse than others. Berkshire, Cardiganshire, Cornwall, Gloucestershire, Kent, Montgomeryshire and Suffolk were virtually cleared of wild rabbits in short order. A survey conducted in mid-1955 indicated that in all the counties of southeast England, except for some small urban areas of Surrey and northeast Kent, 99 per cent or more of the rabbit population had been destroyed.[33] Lancashire, on the other hand, was affected only patchily. The disease appeared along its coastline in September 1954 and initially spread quite quickly. A year later, however, only about one-third of the county had the disease and east Lancashire was virtually unaffected. The relative immunity of some areas often reflected the moderate or low density of the rabbit population. Southwest and east Lancashire were either 'not very rabbity' or virtually free of the animal even before myxomatosis struck. Such an explanation did not apply everywhere, however. Leicestershire, for example, experienced its first outbreak in August 1954 but thereafter 'only small scattered areas were affected'. By October 1955 two-thirds of the county remained disease free.[34] Similar patterns, or lack of them, occurred in Scotland where outbreaks were 'patchy and puzzling'.[35]

Notwithstanding its erratic spread, myxomatosis, with its extremely high mortality rate, had a dramatic impact on rabbit numbers. In the relatively mild winter of 1954–5 the disease 'spread much more rapidly … than anyone expected.' In March 1955 *Farmer & Stock-breeder* predicted that Britain's wild rabbit population would soon hit its lowest level since Norman times. Some reports spoke of near extermination with 99.9 per cent of rabbits killed in some areas. NC surveys indicated that 'most of the larger affected warrens in England and Wales were reduced to roughly 0.5 per cent of the 1953 numbers.' Although numbers recovered in the second half of the 1950s, quantification is difficult. As the NC pointed out, 'no scientifically acceptable method has yet been devised for sampling the numbers of wild Rabbit populations.' In March 1957 Harry Thompson estimated that the original epizootic killed 95 per cent of rabbits, thereby reducing the population to around five million. At about the same time, *Farmers Weekly* claimed that myxomatosis cut numbers from 100 million to about 1 million. Published estimates in 1957, 1958, 1959 and 1960 all put the population at around 10 per cent of the pre-myxomatosis level, that is, between about six and ten million rabbits.[36]

Chapter 4

Accident or Design?

In September 1954 the narrator of a BBC Home Service documentary on myxomatosis observed: 'No one knows, or at least no one has admitted to know how the virus reached England last autumn.'[1] The myxomatosis advisory committee was not asked to investigate the transfer mechanism and its first report virtually ignored the issue beyond observations to the effect that 'there was no evidence to indicate how the disease was introduced in this country' and 'no official attempt has ever been made to introduce myxomatosis on to the mainland of Great Britain.'[2] Subsequently, Lord Carrington has observed that the arrival of myxomatosis in Britain was 'inevitable' once it had become established in France.[3] It is unclear, however, whether he held this view in the 1950s.

Suggestions that an outbreak of myxomatosis in Britain was 'inevitable' once the disease was established on the continent are widespread in the literature. For example, Harry Thompson, of MAF's ICD, wrote in 1954 that it 'seemed inevitable that it would cross from France to England'.[4] Forty years later he observed: 'As the disease spread across Europe it seemed inevitable that it would reach Britain.'[5] In 1965 Fenner and Ratcliffe also considered it 'inevitable', in view of Britain's proximity to the French epizootic, that myxomatosis would cross the Channel. However, the alleged inevitability of the transfer tells us nothing about the mode of transmission or the involvement, intentional or otherwise, of people. Fenner and Ratcliffe said nothing about agency: 'the disease probably reached England from France in August or September 1953, the actual means of entry being unknown.'[6] So what exactly was inevitable? Was it that virus-harbouring insects would reach Britain without human intervention, that returning tourists would unwittingly import the virus, perhaps on their shoes or car tyres, or that somebody would deliberately introduce the disease, perhaps by importing an infected rabbit, once the exercise involved little more than a round trip across the Channel?

One of the earliest published references to the issue of responsibility appeared in a paper by Harry Thompson in 1954. Though a relatively junior official (he was then a senior scientific officer with an annual salary in the £750–£950 range), Thompson was MAF's rabbit specialist; he possessed an insider's knowledge of the ministry's policy towards myxomatosis. He was also 'one of the first people on the scene' at Bough Beech in October 1953 and encountered his first myxoma rabbit on that occasion.[7] Over a period of more than forty years he wrote extensively about myxomatosis in Britain and elsewhere; his observations and reflections about the disease therefore deserve serious consideration.

In 1954 Thompson noted that it 'has frequently been suggested that the virus should be introduced into Britain'. However, in almost the same language as the MAC, he observed that: 'No official effort has ever been made to introduce myxomatosis on to the mainland of Britain.' Such a step was rejected because:

> conditions here are very different from those in Australia; it was not known whether suitable vectors occurred here, nor whether the disease would provide a permanent form of control, and it was not desired to endanger stocks of domestic rabbits without this certainty. The symptoms of the disease are also very distressing.[8]

In a book published in 1956, Thompson (and a co-author) offered a slightly different explanation of why deliberate introduction on the mainland had never been attempted. 'For many years there were suggestions that myxomatosis should be introduced on the mainland of Britain; but this method of rabbit control did not appeal to our national temper and received no official encouragement.'[9] In other words, the authorities eschewed myxomatosis for rabbit control for emotional or psychological, rather than practical reasons.

In the 1970s Thompson confirmed on television that a 'positive government decision had been taken not to introduce myxomatosis … officially into this country [Britain].' The introduction of a disease

> no matter how specific to rabbits [was] quite consciously seen as being a dangerous thing to do … we knew the reaction abroad [presumably the controversy in France rather than the much more positive response in Australia] and the danger it would pose to domestic rabbits; it was not clear how it would develop, that is, if it would operate as a permanent means of control; it was known in some degree that it was an unpleasant disease, though to a lesser extent than subsequently realized.[10]

Of course, rejection of a policy of deliberate introduction implies consideration of the possibility. Late in life Thompson acknowledged in print for the first time that the government had contemplated introducing myxomatosis during the war years, but continued to insist that no action ensued.[11] In 1977 he stated that the disease arrived 'by means unknown to us at the time'.[12] Accidental transmission appeared plausible, for 'Australian experience suggested that the virus could "jump" considerable distances'.[13] Elsewhere he nailed down the possibilities more precisely: 'the means of introduction has not been discovered; although carriage by flying or wind-blown insects, by birds carrying fleas, or by man are all possible.'[14]

Moynahan agreed that the virus was probably introduced accidentally: 'In view of the role of the rabbit flea (*Spilopsyllus cuniculi*) as vector in this country, it is probable that the virus was introduced here from the Continent on fleas which had straggled onto some bird, probably a carrion feeder, from the carcase of a rabbit recently dead from the disease.'[15] Ronald Lockley took the same view. So too, though with slightly less conviction, did Brown et al: 'it is possible that the first outbreaks in England occurred through infected fleas being carried mechanically by sea-birds across the Channel.'[16] C. H. Andrewes, a virologist who served on the Myxomatosis Advisory Committee (MAC) in the 1950s and chaired its scientific subcommittee, absolved scientists of responsibility for bringing myxomatosis to Britain. On the grounds that 'all the earlier outbreaks were in counties opposite the French coast', he thought its introduction was probably accidental.[17] This position was hardly logical, for it was obviously easier for residents of Kent or Sussex to take a ferry across the Channel for the purpose of obtaining a diseased rabbit than it was for those who lived far from the south coast ports. Yet Andrewes, while admitting that there was never likely to be certainty, opted for rabbit fleas conveyed by birds or wind-blown mosquitoes. In the 1970s Stamp, with greater certainty than any of his predecessors, asserted that 'the disease is spread by wheels of cars. It is probably in this way that it was introduced into England.'[18]

For all the differences between these judgements, certain themes emerge: lack of consensus about agency, emphasis on the role of accident and lack of suspicion about government involvement. But these themes have not been universally agreed. James Wentworth Day wrote: 'The disease reached Britain on October 13, 1953, when it appeared in Kent, followed by outbreaks in Sussex and Essex. No one knew how it was introduced. Insects, birds or man may have been the cause. I believe it was deliberately brought here by man.' Twenty-one years later Marchington took much the same line: 'Quite how the virus reached England we will probably never know. Birds or insects may have been responsible, but my own estimation is that it was a deliberate introduction by man.'[19] The 1977 BBC television documentary in which Harry Thompson took a prominent part noted the scientific backing for this viewpoint: 'scientists are almost certain it was introduced by man.' Soon after, C. J. Smith observed that 'myxomatosis was deliberately introduced from France as an early experiment in biological control.' In 1987 Norman Moore, a retired NC scientific officer, agreed that myxomatosis was brought to Britain deliberately.[20]

John Sheail, the only authority to have consulted government records, does not offer an opinion but observes: 'Local gossip, the time of year and the localized nature of the outbreak suggested that the disease had been introduced deliberately. The Ministry's veterinary officers discounted the idea of its being introduced by insect vectors or on the wheels of vehicles.'[21] MAF knew about the local gossip and was quick to note that there might be something in it. Furthermore, government veterinary officers did think it 'most unlikely that it was conveyed by insect vectors on the wheels of cars or, indeed, by any fortuitous route'.[22]

In 1994 Thompson voiced an opinion that contradicted the line he had taken over the previous 40 years: 'A local man brought a myxomatous rabbit from France and the first outbreak was confirmed near Edenbridge, Kent, on 13 October 1953, and a second outbreak on 27 October, in East Sussex.'[23] The only sources cited to substantiate this observation are two 1954 papers authored or co-authored by Thompson. Neither provides any support for deliberate introduction, whether by a man from the Edenbridge area or anyone else. Indeed, the co-authored piece explicitly stated that 'it has not been possible to discover how the infection was introduced.'[24]

In 1994 Fenner and Ross, probably following Thompson's lead, also espoused the idea of deliberate introduction: 'Permanent establishment of myxomatosis in Britain dates from autumn 1953. Deliberate carriage by an English resident, of an infected rabbit from France, and its release near Edenbridge, Kent, resulted in the first observed cases of myxomatosis.'[25] As we have seen, in 1965 Fenner and Ratcliffe had confessed ignorance about the manner in which myxomatosis reached the UK.[26] The only source Fenner and Ross cite in support of their claim for deliberate introduction is Armour and Thompson's 1955 paper in *Annals of Applied Biology*.[27] Obviously, this paper was available in 1965; indeed, Fenner and Ratcliffe consulted it and acknowledged that: 'The spread of myxomatosis in the first outbreak has been reported in detail by Armour and Thompson (1955).'[28] However, Armour and Thompson's paper focuses exclusively on the transmission of the disease *within* the UK; it is silent about the means by which it entered the country. While a change of mind in response to new evidence is understandable, it is hard to see why Fenner reversed his opinion between 1965 and 1994. It is still harder to understand why he adhered to his revised viewpoint for such a short time, for by 1999, this time in collaboration with Fantini, he had reverted to the conclusion that: 'The mechanism by which it [myxomatosis] crossed the Channel has never been determined with certainty.'[29] Notwithstanding this verdict, recent years have seen a definite shift in opinion in favour of deliberate introduction. In 1986 for example, Oliver Rackham wrote: 'In 1953 someone, disapproving of rabbits, introduced the South American myxomatosis virus via France, and promptly killed at least 99 per cent of the rabbits in Britain.' Still more recently Jackie Drakeford has written: 'At about the same time [March 1953], probably deliberately, the virus was let loose in Kent and East Sussex.'[30]

To return to Sheail's point about 'local gossip' concerning the arrival of the disease in Britain, it is hard to establish, at this remove, the extent to which public opinion at the time held that myxomatosis was introduced deliberately. Will Atkinson (born 1908), a former rabbit catcher from northeast England who lost his job as a result of myxomatosis, told BBC Radio Newcastle in 1999 that the disease was 'definitely introduced on purpose' and, furthermore, that the government encouraged it.[31] The veteran gamekeeper/writer Dugald Macintyre also thought the introduction was deliberate. Shortly after the British outbreak began he wrote: 'My own idea, and that of many others, is that (as in Australia and in France) the disease was deliberately introduced into Britain.'[32] He and others raised the possibility of official involvement: 'it is up to our biological experts and others interested in germ-warfare to clear themselves of the uneasy suspicion that they are to blame for the introduction to this country of germ-warfare for animals.'[33] Hundreds of people apparently thought that 'the Government and the farmers worked together on the rabbit disease to keep the price of meat up as it started at the same time that meat was taken off the ration'.[34] Suggestions of government involvement reached the ears of Miriam Rothschild (Mrs George Lane), the celebrated entomologist. Indeed, she refused to accept a place on the MAC before receiving (as she did) an official 'assurance that as far as one can ascertain there has been no deliberate introduction of myxomatosis at Edenbridge.'[35]

To sum up, there have been two main schools of thought about the arrival of myxomatosis in the UK: the first points to accidental introduction, with or without unwitting human assistance; the second argues for deliberate introduction. On occasion, though seldom in print, it has been suggested that the government might have been involved. Over the longer term, official and scientific opinion appears to have inclined to the former interpretation, with popular and journalistic opinion inclining to the latter. In recent years serious scientists and other scholars have espoused the notion of deliberate introduction, but without government involvement. Occasionally other theories have surfaced, for example that myxomatosis '"escaped" from a laboratory in Kent'.[36] This particular suggestion, or journalistic fantasy, can be dismissed because of a total lack of evidence.

One feature of the initial outbreak would appear to undermine the school of accidental introduction. By September 1953, that is the month in which myxomatosis probably broke out at Bough Beech, the disease had reached the French coastal regions of Nord, Somme and Pas de Calais. If it crossed the Channel accidentally, however, whether via car tyres, bird plumage or insects, the first British outbreak would surely have occurred near a port or the coast. As Macintyre wrote in December 1953: 'If the disease had been carried by flies from the Continent to England one would naturally expect to have its first English appearance reported from the seashore.'[37] Its actual occurrence, 28 miles inland would appear to indicate deliberate introduction. However, in a retrospective analysis published in 1987, R. F. Sellers suggested that on the night of 11–12 August 1953 meteorological conditions were such that live specimens of the mosquito, *anopheles atroparvus*, a species present in the coastal marshes of northern France and known to spread the myxoma virus, 'could have been carried across the English Channel' and, as a result of temperature inversion, deposited on the Bough Beech estate where they proceeded to infect wild rabbits. He also speculates that the Robertsbridge outbreak, rather than being an extension of the Bough Beech outbreak, may have been caused by another windborne incursion of mosquitoes from the continent.[38]

For some years mosquitoes were 'not considered to be [myxomatosis] vectors amongst wild rabbits in Britain'.[39] Thus, the MAC's scientific subcommittee judged that fleas were 'the only insect vectors responsible for the local spread' of myxomatosis. 'Contrary to expectations, rabbit biting mosquitoes appeared to have played no part so far in spreading the disease.'[40] Two years later Muirhead-Thompson observed that 'there is no evidence ... to show that this mosquito [*anopheles atroparvus*] plays any major role in spreading the disease among wild rabbits.' He further concluded that mosquitoes of the *aëdes* genus, which predominated in the vicinity of Bough Beech, also were of 'negligible importance as vectors of myxomatosis'.[41]

Service modified these assessments when, in 1971, experimental studies carried out in southern England led him to conclude that 'contrary to previous beliefs mosquitoes in Britain feed to a certain extent on wild rabbits, and therefore are potential vectors of myxomatosis.' However, he made no attempt 'to assess their relative importance in the transmission of the disease' and endorsed the view that in Britain it was 'transmitted mainly by the rabbit flea'.[42] His paper does not establish that mosquitoes brought myxomatosis to Britain from the continent.

Sellers's article, which built upon a substantial literature about windborne viral transmission, raises intriguing possibilities. Ultimately, however, his theory cannot be substantiated. Rather like Thor Heyerdahl's *Kon-Tiki* expedition of the late 1940s, it demonstrated feasibility, not occurrence. It remains the case that we have 'no evidence to show that it [myxomatosis] was introduced in this country [the UK] as a result of disease-carrying insects drifting or blown across the Channel'.[43]

Is it possible to establish whether deliberate infestation took place? Who stood to gain from the elimination or drastic reduction of the rabbit population around Edenbridge or elsewhere? Farmers and foresters were potential beneficiaries in terms of improved yields and higher profits. Farmers, in particular, would have known this by the summer of 1953, for the British press was then reporting big increases in Australian agricultural output owing to an absence of rabbits.[44] The collapse of the rabbit population also suited a government committed to rabbit control and increased domestic food production. The first appearance of the disease far from the coast supports the idea that a local farmer or landowner was responsible. Without suggesting that there is an easy, let alone definitive, answer to this question, the appropriate way of exploring it is to examine the extant government files.

As we have seen, Harry Thompson has written that during the Second World War officials rejected use of myxomatosis for rabbit control. Since Thompson joined MAF (from Oxford University's Bureau of Animal Population) after the war, in 1946, he could not have been party to such discussions (unless as an invited observer). Until his appointment the ministry employed no full-time rabbit biologist.[45] Before and during the war many politicians, civil servants and others supported rabbit extermination (or, at least, vigorous control). But surviving records give no indication that myxomatosis was at any point regarded as a feasible supplement or alternative to gas, traps, guns, ferrets, nets and snares or even that its possible use was seriously discussed. Since conventional methods of control worked effectively during the war years, there was little incentive to consider an unproven biological control. Thompson is now deceased and therefore cannot be asked about the assertion he made in 1994. No files in the National Archives support his claim, however, and no evidence indicates that government, which was not involved in the experiments of Martin and Lockley, explored the potential of myxomatosis either in the 1930s or during the war years.[46]

There is rather more evidence of government attitudes towards the control of rabbits by biological means for the postwar years when rabbit numbers appear to have resumed their upward progress. In 1948, James Scott Watson, director general of the National Agricultural Advisory Service, noted that:

It was at one time thought possible that an infectious and fatal disease organism could be used, but experiments on one of the Western Isles [Skokholm?] were not successful. The finding was that, although an artificial epidemic could be set up, there were a few survivors. Moreover, rabbit populations are rather static, and there was very little outward spread from the centre when the disease was set up.[47]

At about the same time the Committee on Industrial Productivity, concerned about the impact of the rabbit on agricultural and anxious to see an extermination programme, had its secretariat examine Australia's experience with myxomatosis. The resulting report provided a largely negative appraisal of the value of the disease in rabbit control. It 'seems possible that in some parts of Australia under special conditions ... the disease could be used with some promise of temporary control of a rabbit population'. Generally, however, 'field experiments and field trials show that myxomatosis cannot be used to control rabbit populations under most natural conditions in Australia with any promise of success.' The report contained no suggestion that research or trials should be carried out in Britain.[48]

At the end of 1949 the ICD's director, W. McAuley Gracie, expressed equally unenthusiastic views: 'The control of rabbits by the artificial creation of an epizootic is a perennial suggestion, but the scientific evidence is heavily against its success.' He went on to point out that British, Danish and Australian experiments had shown that for various reasons the disease failed to spread. Although

> Some results in Sweden, and recent unofficial claims from Australia, suggest that finality of view has not been reached ... my present view is that even if the introduction of myxamotosis [sic] were a practical solution to the problem of eliminating rabbit colonies in certain environments – particularly in very large areas of unenclosed lands or on small islands it would be unsuited to the physical conditions of land tenure in this country, and further would offend the public conscience as well as produce resistance from those more directly concerned in the rabbit areas.[49]

Around the same time the ARC discussed the possibility of doing some research on myxomatosis. However,

> the general view of the Council was that there was not much point in such research and that if one wanted to do anything about it the best thing would be to start the disease off; but I think all the Council members were against this, for a number of reasons.[50]

A Home Office file, 'Legislation: Prevention of Damage by Rabbits Bill', covering the years 1934–48 carries no reference to myxomatosis.[51] Neither was the disease mentioned in the course of the
protracted discussions within MAF about rabbit control in the late
1940s and early 1950s. Thus, the 1949–50 rabbit control working
party, whose members included Charles Elton of BAP and A. D.
Middleton, agreed that there was 'a clear case for maximum destruction of wild rabbits' but also that 'there is no immediate prospect of
new scientific methods of radical value becoming available'.[52] Neither
does a MAF file on 'Destruction of Rabbits, 1939–1952' include any
mention of myxomatosis until July 1950 when the ICD produced a
paper on the subject. This paper, which identified no ministry-
sponsored work, noted that the 'control of rabbits by artificially
creating an epizootic is a perennial suggestion'. It briefly reviewed several scientific papers (by Sanarelli, Kessel, Bull and Dickinson) as well
as the unsuccessful experiments of Martin, Lockley, Bull and Mules,
Schmidt and Jensen (in Denmark), and the somewhat more promising
work of Hvass, Schmidt and Hensen (in Sweden). Mainly because the
Australians were about to resume their field trials, ICD judged that 'no
useful purpose would be served by further investigations' in Britain 'at
the present time'.[53] When, in 1952, Dr J. W. Evans of MAF reviewed
recent ministry-sponsored and other research on rabbits he did not
identify 'a single biological control project'.[54]

The fact is that until the Australian epizootic commenced, in late
1950, there was little reason to suppose that myxomatosis had any significant potential for large-scale rabbit control.[55] Accordingly, even if
myxomatosis were considered during the war as a means of destroying
Britain's rabbits and, Thompson's statement apart there are no
grounds for thinking it was, anyone with even a passing knowledge of
the subject could have pointed out the impracticality of such an idea.
All other considerations aside, there was scant evidence to indicate
that the disease would work on anything other than a local level. Only
from 1951 was there any reason to suppose that myxomatosis might
provide a practical solution to an intractable problem. Even then, it
was far from clear that the disease would act in the same way in the
temperate northern hemisphere that it had in Australia. Only in 1952,

when the disease took off in France and neighbouring countries did myxomatosis begin to look as if it might have potential in British conditions (though Lockley remained sceptical in October 1953).[56] Only then did officials begin to discuss its possibilities for wild rabbit control.

In June 1952 the North of Scotland College of Agriculture began experimenting with myxomatosis on the Heisker or Monach Islands in the Hebrides. However, these experiments were apparently conducted without government finance, permission or, in the early stages, involvement. Once myxomatosis had broken out at Bough Beech and elsewhere the research group of the MAC's scientific subcommittee agreed that the Hebridean experiments 'should be encouraged'. One of the college's researchers, P. L. Shanks, was invited to attend the group's next meeting in January 1954. On this occasion he described the rather inconclusive experiments he and his colleagues had conducted. They had obtained 'only circumstantial evidence to suggest that ... fluctuations in rabbit numbers [on the islands] were due to myxomatosis'. It was then agreed that Shanks and Harry Thompson 'should produce a programme for research on induced outbreaks in the Hebrides and Shetland Islands for submission to the Committee and the Department of Agriculture for Scotland'. It was also agreed that Shanks should represent Scotland on the research group. The research programme did go ahead in the Hebrides, though not on the Shetlands, but all this occurred after myxomatosis had broken out on the British mainland.[57]

In November 1952 Dr Evans, under the heading of 'Research Needs', briefly discussed use of myxomatosis in a paper on 'The Rabbit Problem'. He expressed little enthusiasm. The public was 'becoming increasingly antagonistic to cruelty to wild animals' and for this reason alone he considered it 'improbable that virus dissemination could ever become a recognized method of control here, even if it were a possible one'. The danger to domesticated rabbits was another consideration. Even so:

as it is certain to be raised perennially as a possible means of control, it is considered that the first essential step of any investigation of its possibilities should be taken. This would be the determination of whether or not adequate vectors (principally rabbit-biting fleas) occur and are well distributed in Great Britain.[58]

It is impossible to imagine that Evans would have expressed these sentiments if MAF had previously considered introducing myxomatosis to control Britain's rabbit population. Neither is it conceivable that he, as deputy chief scientific officer, would have been unaware of such discussion had it taken place as anything more than canteen conversation.

Evans was right to anticipate proposals to deploy myxomatosis. At the end of December 1952, in response to a query from Cheshire's chief pest officer, T. J. Marjoram of the ICD wrote that while MAF was keeping in close touch with Australian developments, 'we are not yet satisfied that such methods would be suitable or appropriate for application in this country, and we are not yet in a position to carry out experiments.' Winch gave the same information to Brecon AEC in February 1953.[59] At the end of March Marjoram informed a correspondent (wrongly) that fleas were not efficient carriers of myxomatosis and that the ministry had yet to follow up Australian experiments in Britain because of concern about cruelty, the danger to domestic rabbits and the continuing absence of a study of insect vectors. Recent evidence of the declining virulence of the virus in Australia and recognition that British conditions were so different from those of Australia (or Sweden) were additional considerations.[60] Towards the end of July Sankey rejected a suggestion from Wales that islands off the coast of Anglesey (the Skerries) might be a suitable location for a myxomatosis experiment. Indeed, he wrote that MAF would not even start investigating the potential of the disease for rabbit control in the UK until the French outbreak had played out.[61]

A few days later, Evans, responding to yet another query about the release of myxomatosis in Britain, wrote that MAF was 'extremely interested in the possibilities offered by myxomatosis' and had 'given much thought to the problems involved'. However, guided by Australian as well as British experts, 'up to the present we have taken no active steps to liberate the virus in this country, nor do we propose to do so unless we are fully satisfied as to the desirability or otherwise of such a step.' This would entail 'long-range research'. The first step would be a study of possible vectors but a study of this sort, far from having begun, was still at the discussion stage. No such study appears to have been initiated until 1954, that is after the Bough Beech and several other British outbreaks.[62] Like Sankey, Evans observed that developments in France, which he was about to visit, would be monitored, perhaps with a British researcher stationed there for a while. 'This is because it will enable a study to be made of its effects under conditions very similar to our own.' But even if it were established that the virus promised success, there remained the problem of public opinion, which, Evans continued to think, would object to myxomatosis on humanitarian grounds.[63] On 14 July 1953 the minister informed parliament that the evidence for myxomatosis 'as a long-term control measure is, I fear, not encouraging'.[64]

One month later, by which time the disease might actually have been present though undiscovered in Britain, MAF's attitude towards myxomatosis remained cautious. Thompson stressed the absence of knowledge about insect vectors and the need for further research on the issue. He too pointed to the importance of public opinion, humanitarian considerations and the danger the disease would pose to domestic rabbits.[65] On the following day Evans informed the head of the ICD that 'we do not wish the disease established in this country until we are satisfied that it would permanently reduce the number of wild rabbits.'[66] He was not persuaded that this would happen. 'Recently it has been noticed in Australia that immunity to the disease occurs among certain individuals in the rabbit population. On this account it may be expected that in a relatively short time the disease will cease to be an effective measure for rabbit control.'[67]

In August 1953 MAF outlined its position to the country's CAECs:

The employment of the virus of myxomatosis against rabbits in this country would present many problems. It is reported from Australia that the disease is spread mainly by a single species of insect. It is not yet known whether vectors which may exist in this country are suitably distributed. Nor is it clear from

Australian results whether the efficacy of myxomatosis as a
control measure could be permanently maintained. Such phe-
nomena as immunity and progressive loss of virulence need
further investigation. Moreover, the virus once established
would be a threat to the domestic rabbit industry and the
symptoms produced in the rabbit are unpleasant to see and
would doubtless provoke some public out-cry. The situation in
Australia, France and elsewhere is being closely followed.[68]

The minister expressed the same opinion, notwithstanding the damage
wrought by rabbits:

The rabbit takes a toll on home food production out of all
proportion to its value and we must clearly do everything
possible to reduce these losses. Nevertheless you can rest
assured that we would very carefully weigh the pros and cons
before considering the use of myxomatosis as a means of
controlling rabbits in this country.[69]

By this time, aware that some wanted to see a myxomatosis
outbreak in Britain, the ministry had become concerned that someone
might take matters into his own hands. Evans asked his head of
division to explore the means available to prevent introduction of the
disease:

At present there is nothing to stop a farmer bringing back a
diseased rabbit from France and placing it in a warren in this
country. I believe it would also be possible for anyone to write
to the Pasteur Institute and obtain a supply of the virus,
together with instructions for its use.
    It is clearly undesirable that our hand should be forced and
the disease established here before we are satisfied as to the
wisdom of such action.[70]

The legal department's advice was not reassuring. It was not illegal to
introduce the virus. Neither would prosecution under the Protection

of Animals Act 1911 be practicable: 'in any case the damage would have been done whatever happened to the initiator, and to threaten possible offenders with prosecution might have the effect of putting ideas into their heads.'[71]

From all this it appears clear that the government was not responsible for the introduction of myxomatosis. In terms of a long-standing desire to reduce the damage done by rabbits it certainly had a motive to act (see Chapter 2). As Evans wrote: 'These animals [rabbits] are the greatest single menace to food production in the country, and cause far greater destruction to growing crops than any other injurious mammal, bird or insect.'[72] The director of the Forestry Commission agreed: 'The rabbit is more than a source of anxiety to foresters – it is one of the deadliest foes of the forest and it should never be permitted to exist in young plantations even in the smallest numbers. Its presence is fatal to good forestry.'[73] Furthermore, there were grounds to think that rabbit numbers were increasing in the postwar years.[74]

To tackle the rabbit menace MAF was ready to consider myxomatosis, but only after the Australian experience initially suggested the disease might have the potential to reduce rabbit numbers. Scott Watson identified 'the Australian approach of introducing epidemic disease' as one of the 'main possibilities' for rabbit control, along with narcotics and poisons.[75] At the same time, however, all interested parties within MAF recognized that such a step would, for reasons already mentioned, be a leap in the dark. Moreover, as Australia's epizootic developed, it soon became clear that myxomatosis did not offer the prospect of the wild rabbit's permanent eradication. As Thompson wrote in September 1953, there were 'weighty' objections to the use of myxomatosis in the UK, 'particularly on humanitarian grounds', but also because of the threat to domestic rabbits. Consequently:

Before embarking upon any campaign to exterminate rabbits by methods that do not easily recommend themselves to our national disposition, it would seem desirable first to become a little more assured that we shall not, in the end, have introduced one more disease that is enzootic but not lethal, so that we are left with this and the rabbits as well.[76]

A month later he informed Lockley unequivocally that 'the Ministry does not intend to introduce the disease [myxomatosis] into Great Britain.'[77] Reginald Franklin was adamant about the absence of official involvement when he responded to Miriam Rothschild's enquiry about whether the Bough Beech outbreak was deliberately induced: 'We have no evidence about how the disease was introduced into England, I can give a definite assurance that it was not introduced through our agency or with our connivance.' Thirty years later John Ross, a MAF scientist, was equally definite that the ministry had not been involved in bringing myxomatosis to Britain.[78] But if the authorities were not involved, where did responsibility lie?

At this remove, it is not possible to establish conclusively whether myxomatosis reached Britain by accident or design. The suggestion that it was initiated by windborne mosquitoes is unconvincing, mainly because the association between mosquitoes and the post-Bough Beech spread of the disease within Britain is so tenuous. Since transmission on car tyres was ruled out at an early juncture, the sole remaining possibility for accidental introduction would seem to be by means of fleas transported across the Channel on birds.[79] If only because of the distance between Bough Beech and the coast, this is little more persuasive than the idea of windborne mosquitoes.

In 1953 C. P. Quick of MAF observed that, though the origin of the Bough Beech outbreak was unknown, government veterinarians deemed accidental transmission 'most unlikely'. In his view, the localized nature of the outbreak pointed to deliberate introduction, for it was unlikely 'that any other agency would have stopped short in the general area of the Bough Beech estate'.[80] In contrast, Sankey, the MAC's secretary, observed three years later that 'there was not the slightest evidence to suggest that the original outbreaks of the disease in this country had been deliverately [sic] introduced.'[81] Later still the MAF scientist, Ieuan Thomas, described the fortuitous arrival of a flea on an animal other than a rabbit as 'a rather unlikely happening'.[82]

The balance of probability is that myxomatosis was deliberately brought from France, probably by means of an infected rabbit, and that the dead or ailing animal was placed in a burrow on the Bough Beech estate, thereby virtually guaranteeing further infection. After all, we know for sure that the disease was deliberately spread within the UK after the first outbreak. Furthermore, Thomas noted that a 'few farmers have from time to time said that they know how, when, and by whom the disease was brought into this country; none, however, is willing to mention names.'[83] Local opinion apparently insisted that 'the virus was deliberately procured by a neighbouring farmer who for some time past had complained of the invasion of his farm by rabbits from the Bough Beech estate, and had declared that by some means or other he would get rid of them.'[84] Before the end of October 1953 *Southern Weekly News* was reporting on the 'atmosphere of rumour and suspicion' hanging over the villages of Four Elms and Bough Beech and on local opinion 'that someone has deliberately planted the virus'. Frederick Feeke was 'sure of one thing. This is a case of sabotage.'[85]

In June 2005, in the hope of clarifying the question of responsibility, the present author appealed in the Kent press for information about the Bough Beech outbreak. Mrs Georgina Coleby (born 1940) subsequently told me that Major Williams, owner of the Bough Beech estate, obtained the virus from France and then instructed her father, the estate's head gamekeeper, Alfred Ottaway, to disseminate it. This single piece of uncorroborated second-hand evidence secured more than half a century after the event cannot be regarded as definitive. In fact, it raises a number of questions. Why was the octogenarian Williams, who was only months from the end of his life, concerned about rabbits, especially as he was a landlord who farmed on his own account only to a very limited extent, if at all?[86] How did the elderly and ailing Major Williams, who travelled little in his last years, import the virus? Why, if he were responsible for introducing the disease, did Williams cooperate with MAF officials who tried to contain it? Why is Ottaway's name completely absent from all MAF documents relating to the Bough Beech outbreak and Feeke repeatedly identified as Williams's only gamekeeper? The author's taped interview with Mrs Coleby shed no light on these questions.[87] However, it appeared that it would be possible for the first time in print to identify individuals who *might* have been responsible for causing Britain's first myxomatosis outbreak.

Then, in December 2005, I made contact with Cyril Skinner (born

1924) who, in 1953, was helping his father run Roodlands Farm near the village of Four Elms in Kent. This farm, also part of the Bough Beech estate, was very close to the site where myxomatosis was first discovered. Skinner, though in no doubt that the disease was deliberately introduced, dismissed out of hand the suggestion that either Major Williams or Ottaway were responsible. Indeed, he denied that Ottaway was ever Major Williams's gamekeeper, head or otherwise, as opposed to a general estate worker (and 'right old rogue'). Instead, he pointed the finger at his old friend Gordon Williams, the tenant of Ivy House Farm, which was later flooded to make way for Bough Beech reservoir. Skinner, though admitting he had no proof, stated that Williams, who was not related to the major, visited France on his motorcycle in 1953 and brought back a sick rabbit or two that he then released. Williams, now deceased, 'hotly denied' these allegations, but Skinner and others were not persuaded.[88]

The case against Williams is entirely circumstantial: he was a farmer who, in common with many others, had a serious rabbit problem (Skinner described the level of infestation in the Edenbridge area in the early 1950s as 'desperate' and Geoff Wicks was unable to grow winter wheat on some fields at Syliards owing to rabbit damage); he had good contacts in northern France from his wartime service there as an army officer in 1944; he made a cross Channel visit shortly before the disease was discovered at Bough Beech; his involvement fits Quick's early suggestion that a local farmer was responsible. Against such tenuous 'evidence' it is right to point out that Skinner's allegation cannot be corroborated. Also one might ask why, if Gordon Williams wanted to rid his farm of rabbits as quickly as possible, he released infected animals on a neighbour's land rather than his own. Williams, who in 1977 appeared anonymously on the BBC television documentary, *Rabbits Wanted: Dead or Alive* never admitted responsibility, though in his short televised interview he emphasized the damage rabbits did and made a case for the disease.

Since the introduction of myxomatosis was not an offence in 1953 and, indeed, was seen by local farmers as a 'godsend', it can be argued that Williams had no reason to feel ashamed for having imported the virus.[89] On the other hand, the moral aspect was less clear; many people were horrified by myxomatosis and disgusted by the thought that it was spread deliberately. The farmer who introduced the disease to Scotland received much abuse, as did A. G. Street after he advocated deliberate transmission.[90] Furthermore, as was widely reported in the British press, Dr Delille was dragged through the French courts by aggrieved parties who sought damages. So if Gordon Williams was the 'guilty' party he was surely wise to deny all allegations.

In conclusion, all that can be said is that Gordon Williams may have brought myxomatosis to Great Britain; Cyril Skinner certainly made a persuasive case for his involvement. However, there can be no certainty. Neither can Major Williams and Ottaway, for all the question marks against their involvement, be unequivocally absolved. Questions might also be asked about the involvement of Geoff Wicks. After all, myxomatosis started on his farm. Wicks also had French connections, his sister-in-law having married a Frenchman and settled in France. But why would Wicks have reported the disease if he introduced it? Moreover, according to his son, Stuart, Wicks seldom left his farm and was 'lost' if he ventured five miles from home. It is therefore hard to entertain the possibility that he visited France to obtain the virus.[91] Many questions remain unanswered and unanswerable. It is even possible that the disease really was introduced by windborne mosquitoes or infected fleas carried from France by birds.

Chapter 5

The Myxomatosis Advisory Committee

On 13 October 1953, the day Britain's myxomatosis outbreak was officially confirmed, the minister of agriculture, Thomas Dugdale, authorized the appointment of an expert standing committee (the MAC) to offer advice and recommendations.[1] The committee was asked to consider whether the disease should be contained, allowed to run its course or deliberately introduced to uninfected areas of the country in the interest of pest control.[2] Lord Carrington, who had been joint parliamentary secretary to MAF since 1951 and was also a Buckinghamshire farmer, had already been selected to chair the committee. After the nature of the position was described to him over the telephone, he 'readily agreed' to take it on.[3]

Peter Alexander Rupert Carington, sixth Baron Carrington since 1938, was 34 years of age and in his first job in government when he became chairman of the MAC. Educated at Eton and Sandhurst, he had served as a major in the Grenadier Guards during the Second World War, seeing action in northwest Europe in 1944–45 and winning the Military Cross. Carrington went on to have a distinguished career as British high commissioner to Australia, first lord of the Admiralty, leader of the House of Lords, defence secretary in Edward Heath's government, and secretary general of NATO. He is perhaps best known for having been Margaret Thatcher's first foreign secretary (1979–82), a position from which he resigned following the outbreak of the Falklands War. Unsurprisingly, given the number of prominent posts he occupied in the course of a long political career, his autobiography devotes little attention to myxomatosis. It does, however, indicate the manner in which he was appointed to chair the MAC: 'Because I was less tied to parliament, because I was freer to travel and investigate and explore, I found myself often with the odd jobs which nobody else wanted or had time for. One of these, I remember, was a study of the myxomatosis problem.'[4]

Several individuals and institutions were quickly identified as potential members of the committee. These included senior civil servants, scientists and representatives from various interested organizations. The possibility of including a woman and another scientist was also discussed. Miriam Rothschild, 'the greatest living expert on fleas', was seen as someone who would fit the bill on both grounds. She also had the additional advantages of being the wife of a farmer and sister of Lord Rothschild, chairman of the ARC. Surprisingly, given the damage rabbits did on woodland, forestry interests were unrepresented.[5]

The original MAC members were:

Professor C. H. Andrewes MD FRCP FRS	Deputy director of the National Institute for Medical Research and a leading virologist
Lord Carrington MC	Joint parliamentary secretary to the MAF (chairman)
H. Collison	Member of the general council of TUC and general secretary of the NUAW
Earl of Dundee	Landowner and farmer, former parliamentary under secretary for Scotland
J. W. Evans MA DSc ScD	Applied entomologist and deputy chief scientific officer in MAF's ICD
Hugh Gardner CBE	Senior under secretary in MAF
Professor R. E. Glover MA BSc FRCVS	President of the RCVS
John Scott Henderson QC	Recorder of Portsmouth and chair of committee on cruelty to wild animals
Lord Merthyr	Chair of RSPCA
G. T. Plumb	Assistant secretary to the Board of Trade
J. N. Ritchie BSc MRCVS DVSM	Chief veterinary officer at MAF

Miriam Rothschild	Eminent parasitologist
J. C. Sandford BA	Author, lecturer on rabbit husbandry, member of National Council for Domestic Food Production
L. R. Sankey	Of the ICD, served as secretary
W. H. Senior FRSE	Assistant secretary, Department of Agriculture for Scotland
R. B. Verney	A Buckinghamshire landowner who later chaired the Nature Conservancy Council
Harold Woolley	Leading Cheshire farmer and chairman of NFU's parliamentary committee

The committee's exact terms of reference were: 'To advise the Minister of Agriculture and Fisheries and the Secretary of State for Scotland on the problems that would be raised by an outbreak of myxomatosis in rabbits in Great Britain and the action that should be taken by the Government.'[6] This was peculiar terminology because myxomatosis had already started and was the reason the committee was appointed in the first place. In late October and early November 1953 it appeared that the disease could be eradicated in the two locations where it initially occurred and prevented from spreading. But Lord Carrington's recall was faulty when he wrote in his autobiography that the MAC 'had first to discuss the point of principle – should myxomatosis be kept from Britain's shores, in the unlikely event that it was possible. ... While we were deliberating, however, myxomatosis arrived. Rabbits started dying.'[7]

Advisory bodies are sometimes appointed to gather information and provide expert advice to government on a specific issue. Their real purpose, however, may be to buy time, thus allowing postponement of a political decision, to appease demands for action, or to legitimate a predetermined policy.[8] In autumn 1953 the government lacked information about myxomatosis and was uncertain about how to respond. Aware that it would come under pressure to act, ministers no doubt understood that they could deflect questions in parliament or elsewhere by stating that they were awaiting the report of a committee of inquiry. At the same time, the government did face a crisis of unknown proportions; it really did need prompt and sound advice from scientific experts and interest group representatives.

The MAC's first meeting took place on 4 November 1953.[9] Sankey prepared detailed notes, amounting virtually to a script, to serve as a basis for Carrington's opening statement. These notes identified the main questions for consideration:

1. Could the disease be eradicated and, if so, should it?
2. If it was impossible or inadvisable to eradicate the disease, should its spread be encouraged?
3. What could be done to protect both domestic rabbits and the fur and hat trades?

The 'urgent' priority was to determine the advisability of continuing the government's containment policy. But the expectation that the disease would remain quiescent until spring did allow 'a reasonable time to hear evidence, consider long-term issues and reach conclusions on policy.'[10]

Since the wild rabbit was widely recognized as a pest, the obvious response to myxomatosis was to welcome it as the solution to a long-standing and intractable problem. The government's failure to do so was regarded in some quarters as absurd.[11] Lord Rennell, himself a farmer, wondered:

> why the Ministry of Agriculture are taking such pains to make British farming safe for rabbits. It is an incredible position; it is Gilbertian. We have something which is a pest. By an Act of God, or perhaps the machinations of somebody, the pest is in process of being exterminated. The Ministry of Agriculture exterminate the exterminator of the pest.

If humanitarian considerations were behind the attempts to contain the disease, Lord Rennell was unimpressed: 'If it is not humane to kill rabbits by a disease, is it not also equally inhumane to kill rats with phosphorus?' These and other reflections were a source of amusement for Rennell and several of his fellow peers.[12] Years later the zoologist, L. Harrison Matthews, expressed similar views. He referred to MAF's 'ridiculous antics' and 'frantic attempts' to stamp out a disease that promised to clear the country of rabbits, an objective that the ministry had spend vast sums of money trying to realize. He too believed that a 'similar pandemic among brown rats would have been welcomed, for rats are "not nice"'.[13]

In his notes for Carrington, Sankey gave three reasons for rejecting these arguments. First, rabbits might acquire immunity so that any decline in their numbers would be temporary. In this event the country, while continuing to be plagued by rabbits, would have acquired a new disease to no purpose. In these circumstances, wild rabbits would lose their economic value and the 'tame rabbit industry' would suffer 'serious damage'. Second, humanitarian considerations – Rennell's points notwithstanding – were important. Third, there was the potential danger of allowing a viral disease to become established, even if it did appear to be confined to rabbits.[14]

When Hugh Gardner read Sankey's paper he believed that an opening statement based on it might sidetrack the committee. Accordingly, he prepared some supplementary notes to encourage it to focus on 'the main item on which we wish to reach an immediate decision'. In his eyes the most pressing question was whether to continue exterminating rabbits in infected areas or allow the disease to run its course. Gardner believed that the committee could resolve this question in short order, for he had already decided, as indeed had Carrington and Sir Reginald Franklin, one of the deputy secretaries at MAF, that the Lewes outbreak could not be controlled. He thought the 'contain and exterminate' strategy, far from having been a waste of time, had served a useful purpose. He foresaw, accurately, that a flare up of myxomatosis in the following year would produce a 'countryside ... littered with rabbits, dead and dying from myxomatosis'. If this upset the public, the authorities would be in a position to say that 'when the disease first made its appearance in this country, we took all practicable steps to stamp it out.' In other words, the containment operation was an important public relations exercise.[15]

So, Carrington's job was not to chair a frank and open-ended discussion but to guide the committee towards the 'right' decision without giving the impression that this conclusion had been pre-ordained.[16] In anticipation, MAF prepared a press release indicating that containment was no longer viable:

> Reports make it clear that it would not be practicable to erect a fence around the area affected [near Lewes] with a view to containing and subsequently destroying the rabbits within it. The Minister of Agriculture has, therefore, reached the conclusion that there is no alternative but to allow the disease to take its course. The efforts being made to stamp out the two earlier outbreaks near Edenbridge, in Kent, and Robertsbridge, in East Sussex, will, in these circumstances, be discontinued.[17]

When the MAC met, however, Carrington did nothing to steer it towards MAF's preferred outcome. Instead, he rehearsed the arguments for controlling the existing outbreaks while ignoring all counter arguments beyond making the obvious and oft-repeated point that the cost of damage inflicted by wild rabbits far exceeded any economic value they possessed. It was left to Dr Evans to make a case, partly on humanitarian grounds, for encouraging the disease and launching 'an active campaign to mop up survivors'. He argued that a swift programme of destruction would minimize suffering. But, with Baylis and Ritchie pointing out that it still might be possible to control the Lewes outbreak, Rothschild and Carrington predicting that the mass demise of rabbits was likely to shock the public, and the scientific experts uncertain about how the disease might develop or whether vaccination would thoroughly protect domestic rabbits, the committee decided that 'every reasonable and practical effort should be made to control the disease'. The committee agreed to review the decision at its next meeting on 10 November.[18]

The minister, persuaded that myxomatosis would spread little during the winter, accepted the MAC's recommendation. MAF's draft press notice was rewritten and Baylis implemented his plan for destroying the Lewes rabbits.[19] With the containment exercises apparently going well, the decision to persist with them was endorsed at the

MAC's 10 November meeting. The committee also discussed the desirability of controlling imports of myxoma virus (without discussion Carrington dismissed this as impractical), rabbit skins and carcasses (this was deemed 'unrealistic' in the present state of the law), and live rabbits (a majority favoured imports only under licence).[20] Otherwise, the main decision taken at the MAC's second meeting was to establish a scientific subcommittee consisting of Andrewes, Evans, Glover and Ritchie, though Rothschild later joined. In the course of the next fortnight each member would prepare papers summarizing the state of knowledge on scientific aspects of myxomatosis. The agreed areas of investigation were:

1. The specificity of the disease to rabbits and the susceptibility of hares.
2. The cause of transmission under natural conditions.
3. Methods of deliberately spreading the disease.
4. The experience of New Zealand and Tasmania.
5. The seasonal incidence of mosquitoes in the UK.
6. The projected impact of rabbit depopulation on British flora and fauna.
7. The inoculation of caged rabbits.
8. The evidence for the development of immunity against the disease.[21]

When the subcommittee next met, on 3 December, it was agreed that:

1. Though hares could very occasionally be infected, myxomatosis was, for all practical purposes, specific to rabbits.
2. The disease could be spread by contact and by insects, but further research was needed on the relative importance of mosquitoes and rabbit fleas as vectors.
3. Consideration of methods of deliberately spreading the disease should be deferred.
4. The experience of New Zealand and Tasmania was of little relevance to the UK.
5. Britain was host to eight species of rabbit-biting mosquitoes. The significance of the flea as a vector required further consideration

(Rothschild submitted notes a few days later) but it appeared that the flea spread the disease locally and was responsible for the virus surviving the winter whereas mosquitoes caused transmission over longer distances in favourable weather.

6. The impact of myxomatosis-induced rabbit depopulation on flora and fauna 'should not be regarded as important enought [*sic*] to influence any decisions that might be made'.

7. MAF's veterinary laboratory had made 300,000 doses of vaccine. However, the risk of infection for tame rabbits was deemed slight and use of protective measures (screens, insecticides, quarantine) was advised.

8. Rabbits might become resistant and were 'most unlikely' to be exterminated by myxomatosis.[22]

The MAC was informed of these verdicts.

The MAC's third meeting took place on 10 December. In the month since it had previously met, five fresh outbreaks of myxomatosis had been confirmed. The disease was now present at eight locations in four counties. The outbreak near Lydd in Kent, confirmed on 5 December, was particularly extensive. Sick rabbits had been found as far as a mile apart, across 5000 acres of farmland, coastal shingle and marsh, and an army tank range. In these circumstances, and in light of the scientific subcommittee's opinion that the disease, even if it died out over the winter, would probably be reintroduced from the Continent in 1954, Carrington suggested that the MAC consider whether the containment measures in Kent and East Sussex remained worthwhile. The committee agreed that while the attempts to control the first outbreaks were 'fully justified', such measures no longer served a useful purpose.[23]

This conclusion was not simply a recognition that the disease was out of control and that its nationwide spread had become inevitable. On the contrary, the committee still believed that the disease might 'die out from natural causes' over the winter.[24] If this were the case, then the question of containment to prevent reinfestation would recur. If, on the other hand, the disease persisted or recurred, two courses of action were possible: to allow it to spread naturally or to accelerate its spread by deliberate introduction at strategic points. Phillips and Collison, representing the interests of farmer and farm worker respectively, advocated 'the spread of the disease in the interests of food production'. On humanitarian grounds the committee could not decide between the options. Accordingly, it accepted Lord Merthyr's offer to discuss the humanitarian issues with animal welfare groups. Senior suggested that the scientists on the committee should provide advice about the chances of spreading the disease in northern parts of the UK. In policy terms, the one area of agreement concerned the need for 'mopping up operations' in the event of further outbreaks, in order to destroy any rabbits that escaped or survived the disease. In addition, organizations interested in the problem would be invited to present their views in writing, and in some cases in person, before any further policy decisions were made. The committee would supply all such organizations with a summary of the scientific evidence prepared by its scientific subcommittee. On this note the MAC broke up, having scheduled its next meeting for 20 January. Not surprisingly, since he had been in favour of it some five weeks earlier, the minister accepted the recommendation to cease attempts at containment.[25]

The MAC invited 22 organizations to submit written evidence; 16, plus two individuals, complied. Most of the evidence came from agricultural and landowning bodies, animal welfare groups and representatives of the rabbit-skin and fur trades. Only Dr W. Lane-Petter, director of the MRC's Laboratory Animals Bureau, represented medical or veterinary opinion, and his evidence dealt purely with the implications of myxomatosis for laboratory rabbits.[26] The MAC apparently considered it possessed sufficient expertise within its own ranks to render the acquisition of additional scientific opinion superfluous.

By mid-February 1954 the committee had received written evidence from UFAW, BFAWS, the RSPCA and Scottish SPCA, various trade bodies, the British Rabbit Council, CLA, and NFUs of Scotland, England and Wales. In addition, members of the committee had taken soundings of their own. For example, Lord Dundee consulted the executive committee of the Scottish Landowners' Federation (SLF), of which he was a member, and 'various prominent farmers'. Lord

Merthyr reported the views of 18 animal welfare societies that met in conference on 10 December. The SLF was not opposed to artificial transmission if it were deemed that myxomatosis was in the national interest. The animal welfare societies, on the other hand, unanimously opposed such a step.[27]

Of the bodies that submitted formal memoranda, only the NFUS advocated the deliberate transmission of myxomatosis. Excited by the prospect of rabbit-free farming and persuaded that there was no risk to humans or other animals, it favoured 'steps being taken by every means possible to spread myxomatosis to the end of exterminating the rabbit pest'.[28] Mainly on humanitarian grounds, every other organization rejected such action – at least in the short term. None of the evidence submitted supported containment. Perhaps surprisingly, no animal welfare group opposed the mass slaughter of wild rabbits. On the contrary, all wrote in support of vigorous rabbit control. For example, UFAW, favoured a campaign of 'unprecedented proportions' by gassing, long netting and other means. The RSPCA favoured rabbit extermination by 'every possible means' except myxomatosis, which it considered 'extremely painful'. It even supported trapping, which both UFAW and the BFAWS wanted to see banned.[29] The evidence of the BFAWS barely addressed the issue of myxomatosis. It used its submission mainly to urge the immediate prohibition of steel traps (on the grounds that they were cruel and did little to reduce rabbit numbers). It favoured neither artificial acceleration of myxomatosis nor a policy of inaction, though it did support rabbit control by unspecified means, on the grounds that fewer rabbits would mean less cruelty through myxomatosis.[30]

The strongest defence of the wild rabbit came from trade bodies whose businesses depended on rabbit meat, fur and skin. They emphasized the economic importance of the animal, including its waste products, which were used both as manure and in glue manufacture. The rabbit, they calculated, contributed almost £15.5 million per annum to the national economy and earned valuable foreign currency, not least in US dollars. They admitted that the cost of rabbit damage to agriculture exceeded this figure. Consequently, 'if ... by the waving of a wand the wild rabbit population of Britain could be completely exterminated, permanently and without counterbalancing disadvantages, there is little doubt that the national economy would benefit, regardless of what might happen to our associated trades.' They argued, however, that myxomatosis was no panacea and that 'use of this artificially cultivated disease' was fraught with uncertainty. The disease might not amount to much in British conditions; alternatively, it might create a race of immune rabbits, decimate domestic animals or upset the balance of nature. The rabbit was already controlled to the extent, so they claimed, that some 40 million were killed every year for meat and pelts at zero cost to farmers or taxpayers. Yet if myxomatosis became established, consumers would cease buying rabbit meat. Since the fur trade depended on rabbits killed for meat, the value of the pelt alone being less than the cost of collection, the trade would collapse. With it would go the entire system of rabbit control. If rabbits survived the epizootic, developed immunity and recovered their numbers, the plight of agriculture would be worse than ever, for with rabbits stripped of their economic value the cost of control would fall entirely on the farmer.[31]

The Board of Trade was impressed by this 'moderate, lucid and comprehensive' testimony. It calculated that the wild rabbit generated about £3.5 million per annum in export earnings; at 'a time when exports are more than ever important to our economy, this is by no means a negligible factor'. Consequently, the evidence of the trade bodies 'ought to be given its full weight in the scales before any decision is taken to encourage the spread of the disease'.[32] Sankey was less impressed and prepared a paper on 'The Economics of the Wild Rabbit' in rebuttal. He calculated that wild rabbits contributed substantially less than £2 million per annum to agricultural incomes. The annual cost of the damage they wrought, on the other hand, exceeded £38 million per annum and was possibly more than £50 million. Such figures dwarfed the rabbit's contribution to the national economy. Sankey's paper influenced the MAC so much that it included the gist of the argument in its first report.[33]

The British Rabbit Council, which represented 6000 individual domestic rabbit breeders and clubs with a combined membership of about 75,000, paid little attention to myxomatosis, at least in the wild rabbit context. Its concern was the protection of domestic rabbits, which in their millions were useful for meat, pelts, wool, laboratory experimentation, pets, exhibition, teaching in schools and furthering social interaction. It urged that cheap vaccine should be widely available. Under most circumstances the council opposed the artificial introduction of myxomatosis. Not only was it inhumane, it might also fail to wipe out wild rabbits and affect other animals. Only if the disease became so widespread through natural transmission that the elimination of 'wild infective stocks' was possible could the council contemplate deliberate introduction.[34]

The CLA 'subscribed to the policy that the wild rabbit is a pest whose destructive capabilities far outweigh its value as meat or fur' and welcomed 'any natural disease' that promised to exterminate rabbits cheaply. On the other hand, it supported the artificial spread of myxomatosis only if this promised to bring the outbreak to a swift conclusion and reduce suffering. Otherwise, nature should be allowed to take its course with serious efforts either to wipe out survivors (by 'orthodox methods') or at least prevent rabbits from again becoming serious pests.[35]

Because it consulted its county branches, the NFU (England and Wales) submitted its views at a comparatively late date (18 February). The union agreed with the CLA that the rabbit was a pest whose damage to food production far outweighed its value. It did not consider how to respond if myxomatosis died out because it did not think this would happen. Instead, it focused on whether the disease should be artificially spread or left to run its course. For humanitarian reasons, and because of the legal and practical difficulties of the alternative, it favoured natural spread.[36]

The MAC also took legal advice. Bazil Wingate-Saul's opinion was that the government had no legal obligation to take steps either to encourage or discourage the spread of myxomatosis. Deliberate transmission would constitute a tort and render the government (or anyone else responsible) liable to compensate those who suffered damage. The inoculation of a rabbit with myxoma virus might constitute an offence under the Protection of Animals Act, 1911, though the infection of other rabbits as a result of the release of the inoculated animal was not covered by the statute. The Diseases of Animals Act, 1950 allowed the government to ban or control the import or internal movement of live rabbits, carcasses and the virus. It also allowed the government to order the slaughter of diseased or exposed animals provided compensation, which could be minimal, was paid. On the other hand, no existing legislation allowed containment measures, such as fencing or the slaughter of healthy animals, without an occupier's consent. Sections 98 and 100 of the Agriculture Act, 1947, which empowered the minister to order the destruction of rabbits to prevent crop damage, were deemed inapplicable if the rabbit population had already collapsed. In short, new legislation would be necessary if the minister wished deliberately to spread myxomatosis, to enter private land to destroy healthy rabbits or take other steps to contain the disease, compel occupiers of land to destroy healthy rabbits, or destroy diseased or exposed rabbits without having to pay compensation.[37]

At its fourth meeting, on 20 January 1954, the MAC considered Wingate-Saul's opinion and discussed amending the Pests Bill, then before parliament, to allow the government to compel the destruction of rabbits wherever myxomatosis outbreaks had occurred. The only decision taken, however, was to recommend a ban on imports of American cottontail rabbits except under licence. The committee reviewed the evidence received to date (from UFAW, Lane-Petter, the British Rabbit Council, the trade bodies and CLA) but postponed further discussion pending receipt of further submissions.[38]

The MAC considered these later submissions at its fifth meeting, which Carrington missed through illness, on 23 February 1954. Collison of the NUAW represented the views of the union he served as general secretary. These were different from those he had outlined at the MAC's third meeting when he and Phillips of the NFU had advocated deliberate transmission on food production grounds. On this occasion, however, he favoured such action only if it could be accomplished 'without causing much suffering', a point with which the chairman of the RSPCA (Lord Merthyr) agreed, and was 'really effective' in destroying rabbits. His members were concerned about cruelty and considered that the disease should be allowed to take its course.[39]

By this time a draft report had been circulated among MAC members.[40] Its main thrust was that for practical and humanitarian reasons myxomatosis 'should be allowed to run it course without let or hindrance'. Follow-up operations to destroy any rabbits that survived the disease should be organized by CAECs in conjunction with farmers, landowners and workers. Farmers reluctant to expend time on 'comparatively costly measures to destroy the few rabbits surviving an outbreak' would have to be persuaded that the effort was worthwhile, for the 'opportunity to reduce the rabbit population to a point of near extermination would be unique and every possible advantage should be taken of it'.[41]

After lengthy discussion and the addition of some amendments, the committee agreed the draft report at its sixth meeting on 15 March 1954.[42] The nine-page report was submitted to the minister on the following day. It recommended that:

1. There should be no attempt either to contain or artificially spread myxomatosis. Instead, it should be left to run its natural course.
2. Rabbits surviving an outbreak should be destroyed to prevent population recovery. While primary responsibility should rest with the occupier of the land, government should consider how it could assist.
3. Imports of live rabbits such as cottontails should be banned on the grounds that they could become pests in their own right.
4. Special consideration should be given to the protection of domestic rabbits.[43]

Senior MAF officials praised the report. Hugh Gardner, the senior under-secretary (and MAC member), thought the government could accept its principal proposal that the disease should be allowed to take its natural course. He believed the report as a whole 'brought together valuable information' and offered useful recommendations.[44] Sir Reginald Franklin, one of the department's deputy secretaries, agreed. The committee, he wrote, has 'done well to get out this very useful and informative report in a relatively short time'. He believed it would do much to educate the general public and farming community about the need to destroy wild rabbits. Consequently, the 'Minister should be advised to accept [all] the recommendations'.[45] Two weeks later Dugdale thanked the MAC for its 'valuable and timely Report' and informed the Commons that he had accepted their recommendations.[46] The report was published, price 9d (about 3.5p), on 9 April 1954.

Once the MAC had submitted its report the question of how to proceed arose. In fact, policy decisions were being taken even before the government had formally accepted the committee's recommendations. Gardner noted that 'we shall do all we can by propaganda and otherwise to supplement' the efforts of land occupiers, who bore the legal obligation, to destroy survivors of the epizootic. A ban on imports of non-indigenous rabbits immune from myxomatosis, which involved consultation with the governments of Northern and Southern Ireland, was also under consideration within a week of the report's submission. Equally swiftly, the ministry's animal health division began looking into ways of protecting domestic rabbits, including through the plentiful supply of inexpensive vaccine.[47]

There was also the question of how to 'stage manage' the report. Sankey was quick to suggest a press release, press conference and broadcast publicity. Aside from coverage on BBC news bulletins, he thought Carrington might be interviewed for the corporation's 'Farm Fare' programme.[48] Carrington, however, was not keen on excessive publicity. He resisted suggestions for a press conference and broadcast and observed 'that there are advantages in playing down the report at this juncture'. Harold White, who had headed the ICD since 1952, agreed that neither a press conference nor an interview would serve much purpose: 'I don't know that there is a lot to say about myxomatosis at this stage beyond what is in the Committee's report.'[49] In the event the only publicity comprised a press notice and a short information leaflet that explained the cause and nature of the disease, the animals susceptible, methods of diagnosis, prevention and control, and details about vaccination.[50]

In March Sankey had referred to the press's 'continuing interest in myxomatosis', yet newspaper interest in the MAC report was limited.[51] *The Times* published a summary and Dugdale's statement to the House of Commons. It then gave a more considered, though notably uncritical, evaluation. This described the MAC as 'fully competent to assess the problem, representing as it does, scientists, farmers, landowners, animal welfare societies, and domestic rabbit keepers'. In line with official thinking, the newspaper urged farmers and foresters to take advantage of 'a great opportunity to rid themselves of a costly pest, and if myxomatosis comes their way this summer they should be ready with a plan to finish the job'.[52] Only in the summer of 1954, when the disease spread dramatically, did press interest mount. The initial lack of coverage perhaps explains why, as late as mid-April 1954, one MP found it necessary to ask a government minister to inform parliament what myxomatosis was.[53]

The principal issue that faced MAF was how to encourage mopping-up and to take advantage of a historic opportunity to eliminate rabbits. The MAC had expressed concern lest a unique chance should be missed, as it seemingly had been in Australia. In the course of its deliberations one member, Lord Dundee, had suggested that extermination should be a government responsibility. Franklin was not averse to the involvement of pest control staff and CAECs but Gardner did not want to see MAF forced into running an extermination programme:

mopping-up *must* be a matter for the occupier and his own labour. We could not contemplate, even if it were practicable, organizing Government rabbit destruction squads on the scale that would be required and carrying the cost on the Exchequer. Such action, apart from anything else, might deprive the occupiers of the local labour on which they will depend for their own efforts. We must give occupiers no excuse for 'leaving it to the Government'.[54]

As he saw it, the role of CAECs was to engage in propaganda and organize 'local self-help'.[55]

Timing was another critical issue. Some officials thought the ministry should have a detailed extermination plan ready when the MAC report was published.[56] Gardner was less certain. In his view 'mopping up action is not an immediate problem'. In the first place, rabbit control was essentially an autumn and winter exercise, when crops had been gathered, grass had ceased growing and rabbits were using burrows. In the second, any control effort needed to take place '*after* myxomatosis had taken its full toll in any given area'. Premature action might inhibit the spread of the disease and therefore prove counter productive. The important thing was to 'start planning now so that everything will be cut and dried in six months' time'. He envisaged approaching the Treasury for an increase in the subsidy on gassing powder. Since such an approach had recently been rejected, no fresh request would be feasible 'until developments this Spring and Summer lend fresh weight to our arguments'.[57]

On 9 April the ministry dispatched a memorandum, along with two copies of the MAC report, to every CAEC in England. It summarized the recommendations and explained how they affected committees. The most important point concerned the need for 'energetic measures' to mop-up survivors. The challenge for CAECs was to persuade farmers to destroy rabbits even where so few remained that they could hardly be regarded as pests. MAF emphasized that it was for farmers and landowners to take the necessary action as soon as the disease appeared to be on the wane in their area, probably in late autumn. The key was to persuade them that the exercise was not only worthwhile but vital to their long-term interests. They had to be convinced that failure to act would result in rabbit numbers again attaining epidemic proportions. CAECs were enjoined to promote local action, perhaps by encouraging a farmer or someone else to act as a local organizer. They might then provide posters urging other farmers to contact him so that concerted measures could be taken with the aid of county pest staff.[58]

Otherwise, the first practical step to implement any of the MAC's recommendations occurred at the end of July when parliament approved an order prohibiting the unlicensed importation and keeping of non-native rabbits such as the American cottontail.[59]

Chapter 6

Deliberate Transmission

The sixth meeting of the MAC took place on 15 March 1954, largely to agree the report.[1] The next meeting did not take place until 20 October, notwithstanding the extremely rapid spread of myxomatosis in the intervening months. By this time Carrington had moved to the Ministry of Defence.[2] His final task with the MAC, in July 1954, was to chair a joint meeting of the MAC and Land Pests Advisory Committee (LPAC) on matters of common interest concerning myxomatosis.[3] Two issues dominated the agenda – deliberate transmission and 'mopping-up'. At this point, let us focus on deliberate transmission, leaving the subject of mopping-up to the next chapter.

The MAC rejected the deliberate transmission of myxomatosis mainly on humanitarian grounds but also because the legal position was unclear. Of the organizations that gave written evidence to the committee, only the NFUS, was supportive.[4] The extent to which the disease was spread artificially is not entirely clear. MAF was confident that the original Edenbridge outbreak, which by October 1954 covered 200 square miles, spread naturally: 'we are as certain as anyone can be that it has not been assisted in any way by human beings.'[5] By the same token, Lord St Aldwyn, who in December 1954 became chairman of the MAC, considered it 'quite wrong to suggest that human agency has been the main factor' in spreading myxomatosis throughout Britain.[6] On the other hand, the NC's annual report for 1953–54 observed that 'deliberate dissemination has been much more rapid and widespread than was anticipated.'[7] The evidence suggests that this was an accurate appraisal. In fact, MAF knew as early as mid-November 1953 that a trade in diseased rabbit carcasses had commenced in the Bough Beech area.[8]

At a Carlisle branch meeting in April 1954 several NFU members advocated deliberate introduction of the disease. The chairman opposed these suggestions on humanitarian grounds but members agreed that it was for individuals to decide.[9] Next month *Shooting Times* reported that four Cumberland farmers had travelled to an area where myxomatosis was present in order to capture infected rabbits for release in their own county.[10] Also in May, farmers and farm workers in Radnorshire and the Cotswolds told Ronald Lockley that myxomatosis had been introduced to their areas by farmers who had collected infected rabbits from Kent and Sussex.[11]

In June *Farmers Weekly* reported:

the case of the Cornish farmer who introduced the disease to his own land from a couple of infected carcasses brought in from another district. So successful was he that people from miles around have been asking him for diseased rabbits with which to transmit myxomatosis on to their farms. Since the supply began to run out ... he has been offered up to £20 for a single infected carcass.[12]

The disease allegedly was introduced by a number of farmers in the Lerryn area. Also in June the League against Cruel Sports announced that since the discovery of myxomatosis in Cornwall (May 1954), 'many infected carcases (of rabbits) have been taken from the infected farms to parts of Somerset and Devon by people who hope to promote outbreaks of the disease in their own areas'.[13] Brigid Longley, who farmed at Cranbrook in Kent, wrote to *The Times*: 'I understand there is a firm market for these horrifying creatures [rabbits infected with myxomatosis]. They sell, we have been told, at a guinea a head.'[14] In many cases the evidence for artificial introduction was anecdotal. Indeed, the minister told parliament on 1 July: 'We have no positive evidence whatever of outbreaks having been started deliberately by individuals, as has been written in the press.'[15] Such evidence was not long in coming.

When myxomatosis broke out in the Deeside parish of Durris in Kincardineshire in July 1954, the story made front-page news in

Aberdeen's daily newspaper, the *Press & Journal.* It was, after all, the first Scottish outbreak. The big question for Alex Munro, the reporter who broke the story, was: 'How did it get there [Durris] when the nearest the disease was last heard of in England was in Westmorland?'[16] Munro's enquiries led him to 'Balrownie', a 250-acre, rabbit-infested farm in the tenancy of William Milne. After some preliminaries during which Munroe ascertained that Milne and his wife had recently returned from a week's holiday in England, where their son was stationed on national service, Munro

> Pointblank ... asked Mr Milne: 'You did not bring up a diseased rabbit from England?' He smiled quizzically and replied: 'Well, I'm nae saying no am I?'
>
> Frankly, he told me he brought home from Bedfordshire ... not a live rabbit but the carcase of one that had died of the disease, and put it down in one of his infested fields.[17]

A photograph captioned '"I Did It" Says Durris Farmer', shows the beaming Milne and his smiling daughter. He is holding a dead rabbit showing all the symptoms of myxomatosis.

Lord Sempill, whose head ghillie had informed him that people were visiting Durris to collect infected carcasses, drew the attention of the House of Lords to Milne's action and to local protest against it. Sempill believed that the MAC's recommendation against deliberate transmission was being 'widely flouted' in northeast Scotland where diseased rabbit carcasses were fetching high prices. He wanted the press and BBC to publicize the government's opposition.[18]

When, on 15 July, the minister of agriculture was asked about 'the deliberate spreading of myxomatosis on a wholesale scale throughout many areas of the country', he no longer denied, as he had a week earlier, that such action was occurring. A week later Dr Andrewes, chairman of the MAC's scientific subcommittee, said 'there could be no reasonable doubt that individuals had taken a hand in the spread of the disease'. Then, on 29 July, Carrington told the House of Lords that there 'seems little doubt that the spread of the disease has been assisted and accelerated by human agency'.[19]

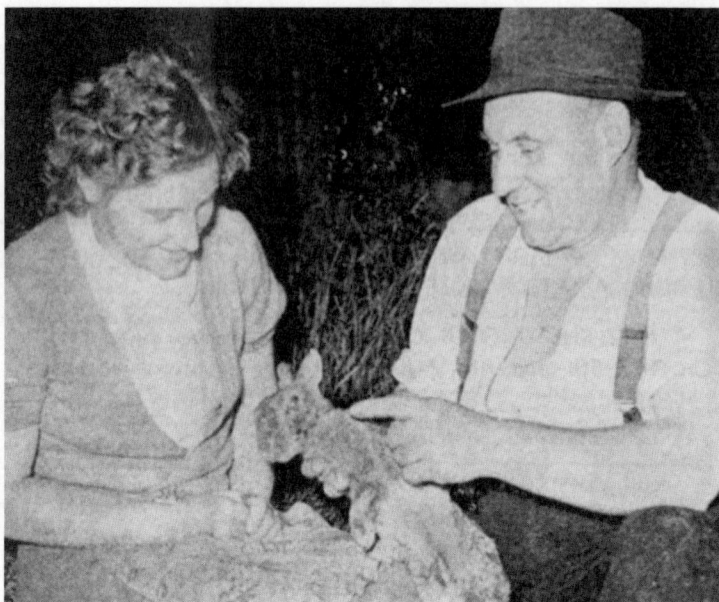

7. William Milne of Durris with daughter, Julia, and diseased rabbit.

Deliberate transmission seems to have been rife in Scotland, which is probably why myxomatosis spread so quickly there, but documented cases also came to light in England and Wales.[20] Durham was affected by the disease in August 1954. Police and RSPCA officers believed that the outbreak in the Billingham area was deliberately induced 'by a person whose identity is known to the authorities'. Infected carcasses were handed over to the police and prosecution was considered.[21] Also in August the Isle of Man Board of Agriculture announced that its recently-discovered outbreak of myxomatosis 'had been deliberately introduced'.[22]

As early as May 1954 'Tower-Bird', in *Shooting Times*, expressed disappointment that 'drastic steps' were not being taken against farmers and others who spread the disease.[23] Then in early July, the RSPCA announced its intention to seek an order prohibiting deliberate transmission.[24] It subsequently placed advertisements in newspaper personal columns:

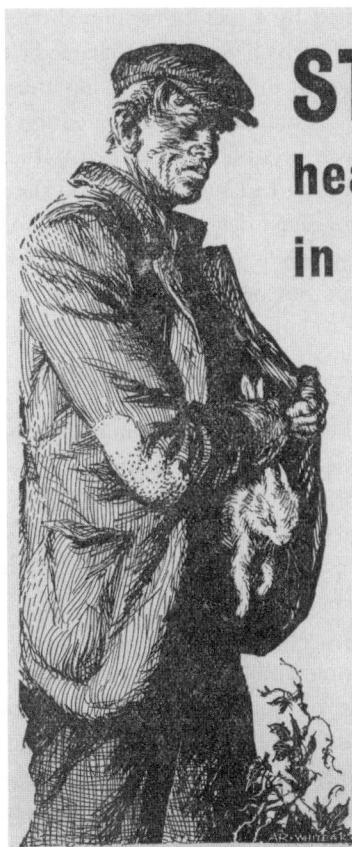

STOP this heartless traffic in MYXOMATOSIS!

STOP the deliberate spreading of MYXOMATOSIS! Victims of this horrible disease—blind, misshapen, tormented —are being caught for sale as carriers, to be let loose in infection-free areas. Effective rabbit-control can be maintained by humane methods; myxomatosis kills only after intense, prolonged pain and misery. Nothing can justify this callous encouragement of animal suffering, and the R.S.P.C.A. appeals for your moral and material support in demanding an immediate legal ban. **Volunteers in infected areas, who must be expert shots, apply please,** to the Chief Secretary, R.S.P.C.A. (Dept. T.) 105 Jermyn Street, London, S.W.1 or to the nearest R.S.P.C.A. Inspector.

Remember the **RSPCA**

8. *The Times*, 17 September 1954.

Stop the deliberate spreading of MYXOMATOSIS! – Victims of this horrible disease – blind, misshapen, tormented – are being caught for sale as carriers, to be let free in infection-free areas. … Nothing can justify this callous encouragement of animal suffering, and the RSPCA appeals for your moral and material support in demanding an immediate legal ban.[25]

Sometimes this text was accompanied by a picture captioned: 'Stop this heartless traffic in myxomatosis', which featured a character of sinister, not to say brutish appearance in the act of extracting a dead rabbit from the inside of his jacket, presumably with the intention of leaving it in the undergrowth in which he stood.[26] Even before these appeals began the villagers of Cranbrook had submitted a 200 signature petition to their MP protesting against deliberate transmission.[27] In contrast, A. G. Street argued that it was 'high time that the Ministry of Agriculture ceased havering, came out definitely against the wild rabbit, and *helped* British agriculture to spread myxomatosis throughout the country'.[28]

When the issue arose at the MAC/LPAC meeting on 26 July Carrington said that the matter had been raised with the minister who, while still accepting the MAC's advice against artificial transmission, had requested the committee to reconsider the issue.[29]

Lord Dundee thought the degree of suffering inflicted was an important consideration. The joint committee agreed that the disease did cause suffering and Carrington suggested that it had to settle two questions. Should it 'come out openly against people spreading the disease'? And, if it did, should it recommend legislation? It was agreed that existing legislation (the Diseases of Animals Act, 1950 and Protection of Animals Act, 1911) did not apply and therefore that new legislation would be necessary. Carrington pointed out that nothing could be done until parliament reconvened in October, the assumption being, perhaps, that with myxomatosis spreading so rapidly, the disease might have covered most or all of the country by then. If this happened the issue would have become largely irrelevant.[30]

Every speaker, even Lord Merthyr of the RSPCA, wanted to be rid of rabbits as quickly and humanely as possible. The two scientists who contributed to the debate, Andrewes and Evans, said there was a humanitarian case in favour of deliberate transmission while the disease remained at its most virulent, for such action would eliminate, or virtually so, the wild rabbit, thereby avoiding a situation in which an attenuated form of the virus caused suffering for the indefinite future.[31] For Evans, such a step was also preferable from the rabbit control perspective. Phillips, Verney and Collison, perhaps reflecting mainstream farming and landowning opinion, deplored deliberate transmission, but thought that any legislation prohibiting it would be unenforceable. On a split vote (of seven to three) the committee agreed that deliberate transmission should not be made an offence. It also agreed to review the issue in the autumn.[32]

The MAC's seventh meeting took place on 20 October 1954. G. R. H. Nugent, joint parliamentary secretary to MAF, took the chair following Carrington's departure and Dr Ieuan Thomas, deputy director of the ministry's plant pathology laboratory, replaced J. W. Evans who resigned at the end of August before returning to Australia (where he had worked between 1926 and 1944) to become director of the Australian Museum in Sydney.[33] Otherwise, the only change of personnel involved G. D. Sharman of the DAS replacing W. H. Senior. The issue of deliberate transmission again loomed large. Nugent stated that 'in the light of recent developments', presumably press reports that myxomatosis was being spread deliberately and the 'widespread and extremely vocal demand that action of some sort should be taken against anyone who knowingly spreads myxomatosis', the government, wanted the committee to reconsider whether such activity should be criminalized.[34]

Not least because they deemed enforcement impossible, every member rejected criminalization. Only Scott Henderson was at all sympathetic. The chief veterinary officer presented the most cogent arguments against criminalization: the disease would soon be so widespread that the incentive to spread it artificially would cease, the law would be unenforceable because it would be impossible to distinguish between natural and induced outbreaks, and in the event of attenuation of the virus, reintroduction of the more virulent strain would be the best course for both humanitarian and economic reasons. Others considered it inappropriate to protect a pest or encourage 'snooping in the countryside and widespread recriminations against farmers'. After further discussion Scott Henderson proposed that 'no attempt should be made to assist the spread of myxomatosis' but also that 'no good purpose will be achieved at present by making it an offence for any person to take steps to spread the disease.'[35] The proposal was agreed unanimously. Expert opinion was swiftly set aside, however, as the issue of deliberate transmission became politicized. In order to understand this development it is necessary to go back to late 1953.

On 10 December 1953 a Pests Bill was introduced and received its first reading in the House of Lords. It sought 'to make further provision with respect to the destruction or control of rabbits and other animals and birds and to the use of spring traps for killing or taking animals'. In fact, the bill focused 'almost exclusively' on rabbits. Its first part envisaged, *inter alia*, compulsory rabbit destruction in clearance areas and the establishment of a ministerial power to require the clearance or fencing of land where it was impracticable to kill rabbits. The ministry would continue to subsidize gassing powder and begin providing discretionary grants towards the cost of rabbit destruction. The second part of the bill dealt with trapping and endorsed one of the recommendations of the Scott Henderson Committee on Cruelty to Wild Animals, to ban the sale and use of gin traps, effective from July 1958 or a later date fixed by the minister.[36] Such was the consensus about the depredations of the rabbit that the bill was 'quite uncontroversial', aside perhaps for the delay before the gin was banned. Opposition leaders in the Lords generally conferred their approval and the bill passed through the upper house on 1 April 1954.[37]

The minister of agriculture, Derick Heathcote Amory, 'an easygoing west-country squire', moved the bill's second reading in the Commons on 22 October.[38] In opening the debate, he described the bill, notwithstanding its 'unromantic title', as 'small' but 'useful'. He reviewed the progress of the myxomatosis outbreak and the need for farmers and landowners to take vigorous action to destroy surviving rabbits. On the issue of deliberate transmission, he summarized the MAC's recent deliberations and described its conclusion as 'sensible'.[39] MAF's joint parliamentary secretary, who thought convictions would be 'virtually impossible', agreed:

we do not approve of the deliberate spreading of the disease. It is something we would not do ourselves and we think it is a thing which should not be done. But there are many things in life of which we do not approve personally and which, nevertheless, we do not think are suitable to make criminal offences. This in our judgment [*sic*] is one of them.[40]

Most contributors to the debate supported the bill without touching on the issue of deliberate transmission, but Archer Baldwin, the veteran Conservative MP for Leominster, hoped the government would not make the practice illegal, for in his eyes myxomatosis was no crueller than ferrets, traps or snares.[41] Denys Bullard, Conservative MP for southwest Norfolk and parliamentary correspondent of *Farmers Weekly*, said that deliberate spreading was less common than some thought. Furthermore, though immoral, it could not be stopped by legislation. Other considerations aside, its criminalization would discourage the removal of dead and dying rabbits.[42] On the other hand, the Labour backbencher, Dr Horace King, had serious concerns not only about the delayed abolition of the gin trap, as did many others, but also about deliberate transmission. In a highly emotional speech he likened myxomatosis to 'the Nazi crimes at Auschwitz' and begged the House to modify the bill by adding a clause making deliberate transmission illegal:

> I would urge this House to range itself behind the Christian Church, and to follow, since it has refused to lead, the mass of public opinion, and say that we shall have no further part, as far as we are concerned, in myxomatosis, but that we will use this Pests Bill to prevent anyone at least from deliberately adding to the trail of misery and cruelty which is so ugly a blot on our country in 1954.[43]

Before the bill reached the committee stage more than 40 MPs of all parties signed a parliamentary motion, drafted by Victor Raikes MP and James Wentworth Day, deploring deliberate transmission.[44] King and Frank Hayman, Labour MP for Falmouth and Camborne, then declared their intention to move an amendment.[45] Hayman kept up the pressure by presenting to the House of Commons a petition organized by the Garby-Turner family. 'Deeply moved by the widespread and protracted suffering inflicted on the rabbit population through the deliberate spreading of myxomatosis and by the dangers implicit in this type of germ and virus warfare', they secured 126,000 signatures in the space of a few weeks in favour of legislation banning the deliberate spreading of myxomatosis.[46] On 10 November, further encouraged by members of the public, including a vet, a farm worker and even a local Conservative association, King brought forward a new clause: 'A person shall be guilty of an offence if he knowingly uses or permits the use of a rabbit infected with myxomatosis to spread the disease among uninfected rabbits.'[47] He delivered another impassioned speech, which concluded:

> what is it that we hold against the Nazis? Not that the Germans fought us in the last war on the battlefield, but that at Belsen little children were tortured to death, at Auschwitz old men and women were tortured to death, and just because the Nazis regarded the Jews as inferior creatures as we regard the rabbit.
>
> Let us have a Geneva convention in our rabbit war. If we excel all other animals in our scientific might, let us use that giant strength cleanly and decently. ... I suggest we should accept this new Clause and end bacteriological warfare against the rabbits. Let us kill them by all means, but let us do the job decently and cleanly.[48]

In response, Amory repeated the standard line against criminalizing deliberate transmission: it was pointless and unenforceable. He also referred to the advice twice proffered by the MAC. This advice 'seemed to me to be sensible at that time, and it still does'. Nevertheless, impressed by the strength of feeling displayed in various quarters, the minister was persuaded that 'something more should be done to discourage the deliberate spreading of the disease than by a statement of the Government's disapprobation.' To loud cheers from MPs on both sides of the House of Commons, Amory announced that the government accepted the clause.[49]

Although a letter in *Farmer & Stock-breeder* applauded Amory's humanitarianism, approbation for King's amendment was far from universal. Some Cornish NFU members, for example, announced their intention of doing all they could to spread myxomatosis before the bill became law.[50] On the grounds that Britain might sometime need to deploy a virulent strain of myxomatosis if rabbits were to be exterminated, an editorial in *Country Life* accused parliament of making a 'mistake'.[51] In his maiden speech in parliament (which earned him the sobriquet, 'Bunny'), Lord Dundee expressed his contempt for a decision made:

> after the most perfunctory discussion ... lasting only some twenty minutes and in complete disregard of the carefully considered and unanimous advice which had been repeatedly tendered to the Government by all those who were most qualified to advise ... on this subject and who had, indeed, been appointed by the Government for the specific purpose of doing so.

He then made a scathing attack on the illogicality of a clause replete with contradictions, double standards and sentimentality that would serve little purpose beyond placating the 'well-meaning' but uninformed.[52] Amory, he informed the ministry, had been 'incredibly weak and foolish' to accept it.[53] Other peers were also critical. To no avail, the Pests Act, with King's new clause slightly modified but essentially intact, received the royal assent on 25 November 1954. The fine for deliberately spreading myxomatosis was set at £20 for a first offence and £50 for subsequent convictions.[54] Dundee and Harold Woolley resigned from the MAC in protest. 'No one mourned their passing,' one observer wrote unkindly.[55]

Why, against all expert advice, did Amory accept King's amendment so readily? An editorial in *Farmer & Stock-breeder* expressed bewilderment.[56] Amory admitted that the arguments in favour had little merit; he claimed he was moved by the strength of feeling on the matter. While this may be true, prime ministerial pressure, also driven by emotion, may have been the important consideration.

News that myxomatosis was being spread deliberately had reached the office of the prime minister by early July 1954. Almost immediately one of Churchill's private secretaries, David Pitblado, contacted the Home Office to enquire whether action could be taken, on cruelty to animal grounds, to curtail the practice. He was informed that the home secretary could not order a prosecution and that magistrates were unlikely to convict under the terms of the Protection of Animals Act. The minister of agriculture had been consulted and had referred the matter to the MAC.[57] There the matter rested until the joint meeting of the LPAC and MAC again rejected the idea of criminalizing deliberate transmission. John Colville, another of Churchill's private secretaries, then took up the matter with MAF. The prime minister, Colville wrote, thought the government had paid insufficient attention to the cruelty issue. He wanted information about the composition of the MAC and the line it had taken on deliberate transmission. He was also pondering whether to make a donation to the RSPCA, which was soliciting contributions to support 'mercy squads' intent on putting diseased rabbits out of their misery. If he did so it would be 'deliberately ear-marked for this purpose' and given 'full publicity'.[58]

In reply G. R. Wilde of MAF gave a succinct account of the official response to myxomatosis since the disease was discovered in Britain, giving due weight to the attention the MAC had paid to humanitarian considerations. He emphasized the presence on the MAC of Lord Merthyr (chair of the RSPCA) and Scott Henderson, as well as the ministry's initial efforts to contain the first outbreaks in Kent and Sussex. He also stressed, however, that the committee adhered to its opinion that deliberate transmission, though deplorable, should not be made a criminal offence. Wilde thought that a prime ministerial contribution to the RSPCA would probably be popular with the general public but cautioned that farmers were unsympathetic to the society's 'mercy squads', which trespassed and caused crop damage.[59]

Although there was no further correspondence on this matter between the prime minister's office and MAF, on the day King's amendment to the Pests Bill was due to be moved, the cabinet discussed the matter. It agreed that 'public opinion throughout the country was strongly opposed to the deliberate spreading of this disease and would welcome a statutory prohibition of the practice, even though it could not be uniformly enforced.' The general view of the cabinet was that the government should 'bow to public opinion' and accept the new clause. Thus, Amory, far from making a decision to accept the King amendment on the spur of the moment in response to the feeling of the House of Commons, as MAC members suspected, was actually complying with a cabinet decision and the prime minister's personal wishes.[60]

The criminalization of deliberate transmission made little difference to farmers or others who wanted to introduce myxomatosis on their land. There was, after all, no way of policing and enforcing the law and by mid-1957 Amory was aware of only one, unsuccessful, prosecution. The first conviction dates from April 1958 when an Essex farmer was convicted and fined £5 with 10 guinea costs.[61] The real significance of the King amendment was in preventing MAF from deploying virulent strains of myxomatosis strategically in order to wipe out rabbit colonies that survived an original outbreak. As a result the chance of exterminating the wild rabbit was lost.

Chapter 7

After the Deluge

The Second Report

As a standing committee the MAC continued to meet after submitting its first report, albeit with some changes of personnel (see p.101 above) and at a considerably reduced level of activity. After its joint meeting with the LPAC in July 1954, it met only twice more before submitting a second and final report on 6 January 1955; its meeting of 8 December 1954, mainly involved discussion of the draft report.[1]

The MAC's second report, published on 27 January, reviewed developments since spring 1954 and assessed future prospects. Topics addressed included the geographical spread of myxomatosis, cruelty, methods of spread, immunity, protection of laboratory and domestic animals, imports of non-indigenous rabbits, risk to humans and other animals, implications for the rabbit trade, the impact of declining rabbit numbers on flora and fauna, and developments in Australia and continental Europe. Perhaps because it was too early to make an informed assessment, the committee virtually ignored the economic benefits of myxomatosis for farmers and foresters.[2]

Unlike its predecessor, the second report offered few recommendations. It deplored the inoculation of wild rabbits against myxomatosis, some instances of which had come to light, but did not propose that the practice should be made illegal. It also raised the possibility, on humanitarian grounds, that if an attenuated form of the myxomatosis virus became established, killing fewer rabbits but causing widespread suffering, it might be appropriate to reintroduce the virulent strain in certain areas. However, it reserved judgement on this issue and noted that 'express statutory sanction' would be needed before such a step could be taken.

On the question of mopping-up survivors, the committee welcomed the steps being taken by CAECs, farmers, landowners and agricultural workers. At the same time, it doubted whether existing arrangements would suffice and recommended, again without offering specific suggestions, that the government should consider providing further help. The committee stressed that the winter of 1955–56, when rabbit numbers would be at their lowest for over a century, would be the critical period in the extermination campaign. Experience gained in the interim would therefore be valuable.[3]

Mopping Up

Regardless of their attitudes towards the morality of animal control by biological means, many believed that myxomatosis, though unlikely to exterminate rabbits, offered an opportunity to eradicate them by other means and thereby boost agriculture and forestry at a time of national economic hardship.[4] As the MAC's first report pointed out, 'every effort should be made to eliminate [rabbits] before they repopulate. ... This opportunity will be unique and every possible advantage should be taken of it.' In some quarters extermination, or at least the end of the rabbit as a serious pest, was confidently expected. For example, Lord Dundee believed that if 95 per cent of rabbits were eliminated by myxomatosis 'it would be comparatively easy to deal with the remaining 5 per cent'. The MAC report was less sanguine; it predicted that landholders might be reluctant 'to take prompt and energetic measures to destroy the surviving few' rabbits. Even so, 'all concerned should be convinced that the effort is absolutely essential'.[5]

MAF began preparing the ground for a mopping-up campaign as early as January 1954, at which point myxomatosis had affected only four English counties and no other parts of Britain. Discussions with representatives of the NFU, Royal Forestry Association, Forestry Commission, CLA, NUAW, TGWU and British Railways yielded promises from each organization to cooperate with CAECs, each of which would appoint myxomatosis (mopping-up) committees with local representatives. MAF undertook to publicize the campaign, which would begin in late October or early November once the harvest was in and undergrowth had died back, by preparing leaflets and posters on rabbit clearance and mounting exhibitions at agricultural shows. Mopping-up committees were asked to engage in propaganda of their own through such means as newspaper articles and lectures to Young Farmers' Clubs.[6] Indeed, propaganda, rather than legal sanction or direct action in the field by its own personnel, formed the ministry's prime weapon in the mopping-up campaign.

An early practical step involved the creation of mandatory rabbit clearance areas (RCAs) to supplement the voluntary schemes that had been established in England and Wales, but not Scotland, following the July 1950 rabbit conference (see Chapter 2). The Pests Act, which received royal assent in November 1954, made 'further provision with respect to the destruction or control of rabbits and other animals and birds', and prohibited use of the gin trap. It also banned deliberate transmission of myxomatosis (see Chapter 6), but the first objective was rabbit control.[7] The act obliged occupiers of land within designated RCAs to destroy wild rabbits 'so far as practicable' and then keep their land rabbit free. In an extension of the Agriculture Act, 1947, and its Scottish equivalent, landholders were also required to destroy breeding places and rabbit cover or, where this was impracticable, erect rabbit-proof fencing to prevent rabbits from spreading. As in the past, Treasury grants were available. This could mean that 50 per cent of the cost of destruction and prevention of reinfestation was borne by the taxpayer.[8] Conviction for failure to comply was punishable by fines in line with those specified in the Agriculture Acts of 1947 (England and Wales) and 1948 (Scotland). Non-compliance could also mean that official rabbit destruction squads would intervene, with the costs of such intervention recoverable from the landholder.[9]

An article in the *Field* termed these 'sweeping ... provisions'.[10] In many ways, however, the requirements resembled those already in place. In England and Wales s.98 of the Agriculture Act, 1947, which empowered the minister (in practice CAECs) to serve notices requiring landholders to eliminate the pest, remained the basis of rabbit control. In reality, the Pests Act 'was largely an administrative measure to further the policy laid down in the Agriculture Act'.[11] Its main novelty was to allow the establishment of RCAs within which the occupiers of land, without personal notification, were legally obliged to destroy rabbits. In the course of debate on the bill, Lord Carrington assured the House of Lords that the government would 'most certainly' use its powers to compel occupiers to deal with rabbits on their land. Yet, nothing in the Pests Act obliged the minister to proceed against backsliders and, hitherto, the enforcement records of both Labour and Conservative governments were decidedly unimpressive.[12] When the enforcement issue arose at the joint meeting of the LPAC and MAC in July 1954, Lords Merthyr and Dundee emphasized that CAECs should not hesitate to take action against those who did not comply. However, Harold Woolley of the NFU objected, stating that 'farmers would not take kindly to undue pressure being brought to bear on them'. Harold Collison of the NUAW also thought it important to obtain the cooperation of farmers, though accepting that sanctions against the uncooperative should be used without hesitation.[13] So, even within the MAC, views differed about the use of enforcement powers.

From the first some MPs were sceptical about the government's rabbit clearance strategy:

> In the task of trying to eliminate the rabbit the Minister has a terrific job. I do not think it is recognized by the House what an extensive and difficult job it is. When myxomatosis has run its course, and all the other instruments of elimination have been applied, there will still be pockets of rabbits in different parts of the country that will spring up to spread the rabbit population again. It will be one continuous fight all over the country if the rabbit is to be eliminated. That is why I have no faith in rabbit areas. The whole country must become a rabbit clearance area.[14]

Denys Bullard, on the other hand, thought 'the basic attempt to clear the rabbit population by [designating RCAs] is justified.' He also thought it appropriate to tackle 'the really bad areas' first, for any attempt to 'spread our efforts over all the country … might lose our effort in the total size of the problem'.[15] In the event, and with little delay, most of the country was swiftly included in an RCA. But would designation of all or most of the country make any difference? A correspondent in *Farmer & Stock-breeder* thought not. He termed it 'just plumb crazy' to suppose that rabbits could be exterminated from terrain covered with rocks, dry walls, stone drains, gorse, heather and bracken.[16]

Apart from common land and areas controlled by the War Office or other government departments, where public funds would bear the expense, responsibility for killing rabbits rested with landholders rather than with MAF or CAECs. Prominent local farmers or land-owners were expected to organize action at local level and agricultural workers were expected to play an active part in tracking down rabbits. CAECs were required to 'assist and advise' local effort but not to 'assume responsibility for destroying rabbits'.[17]

Ronald Lockley judged that 'Nothing short of the Ministry being prepared to bear the full cost of rabbit clearance is likely to achieve the hoped-for reduction of [rabbits] to the point of extermination.'[18] But suggestions that the state should finance or even assume full responsibility for eliminating rabbits were repeatedly rejected. In the first place, it was not deemed feasible 'for the Government to set up a large organization with powers of entry' in order to kill rabbits. As Harold White, head of MAF's ICD wrote, the nationwide destruction of rabbits was 'too big a job for the Ministry to tackle with its present organization and resources'.[19] Lord St Aldwyn, Carrington's successor as chair of the MAC, rejected state intervention on the grounds that it would undermine individual initiative. Every farmer would say, 'I shall wait till the Government men come in and do the work for me.' He believed that the 'job cannot be better done than by the farmer and the farm workers: they are on the job; they know the lie of the land; they know their farms; they know where the rabbit is likely to be'. The prospect of better harvests would be incentive enough for farmers to act independently.[20] Throughout the entire mopping-up campaign voluntary action remained the order of the day.

A MAF press release in January 1955 observed that mopping-up operations were 'rapidly gaining momentum'; Hugh Gardner noted that 'we are doing pretty well'.[21] Even so, with the Pests Act on the

statute book, the ministry increased its propaganda. A publicity working party was appointed and White obtained approval for a 'series of
inspired articles' in the farming press. *Farmer & Stock-breeder*'s news
editor, Gordon Gynn, was persuaded to publish a series of ministry-
inspired articles extolling the virtues of mopping up. Gynn visited the
ICD to obtain material and the first of his articles, an illustrated
double-page spread, appeared on 18–19 January 1955. Collison was
also cooperative. Not only did he pledge the support of the NUAW's
3740 branches and individual members (subject to the consent of their
employers), he also:

> proposed to send out a letter to each branch and would also
> arrange for articles to be published in the monthly journal
> [*Land Worker*]. Both the letter and the article would be based
> on drafts supplied by the Ministry. The article should explain
> the cost of the rabbit to agriculture and forestry and the danger
> – unless full advantage is taken of myxomatosis – of the
> country being left with both rabbits and the disease.[22]

The ministry was equally keen to obtain coverage in the provincial
press. Its efforts did not go unrewarded; in January 1957 24 CAECs
gained publicity in local newspapers for the drive against rabbits.
Radio and television were also targeted. White wished to secure coverage on 'The Archers', the BBC's immensely popular early evening
radio drama serial about farming and country life. The ministry's press
officer, Desmond Bird, doubted whether he 'would get very far' with
such an approach, but in fact references to the anti-rabbit campaign
featured in scripts on several occasions between 1955 and 1957.[23]
Unfortunately, these references did not always push the official line.
Indeed, MAF thought:

> too much weight is being given to the view of the gamekeeper,
> and many of the sporting types, that myxomatosis was a
> dreadful thing because it got rid of the rabbits, and everything
> should be done to encourage them back. We ... feel there
> ought to be some counter to it ... conveying the benefits of

increased crops so apparent this year, so that a balanced picture can be presented to listeners.[24]

A year later Geoffrey Baseley the Archers' editor was still being urged to emphasize the importance of rabbit clearance (on this occasion by the BBC's own agricultural liaison officer, Harry Hunt) though with what success is unclear. Other BBC programmes, including 'Farming Today', 'Farm Fare' and 'Woman's Hour' did cover myxomatosis, but extant scripts give no indication that they publicized and endorsed the ministry's mopping-up campaign.[25]

Notwithstanding the BBC's unhelpfulness, White considered the publicity campaign a 'conspicuous success'; 'propaganda in the provincial press has exceeded all expectations.' MAF's rabbit policy group, set up in 1957 because of increased rabbit numbers to review existing approaches and make recommendations, observed that the rabbit control campaign could not have achieved 'more or better publicity'; Amory and Lord St Aldwyn expressed similar sentiments.[26] Of course, not everyone received the message. Many farmers apparently were 'unaware of the 50 per cent grant offered on the clearance of rabbit harbourages'; others heard the propaganda and chose to ignore it.[27] But for the great majority who took a newspaper or listened to the radio the publicity campaign must surely have made its mark.

By March 1955 mopping up was underway on 4.5 million acres spread across 37 counties. There was little difficulty in finding leading farmers and landowners to act as local organizers; NFU and CLA members in particular displayed 'real enthusiasm'. Some farmers were even willing to offer workers as much as £2 for each healthy rabbit destroyed.[28] Initial operations concentrated mainly on southern England and Wales, where myxomatosis had run its course, but by May 1955 arrangements were 'well in hand' for a campaign in the Midlands and North later in the year.[29] The designation of RCAs also proceeded apace. By October 1955, starting with Anglesey back in mid-June, 7 million acres had been designated with 7.75 million more earmarked for England and Wales. Scottish areas had also been established.[30] Amory regarded the battle against the rabbit as more or less won: 'Throughout the whole country farmers are co-operating in the campaign for the mopping up of surviving rabbits' and the animal was virtually absent from the countryside; 'we may well be approaching a new phase in British agriculture.'[31] Such pronouncements were too optimistic, if not hubristic. Though a regional survey in mid-1955 indicated solid interest in mopping up in some regions, the position elsewhere was variable. In some areas of South Wales, for example, it was 'difficult to arouse enthusiasm among farmers'; in mid-Wales there was little coordinated effort.

As early as May 1955 healthy rabbits were spotted in areas apparently cleared by myxomatosis.[32] In June *Farmer & Stock-breeder* reported 'concern … in many parts of the country that a considerable number of rabbits are reappearing', and in August its regular columnist, 'Blythe', reported quantities of rabbits in southern England and the Midlands.[33] In May 1956 a *Farmer & Stock-breeder* correspondent from Devon claimed there was 'no doubt' that rabbits were on the way back; soon reports 'from all over the country' were speaking of reinfestation. In Kent, where mopping up was initially tackled with enthusiasm, some farmers and landowners were said to be 'sitting back and waiting for a further outbreak of myxomatosis to do the work for them'. The county's agricultural officer reported the 'rabbit population … increasing at an alarming rate'.[34] In September 1956 *The Times* declared that 'one thing is certain: the rabbit has won the day – it will never be completely exterminated.' The best hope was that numbers would remain low for many years.[35]

Ronald Lockley blamed 'apathetic … land-users' who failed to take the appropriate action at the critical moment of minimal population during the winter and spring of 1955–56.[36] But farmers' enthusiasm for mopping up may have been sapped by Amory's announcement that agricultural subsidies could be trimmed to reflect the higher farming profits resulting from the decline in rabbit numbers.[37] Amory's timing was unfortunate, for his announcement coincided with the ministry's launch of the 1955–56 mopping-up campaign. In the hope of fostering cooperation, MAF established a rabbit clearance committee, with strong farming representation, to coordinate action against rabbits across the country. But at its first meeting the NFU, though pledging to back fully the rabbit extermination campaign,

warned that a price review that put 'undue emphasis on the financial
benefits to the farming community accruing from the disappearance
of rabbits' could 'damp farmers' enthusiasm and render more difficult
the task of maintaining co-operation'.[38]

In November 1956, aware that rabbit numbers were greater than
they had been a year earlier, the ministry launched another 'all-out
drive against rabbits'. At the press conference called to launch it, St
Aldwyn expressed confidence in the outcome. Amory was less upbeat:
'the campaign this winter is crucial if we are to stand a reasonable
chance of controlling the numbers of rabbits in the future, and I
would appeal for the co-operation of all who work or live in the
countryside to help in this important job.' If not eradicated, the rabbit
would again 'build up to menace our farms'. The prognosis for
Scotland, where the rabbit already 'has built up a breeding stock large
enough to raise a plague', was gloomier still. MAF, which decided to
assume clearance responsibility on derelict as well as common land,
began offering increased grants of up to 75 per cent of costs for scrub
clearance on non-agricultural land where there was little incentive to
voluntary action.[39]

The winter campaign of 1956–57 did not halt the rabbit's revival.
A MAF press release in February 1957 said that 'all country men
should realize the seriousness of the situation'. Similarly, an editorial in
Farmers Weekly in April 1957 noted that rabbits were still returning,
that it was 'now or never' in terms of curbing their comeback and that
farmers needed to help themselves.[40] MAC and Rabbit Clearance
Committee reports told a familiar story of more rabbits and ineffective
action in the field.[41] The Rabbit Policy Group anticipated that 'unless
some additional action can be taken, rabbit numbers will continue to
increase and in 5 years' time may reach about 30% to 50% of pre-
myxomatosis numbers.'[42] Similar messages were conveyed in parliament and the tone of Amory and his junior ministers grew increasingly
pessimistic. In July 1957, though not prepared to accept 'the failure of
his campaign', the minister was 'increasingly worried about rabbits'.
He believed that 'many occupiers' could take 'much more vigorous
action' and that if they did so 'it should be possible to prevent the
rabbit from again becoming a major pest'. As it was, 'present methods'

were not working and MAF recognized the need for another strategy.[43]

In public, ministers continued to claim that CAECs were taking enforcement action whenever rabbit control responsibilities were shirked. Amory, for example, told parliament: 'Where, after due warning, occupiers fail to carry out their responsibility to deal with rabbits on their land, my officers are instructed to enter and take action under my statutory powers. I shall not hesitate to take vigorous default action as required.'[44]

CAECs frequently investigated rabbit infestations and dispatched warning letters. 'Too often, however, the recipient of a warning letter takes the minimum measures necessary to avoid default action and rabbits on his land become a recurring source of trouble.'[45] Rabbit destruction squads were deployed in 'comparatively few cases'; in 1957 only 12 farmers in England and Wales were compelled to pay for rabbit clearance after failing to comply with orders to clear their land. Until 1961, when Messrs Willows & Willows were fined £40 plus ten guineas costs for failing to control rabbits, prosecutions for non-compliance simply did not happen. Although MAF thought this conviction would serve as a warning, any rational farmer would surely have concluded that the chances of being penalized were vanishingly small.[46]

Ten years after its enactment the ICD described the 1947 Agriculture Act, which still governed pest control enforcement, as 'quite ineffective for implementing a policy of rabbit clearance because farmers resented being placed under notice, whether at the instigation of their neighbours or on the initiative of the [county agricultural executive] committee and there was considerable reluctance to serve notices'. Even the NFU thought that, 'despite protestations to the contrary from the Ministry, the task of enforcement is not at present taken seriously enough' and wanted 'more vigorous action'. As an executive committee member of its Herefordshire branch observed, 'unless already existing powers for rabbit clearances were used more stringently against uncooperative farmers, there would be no solution of the rabbit-pest problem.' But, in practice, rabbit control continued to depend on the 'willing and informed co-operation' of landholders.[47]

During 1957 various ways of reinvigorating the mopping-up campaign received consideration. Possibilities included decriminalizing the deliberate transmission of myxomatosis, banning all trade in rabbit products and compelling landholders to join a rabbit control group, stepping up the publicity campaign, 'more vigorous action' against those who failed to clear rabbits from their land, or adoption of the New Zealand system.[48] In the end MAF rejected all these options and proposed, somewhat lamely, that 'we should do something more to help and encourage occupiers who are willing co-operators.' The idea was 'to put the national anti-rabbit campaign on a coordinated basis, and step up the elimination process which has hitherto been left to myxo, natural predators and individual effort'. By offering £-for-£ grants to groups of occupiers, the government sought to encourage the formation of rabbit clearance societies able to equip and employ professional rabbit catchers.[49] The resulting scheme was later termed 'a poor imitation of the New Zealand idea'.[50]

In effect, MAF proposed offering inducements for work that was compulsory anyway. Logic suggests that landholders would have been delighted at the prospect, but when MAF sounded out various parties it discovered little enthusiasm. The NFU was 'very luke-warm' and the CLA 'advise[d] against our proposals', preferring a compulsory scheme. CAEC chairmen also expressed misgivings. As Basil Engholm of MAF wrote, 'our proposals about rabbit clearance societies have had a very mixed reception from the Chairmen of CAECs.' These were inauspicious omens but, buoyed by support from the various Scottish organizations, the government decided to proceed and the scheme began in February 1958. An advisory committee on rabbit clearance (ACRC), chaired by Lord St Aldwyn, was appointed to oversee it.[51]

The first registered society was at Easter Ross in Scotland. In England and Wales the Carmarthenshire rabbit clearance society (RCS) led the way.[52] By the end of April 1958 plans for societies were under consideration from the Scilly Isles to Cape Wrath. One of the first, at Ashford in Kent, the inauguration of which attracted television coverage, began with about 100 members who occupied 13,000 acres. It charged an entrance fee of 10s (50p) and an annual subscription of 1s 6d (7½p) per acre. With this income matched by government grant, the society planned to equip and employ two rabbit killers.[53] By the time a conference of rabbit clearance societies convened in London in early February 1959 nearly 100 RCSs had been set up in England and Wales and more than 50 in Scotland, with many more under consideration.[54]

With the scheme underway the farmer/writer and regular *Farmers Weekly* columnist, A. G. Street, identified two difficulties. First, the

> small minority of farmers who still believe that a wild rabbit at today's price of 4s. 6d (22½p) more than pays for its keep. If they can go for a stroll with a spaniel, shoot say a quid's worth of rabbits, and pocket the money in cash as a fortuitous receipt not concerned with income tax, they are happy men. They don't care one bit for the serious financial damage they are doing their neighbours who, being real farmers not fiddlers, hate the rabbit and all his works.

Second, the traditional countryman, regardless of wealth or social class, 'will never forgive you ... if you interfere with his rural sport'.[55] In other words, he too wanted the rabbit to survive. By July Street had honed his critique. Because public money was involved the regulations for societies were 'rather complicated and require no little secretarial work'. Hence, 'any farmer who shoulders the burden ... is a hero deserving public honour.' He also foresaw 'lashings of other difficulties', though he identified only two: high set-up and running costs plus the likelihood that in any locality some farmers, for one reason or another, would refuse to join.[56] In *Country Life* Esmond Lynn-Allen considered the scheme too bureaucratic and too reliant on unpaid volunteers. Nevertheless, he thought there was 'no essential reason why rabbit clearance societies should not succeed provided that the plan is administered with tact and realism and carried into effect with keenness and the will to win'.[57] The agriculture correspondent of *The Times* was also hopeful. He attributed the failure of most rabbit clearance work to occupiers' lack of skill and patience in dealing with isolated infestation or the reinvasion of rabbits from neighbours' land. He saw group action as 'the most practicable and economic remedy'.[58]

The conference of RCSs in February 1959, which agreed that a national federation of societies should be formed, heard upbeat appraisals of the new initiative. It learnt that the 'scheme has leapt ahead in the last few months', that new societies were being set up 'every week', and that some existing societies were enlarging their fields of operation. Furthermore, in areas 'in the van of rabbit clearance' such as Scotland, where some societies predated the availability of the £-for-£ grants, 'rabbits are reported to be completely under control and there is no danger of any serious reinfestation'. Overall, however, societies covered only 2 million acres, leaving around 38 million uncovered. Most societies were concentrated in areas such as Cornwall and west Wales, where rabbits had been most prolific before myxomatosis struck. In many places, including the whole of Lancashire, Leicestershire, Glamorgan and Somerset, there were no societies and no plans to create any. Even where societies did exist, some landowners, as Street had anticipated, refused to join.[59] In January 1960 the naturalist Robin Lockley declared that the war had been lost: 'It is now evident that there is no likelihood of the wild rabbit being exterminated, as was hoped by many farmers, foresters, and other landusers. Brer Rabbit has won the battle.'[60]

The scale and scope of rabbit clearance societies, which from 1959 were also concerned with wood pigeons and then other pests, continued to grow. At the end of 1964 the 717 rabbit clearance societies in England and Wales covered nearly nine million acres and received grant income of £350,000 per annum. But the territory they covered still excluded about 73 per cent of the nation's farm and woodland.[61] An article in *The Times* pointed to landholders' 'apathy' and before long members of the Advisory Council on Rabbits and Other Land Pests (ACROLP) bemoaned the lost momentum of the rabbit clearance society movement. It was, said one, difficult 'to keep societies in being at all'.[62] A 1961 article in *The Times*, 'More Wild Rabbits than at any Time Since 1955', referred to 'a marked reluctance to form or join societies' and a host of lapsed memberships. Unpalatable as the prospect was, the newspaper thought the ministry needed to step in. 'Nobody wants to see compulsion so far as joining is concerned. But the Ministry of Agriculture might well be justified in bringing in a form of coercion to deal with some of the apathy which is present.'[63] But the government remained as reluctant as ever. As Lord St Oswald, one of MAF's parliamentary secretaries pointed out to ACROLP in 1963, 'Ministers had decided against compulsion on political ... grounds. The feeling, strengthened by opinion expressed quite recently in the industry itself, was that compulsion would provoke ill-feeling.'[64]

In 1964 the AGM of the federation of rabbit clearance societies, frustrated 'by the lack of power under the 1954 Pest [sic] Act to deal effectively with persistent harbourers of rabbits', passed a resolution calling for compulsory membership of RCSs. MAF again rejected the suggestion, claiming that 'many important sections of the [farming] industry would be opposed' and also that there was 'little prospect' of securing the necessary legislation.[65] Amidst continued 'widespread concern about the future viability of societies', the government set up a review to investigate the organization and work of societies and make recommendations to improve the strength and efficiency of the rabbit clearance movement.[66]

The resultant report, compiled by F. J. Smith, emphasized the problems of some societies and offered 13 recommendations. These included banning the sale of wild rabbits and their skins and continuing voluntary, grant-aided RCSs with staff skilled in control methods. A similar review in Scotland proposed compulsory membership. The government was slow to respond. When it eventually did the outcome involved little change: societies were to remain voluntary; subject to evidence of efficiency they would remain eligible for grants on the same basis as before; trade in rabbit products would not be banned. The most significant change did not even concern rabbits but involved the extension of grants to mole control.[67] Evidence from the field failed to prove the value of RCSs in rabbit control, for the ICD's west Wales rabbit survey of 1961–65 demonstrated that the 'occurrence of rabbits on holdings of members of Rabbit Clearance Societies was higher than on non-member properties'.[68]

In 1968, by which time RCS numbers were down to 664 in England and Wales, ACROLP received a familiar message – voluntary rabbit clearance societies 'were flagging, and should be wound up or given a new incentive'.[69] In the event, grant-aided societies limped on until 1978, 25 years after myxomatosis had reached Britain. *The Times* agriculture correspondent expressed bemusement at their passing; myxomatosis was losing its effect, rabbit numbers were increasing, and gin traps and poisons were banned. As a result, landholders were virtually defenceless. Yet MAF appeared more concerned to cull badgers and a few thousand coypu in East Anglia than to deal with 'one of the most resilient and damaging pests of all'.[70]

Attenuation

When myxomatosis broke out in the United Kingdom, virologists and veterinarians already knew, from laboratory experiments and natural outbreaks elsewhere, that the disease could produce an initial mortality rate of 99.5 per cent or even more. They also knew that, as attenuated strains of virus developed, ousted virulent strains and conferred immunity against the virulent form on recovered rabbits, subsequent outbreaks might cause a significantly lower rate of mortality. Thus, it was recognized in 1953 that 'it was most unlikely that rabbits would be exterminated by myxomatosis.'[71]

Studies of the original outbreak at Bough Beech and elsewhere indicated, as of May 1955, a mortality rate in excess of 99 per cent that showed 'no sign of declining'. Although some of the first areas infected seemed to have been rabbit free for some time, a 'rigorous search occasionally revealed odd survivors, most of which were found to be susceptible'. Furthermore, the disease seemed to persist in cleared areas with the result that rabbits that subsequently appeared were infected. Research in other parts of the country where the disease had been present for some time revealed that only about 10 per cent of the small number of survivors had antibodies to myxomatosis. The remaining 90 per cent remained susceptible to the disease.[72] Hence, at the end of 1956 the mortality rate in most parts of the country remained in the region of 99 per cent.[73]

All of this was good news for those who hoped to wipe out or drastically reduce Britain's rabbits. However, beginning at Horn Heath, Suffolk, as early as September 1954, and then in a few other parts of England and Scotland, some rabbits were found to be affected by an attenuated strain of myxomatosis. In April 1955 such a strain was isolated from a rabbit caught in Clumber Park, Nottinghamshire. Then, three similar strains were found in the same locality. A survey carried out in July revealed that the area possessed 'a high proportion of immunes'. In June 1955 Amory informed parliament that of all the live rabbits from various parts of the country examined by MAF scientists, 39, or about 10 per cent, had acquired immunity to myxomatosis. But it was becoming clear that in Sherwood Forest (The Dukeries), a high proportion of rabbits (50 per cent) were surviving myxomatosis and hence acquiring immunity to subsequent infection, no matter how virulent.[74]

The Dukeries, an extensive area of mixed woodland and farmland, took in parts of three private estates plus land owned or occupied by the Forestry Commission, National Trust and War Office. Most of the region's recovered rabbits were found on the National Trust's Clumber Park estate but they were present in all areas. In autumn 1955 Nottinghamshire's AEC was contemplating designating the whole county a rabbit clearance area, but it was uncertain how to deal with The Dukeries because of the wide extent of woodland, bracken and other cover for rabbits and the involvement of 'very great sporting interests'.[75]

The ministry was 'seriously perturbed' by news of significant attenuation in The Dukeries 'because if news of the immune strain of rabbits ... should "get abroad" it could seriously affect the national efforts to keep rabbits under control and possibly "friends" of the rabbit from other parts may be tempted to collect from this area.' A serious problem would arise if immune rabbits got about the country because Australian experience showed that when attenuated and virulent strains of the disease existed side by side the virulent one died out.[76]

Officials obtained the cooperation of major Dukeries' landholders for a survey to ascertain the extent and exact location of the problem – a 6000-acre wedge of land thought to contain around 5000 rabbits – and for their participation in the eradication effort.[77] But MAF wanted more than the 'normal and reasonable steps' that the owners were in a position to offer; it favoured 'an all-out, intensive drive to destroy the last rabbit in a most difficult area'. Such an effort would involve 'a substantial staff of skilled men going over the area again and again for a period of about four weeks and using all legitimate means for rabbit destruction'. To implement this plan MAF sought government funding for 20 fully-equipped pest officers and operators to be brought in from other counties at a cost of up to £2500.[78]

The Treasury approved the plan and operations commenced in snowy conditions on 6 February 1956 with numerous dogs and up to 100 men wielding shotguns and gassing equipment. Most operatives were local farmers, estate workers or Forestry Commission employees, but some of the CAEC pest control officers came from as far afield as Essex, Pembrokeshire and Northumberland. The extermination exercise, scheduled to last five weeks, received widespread press coverage after reporters were invited to accompany operatives for a day to check on progress. Inevitably, subeditors had a field day with Robin Hood and Blitz allusions; the *Manchester Guardian*, for example, headlined its report, 'With the Ministry's Merry Men in Sherwood Forest'.[79] The effectiveness of the campaign was disputed. A local man involved in the initial effort claimed that a 'miserable' 25 rabbits were killed on the first three days. MAF, on the other hand, claimed that hundreds were gassed and scores shot over the first nine days.[80]

When the exercise was completed in mid-March, within budget but somewhat over schedule owing to illness and bad weather, MAF claimed that 500 rabbits had been shot and thousands gassed in their burrows with 2¼ tons of cyanide powder. Such an outcome was regarded as a success.[81] It was clear, however, that the aspiration to destroy the last rabbit in Sherwood Forest had not been realized. More encouragingly, no rabbits affected by the attenuated strain of myxomatosis were in evidence and it appeared that 95 per cent of all the rabbits in an area of 20 square miles had been killed. This was thought to approximate to the position that would have existed if attenuation had not occurred. It was 'up to the occupiers' to deal with the remaining few.[82] But the extermination of rabbits in The Dukeries was as unlikely as it was in any other part of the country. Neither can the goal of wiping out the attenuated virus be considered a long-term success. When a secondary outbreak of myxomatosis occurred in The Dukeries, the strain was found to be mainly, but not exclusively, of the virulent form. Furthermore, in 1957 attenuation was found to have occurred 'in widely scattered parts of Great Britain' including Argyll,

Dorset, Essex, Hampshire, the Isle of Wight, Kent, Lanarkshire, Nottinghamshire, Stirlingshire, East Suffolk and Surrey.[83]

J. B. Godber, parliamentary secretary at MAF, told the Commons in December 1957 that attenuated myxomatosis had become widespread. Blood tests indicated that 'a fairly large proportion of the rabbit population may already be immune to myxomatosis'.[84] Ten months later Sankey noted

Weakened or attenuated strains of myxomatosis have been found in fifteen English counties this year and in some areas of Scotland. Scientific opinion is that attenuation is likely to increase and this is in accord with Australian experience where attenuated strains are now dominant. In brief, this means that myxomatosis is likely to be an ever decreasing factor in keeping rabbit numbers down.[85]

By December 1958 80 per cent of rabbits in some parts of the country were showing immunity and all the indications were that the proportion of recovering rabbits would grow while the virulence of the disease would 'progressively diminish'.[86] Research by Dr A. R. Mead-Briggs and Dr P. J. Chapple into virus strains revealed 'a marked decrease in the virulence of the myxoma virus' between 1953 and 1962; in 1965 Thompson informed ACROLP that 'the numbers of immune rabbits had increased'. More rabbits were surviving myxomatosis and breeding resistant litters. In some areas, Easter Ross and Hampshire among them, myxomatosis 'appeared to be completely attenuated'.[87] The Dukeries campaign had not worked; the days of 99.5 per cent fatality rates, or anything approaching them, were long gone.

Restocking and Reintroduction

As a 1955 editorial in *Farmer & Stock-breeder* observed: 'Not everyone wants to see the rabbit disappear.'[88] Rough shooters and others supported their perpetuation even if it meant their deliberate reintroduction on land where they had either disappeared or become scarce. In January 1955 a veterinarian from mid-Wales reported that 'serious minded landowners and their veterinary surgeons' were collaborating to immunize rabbits in order to protect the balance of nature.[89] A few days later *Farmers Weekly* reported that immune rabbits had been sent from Scotland to restock land in Gloucestershire.[90] In the following May an advertisement in a gamekeeping magazine offered £5 for three does and three bucks to restock a shoot in Sussex. Other publications carried similar requests and in August 1955 C. W. Hume of UFAW wrote of the 'pernicious campaign' to bring back the rabbit. In Derbyshire, Northamptonshire and elsewhere in the Midlands there were reports of 'misguided persons enclosing healthy rabbits with a view to releasing them later in areas cleared' by myxomatosis. In Warwickshire shooting people were trying to convince farmers that the return of the rabbit would be no bad thing.[91]

Although the ministry knew of isolated cases of restocking for sporting reasons and was empowered to order the destruction of any wild rabbits, it had no powers to prevent reintroduction.[92] The LPAC recommended legislation to prohibit the practice and Lord Merthyr, to the disgust of the *Shooting Times* and some of its readers, introduced a government-inspired private members bill.[93] The measure made some progress but to the dismay of the MAC and UFAWS it was 'talked out' in the Commons. The question continued to be kicked about, though to no great effect, until 1957. A. G. Street expressed amazement that nothing was done:

> How much longer is the Ministry of Agriculture going to countenance the present absurdity – official public ballyhoo about killing rabbits as noxious vermin, and at the same time permitting restocking of land with these animals? Was there ever a more Gilbertian example of absurd government?

However, probably because there was little evidence that the practice was widespread and little hope that such a law could ever be enforced, no legislation ever ensued.[94] Neither was the vaccination of wild rabbits against myxomatosis ever criminalized, though MAF prevailed upon the *Veterinary Record*, the organ of the professional body, to counsel veterinarians against engaging in such practice except for scientific purposes.[95]

Once it dawned upon farmers and others with an economic interest in the permanent disappearance of the rabbit that neither myxomatosis nor follow-up campaigns of destruction would rid the country of an extremely troublesome creature, the question of relaxing the ban on deliberate introduction of myxomatosis resurfaced.[96] In fact, the Scottish NFU's Aberdeen and Kincardineshire area executive was lobbying for this outcome as early as mid-1955. Other Scottish farming organizations were not far behind.[97] With the Scottish NFU, the only body to submit evidence to the MAC in favour of deliberate transmission, 'pressing very hard' for the controlled use of myxomatosis to exterminate rabbits, the MAC's scientific subcommittee further considered the issue.[98]

The subcommittee's scientific secretary, Harry Thompson, said that while myxomatosis 'could be an excellent means of rabbit control' and a useful means of combating restocking, there were 'valid medical and veterinary objections to the use of any disease for pest control'. He also had humanitarian concerns and fears that deliberate transmission could lead to further attenuation of the virus. On balance, therefore, he was not in favour of any change in the law. After further discussion the subcommittee agreed that the rabbit population was too low to allow the rapid spread of introduced disease; the introduction of virulent strains could promote attenuation and undermine mopping-up operations, and myxomatosis would never exterminate the rabbit. In sum, the subcommittee unanimously rejected the deliberate transmission of myxomatosis for rabbit control. Only if the rabbit defeated all other control methods and greatly increased in numbers should such a step be reconsidered. The MAC unanimously accepted this recommendation; it recognized that, scientific considerations apart, it was 'unrealistic' to think that parliament would change the law on 'this controversial subject'.[99]

In March 1957 Sankey informed the Rabbit Policy Group of his conviction that 'when rabbit damage again became widespread, a vigorous demand would arise for reintroduction of myxomatosis.' The Scottish NFU had already requested the retention of a virulent strain for this purpose.[100] Shortly afterwards, a survey of 12 English and Welsh counties revealed that every county expected a 'substantial increase' in rabbit numbers over the next five years. The most pessimistic evaluation, by Essex, anticipated that within this period its rabbit population would be 80 per cent of the pre-myxomatosis level.[101] Sankey's prediction proved accurate; in August Lord Dynevor introduced a Pests Act, 1954 (Amendment) Bill that proposed the repeal of section 12 of the Pests Act, which, controversially, had made the deliberate transmission of myxomatosis a criminal offence. Given the circumstances that had surrounded enactment of the clause, MAF anticipated 'great controversy and considerable embarrassment for the Government'.[102]

At meetings on 3 December both the MAC and its scientific subcommittee reconsidered the issue of deliberate transmission. The subcommittee reaffirmed its opposition to Dynevor's bill, but judged that deliberate transmission might be appropriate 'if rabbits should greatly increase in numbers despite the proper application of conventional methods of control'. It also believed that local circumstances, namely dense populations in circumscribed areas, might justify carefully controlled reintroduction of virulent myxomatosis. For its part, the full MAC was mainly concerned that farmers might spread attenuated strains of the disease and relax efforts to control rabbits in the misplaced expectation that the virus would do the work for them. So even though members doubted the enforceability of section 12 of the Pests Act, they endorsed the opinion of its subcommittee that no change in the law was justified.[103]

Thereafter, demands to legalize deliberate transmission of myxomatosis ceased. The authorities had never been in favour and the climb down over Horace King's amendment to the Pests Act, 1954, made it politically impossible for a Conservative government, in power till October 1964, to change the law. As Lord St Aldwyn told a meeting of the ACRC in 1958, it was not 'a practical prospect politically at the present time to seek statutory powers to use myxomatosis as a method of rabbit control'. In any case, Australian experience argued against such a step because there the disease was proving a less and less effective control. Stocks of virulent virus were held in British laboratories and could be made available in large quantities if required, but Ritchie remained concerned that their deployment could advance attenuation.[104] In contrast with Australia, virulent myxomatosis remained widespread in Britain into the 1960s. Harry Thompson predicted in 1961, a year in which myxomatosis was 'more widespread than at any time since 1955', that the disease 'would probably continue to be a major factor in [rabbit] control for many years', though not indefinitely.[105] Though this forecast was not altogether accurate, some of those whose land was overrun by rabbits no doubt continued to deploy myxomatosis, as they had since 1954 if not earlier, as a quick if illegal, inefficient and short-term solution to a problem that otherwise demanded a great deal of time, skill and patience.

Conclusion

At a press conference in October 1955 the minister of agriculture mentioned the possibility that the attenuation of myxomatosis 'might well result in our having both the rabbits and the disease; something that no one wants, whether he be farmer, sportsman or animal lover'. Such a prospect:

> adds emphasis to the importance of eliminating any rabbits that have survived outbreaks of the disease. In fact, the only way to get rid of myxomatosis is to have no rabbits. I often see suggestions that there is no harm in having a few rabbits about the place, but I regard this as a most dangerous doctrine. Whoever heard of having only a few rabbits! Ask any Australian.[106]

As one observer wrote in January 1956, the 'Ministry of Agriculture has plumped for extermination'. Weeks later Amory confirmed that his policy was 'to do everything I can in an attempt to exterminate rabbits'.[107]

Even at the time, some recognized the futility of the aspiration.[108] More than half a century later, with tens of millions of rabbits again present in Britain, it is difficult to imagine how extermination could ever have been regarded as anything but a forlorn hope. The animal's remarkable capacity to survive in hard times and flourish in good is and was well known. Sexually mature at between three and six months of age and not subject to breeding seasons, in favourable conditions does can produce litters of five, six or more at intervals of a month or so. Potentially, a breeding pair can produce hundreds of direct descendants in a year. Indeed, it has even been suggested, albeit somewhat fancifully, that 'if left undisturbed for three years, the progeny of one pair of rabbits would amount to no fewer than 13,000,000.'[109]

Even on accessible terrain with consensus on the need for extermination the task would have been well nigh impossible. But many rabbits inhabited inaccessible areas on rugged or overgrown land that was extremely difficult, if not impossible, to clear. The strategic and timely reintroduction of a virulent strain of myxomatosis in areas such as The Dukeries where pockets of rabbits survived the first onslaught of the disease might have been effective.[110] But such moves became impossible once the King amendment criminalized deliberate transmission. Otherwise, cyanide gas was the key to rabbit clearance, especially following the abolition of gin traps in 1958; but gas was of limited utility on light soils and useless against surface-dwelling animals. In any case, the attractions of gas diminished as its threat to the health of operatives came to be appreciated. Practicalities aside, it is clear that many people, not necessarily a small minority, wanted the rabbit to survive (whether for the pot, sport or sentimental reasons). As A. G. Street recognized, 'there is no getting away from the fact that the great majority of people in Britain do not want to see the wild rabbit exterminated.'[111]

Even a well-equipped, generously-funded and universally-supported army of rabbit control specialists would surely have failed. The intensive clearance operation in The Dukeries, which involved large numbers of men deploying vast amounts of gas within a comparatively small area for a lengthy period, failed to eliminate all rabbits. Unless an extermination campaign was completely successful, survivors and immigrants would 'breed on a magnificent scale', so that the position was soon as bad as ever.[112] An attempt to clear Skokholm's rabbits in the 1930s destroyed thousands of animals and was 'almost completely successful', but by the 1960s rabbits were 'as numerous as ever'.[113] So the failure to exterminate the animals across the UK should cause no surprise. Indeed, the surprising thing is that extermination was ever seen as a possibility. Lord Merthyr surely hit the mark when he said 'now is the time to join together to reduce the rabbit population so far as we possibly can – I am not going to say "eradicate", because I think nothing but a miracle would achieve that.'[114]

Some, A. G. Street among them, argued that elimination of the rabbit did not require a miracle, merely the prohibition of all trade in rabbit products, as observed in New Zealand, for 'when rabbits don't pay anybody; then nobody loves them.'[115] As we have seen, the 1965 Smith report recommended such a ban, though for various practical reasons the government was not persuaded.[116] Whether trade prohibition would have had the effect that Street and others anticipated is debatable, for too many people approved the wild rabbit's presence. Leaving aside so-called sentimentalists who enjoyed seeing them in the countryside, rough shooters prized them because they provided relatively cheap, accessible and challenging (but not too challenging) sport. Sportsmen no doubt liked to eat, sell or give away some of the animals they shot. A ban on sales could hardly have prohibited personal consumption and donation. Accordingly, it is highly likely that shooters would have pursued their sport, and preserved the rabbits that enabled them to do so, notwithstanding a ban on sales. By the same token, landholders who derived rental income from shooters would also have preserved the rabbit. Take the case of coarse fish, which have next to no economic value as food, at least in Britain, and provide no usable by-products. But coarse fish are zealously preserved and coarse fishing is of considerable economic significance in terms of rents for fishing rights and expenditure on clothing, equipment and licences. In any case, as a *Farmers Weekly* correspondent pointed out, the prolonged destruction of two unsaleable, unprofitable and widely reviled creatures, the rook and the rat, had failed to eliminate either.[117]

Government policy to exterminate the rabbit was probably doomed from the start, regardless of the strategy adopted. If failure were guaranteed, it may seem superfluous to evaluate the manner in which rabbit clearance was implemented. Yet, time and again it appears belated, half-hearted, cheese-paring and inconsistent. Reluctant to assume responsibility for control itself or fully to fund the actions of others, government had legal powers to compel landowners to take the necessary measures. Those who did not act could be prosecuted and, if convicted, fined. Yet, rather than hauling apathetic farmers before the courts, MAF promoted rabbit control almost exclusively through persuasion and propaganda.

At first sight reluctance to prosecute appears puzzling. In fact, this reluctance was consistent with the behaviour of British regulatory agencies as developed over the preceding century. These agencies tended to eschew prosecution, or treat it as a rarely-used weapon of last resort. The reasons for such an approach include the high cost of bringing prosecutions; concern that acquittals or convictions resulting in low penalties will demonstrate to the regulated that the law can safely be ignored; belief that more can be achieved by negotiation, cajolery or even threat than by force of law; and, some argue, reluctance to stigmatize the respectable by taking them to court.[118] Do these explanations fit the rabbit control context?

When, in May 1957, the Rabbit Clearance Committee discussed whether 'the prosecution of non co-operative occupiers would help CAECs to obtain fuller compliance with the Pests Act', its chairman, Basil Engholm, pointed out that 'prosecutions took time and would only be successful if Courts were satisfied that there was no element of doubt in a defendant's favour.' The committee agreed that prosecution should be restricted to 'those cases where legal advisers were satisfied that there was good hope of success ... unsuccessful prosecutions might bring the Pests Act into disrepute and do harm to the [rabbit clearance] campaign.'[119] An additional problem concerned the reluctance of 'magistrates' courts ... to convict private individuals at the instance of a Government Department, and even where they do so the fines are usually very small'.[120] A few months later, at a meeting of CAEC chairmen, Lord St Aldwyn enquired 'whether a more rigorous enforcement of the Pests Act would not ... secure better control of rabbits'. He then answered his own question:

> successful legal proceedings would depend upon proof that there had been consistent default on the part of the defendant, and unless a reasonably severe penalty was imposed by the Court prosecution might do more harm than good. More

rigorous enforcement of the Act would also require considerably more staff for inspection work.[121]

While MAF's approach to the enforcement of rabbit control con-
formed to the norms of regulatory behaviour, its avoidance of robust
enforcement procedures may have another explanation. Michael Winter
has argued that the Crichel Down affair 'almost certainly convinced
the government of the need to reduce the powers of the Ministry' of
Agriculture and CAECs. The Agriculture Act, 1958, left CAECs in
place but terminated their powers of sanction.[122] But even before this
enactment MAF had become reluctant to throw its weight about. It is
likely that this reluctance accounts, at least in part, for its unwillingness
to prosecute farmers for their perceived failings in rabbit control.

'Negotiated compliance' whereby regulators seek to encourage the
observance of laws through non-coercive means can be an effective
way of implementing regulations.[123] In the rabbit control context,
using the eradication of rabbits as an index of success, it is arguable
that it failed. However, far more significant an explanation for the
survival of the rabbit is the futility of the extermination exercise in the
first place.

Chapter 8
Agriculture and Environment

Agriculture

By the 1950s it was well known that rabbits destroyed crops and young trees, reduced the stock-carrying capacity of land, assisted the spread of moss and unpalatable weeds, damaged banks and fields with their burrows and scrapes, diverted human effort and scarce materials from productive work to the tasks of fencing and trapping, and frustrated efforts to control animal diseases such as liver fluke.[1] Their impact on agricultural production had been a matter of speculation for years. In 1936 Ronald Sperling estimated £70 million a year (see Chapter 2), but in 1940 A. D. Middleton referred to 'oft repeated and quite unauthentic estimates of ten, fifty, or seventy million pounds as the measure of rabbit damage annually in this country'.[2] Lord Rothschild, chairman of the ARC, took a broad brush approach; he thought merely that 'a devil of a lot of money' was involved.[3]

Once myxomatosis reached Britain questions about the economic importance of rabbits were resurrected. At first Lord Carrington stated that there were 'insufficient data on which to make a reliable estimate of the total damage caused by wild rabbits to agriculture and forestry in this country'. Before long, however, he was prepared to suggest a figure of £50 million a year or more. Sankey's study of the 'economics of the wild rabbit' for the MAC also endorsed 'the frequently quoted figure of £50 million [per year]'. The Labour peer, Lord Archibald, however, estimated the much smaller sum of £20 million a year and others produced still lower figures.[4]

The MAC was influenced by Sankey's report but could find 'no reliable basis for calculating the total annual damage'. It considered wild rabbit consumption of grass and crops 'very great' and cited survey and experimental evidence indicating £15 million a year for cereals, £21 million for grass and unknown further amounts for vegetables and fruit trees. No monetary value could be placed on losses to forestry and woodland, but over £2 million a year was spent on protection measures alone. The committee calculated that rabbit products generated income in the order of £15 million a year but had 'no hesitation in suggesting that the loss or potential loss caused by the depredations of the rabbit to agriculture and forestry is three or four times as great', namely between £45 and £60 million.[5]

A little later Harry Thompson and Alastair Worden observed that it was 'impossible to assess the total damage done by rabbits … because the losses are spread over a large area and, while sometimes obvious enough, are frequently confused with those caused by other pests, or are attributed to adverse conditions of soil or weather.' However, they were not deterred from producing various estimates of their own, including one of £40–£50 million a year for damage to farm crops, offset against a profit of up to £15 million a year in rabbit products, of which less than £2 million actually went to agriculturalists.[6]

All these estimates have been challenged. C. J. Smith, Wentworth Day and others regarded the figure of £50 million a year variously as an 'absurdity', 'a gross exaggeration', 'utterly false' and 'sheer bunkum'.[7] Years later John Marchington, while conceding that rabbit damage to agriculture was very serious, viewed 'all round figures and unproven estimates with suspicion, for if anyone has an axe to grind, a benefit to be won, or a bias to push further, then estimates, opinions and forecasts glow brightly in the fires of their enthusiasm'.[8] Yet, in 1994 Harry Thompson, doyen of rabbit researchers, still believed that the 'total cost of rabbit damage before myxomatosis is likely to have been some £50m annually'.[9]

Not least because Australian 'rural production' was reported to have increased by £50 million in 1952–53, many thought that MIRD (myxomatosis-induced rabbit depopulation) would lead to substantially higher crop yields, greater productivity and improved profitability for Britain's farmers and foresters.[10] Why else did farmers spread the disease if not for the extra income they anticipated? But to what

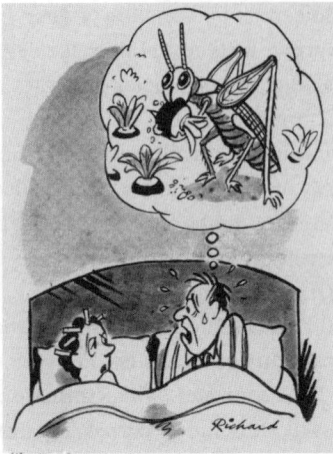

9. 'Dreamed some crank introduced something to replace the rabbit!'

extent, in the short, medium and long terms, did MIRD benefit agriculture and forestry?

During the 1954 growing season much of Britain remained heavily infested with rabbits. It was too early, therefore, to estimate the impact of MIRD on farming. In 1955 reports of bumper crops and the cultivation of land previously not worth farming owing to rabbit damage began to appear at an early stage. In March, for example, Norfolk farmers claimed improved yields from winter cereals wherever rabbits were absent; it was estimated that the county's agriculture production was already worth an additional £1 million per annum.[11] In May, Sankey informed the MAC that 'reports had been coming in from all over the country of significant improvement in crops – mainly cereals and grass – due to the absence of rabbits.' Corn was growing to the edge of fields; the quantity and quality of grass had improved; trees were being planted without wire protection and 'old rabbity grass was being confidently ploughed up for crops.'[12] These were promising signs but the summer and autumn harvest provided the first real opportunity to assess the myxomatosis premium; not for decades, perhaps centuries, had the crops been brought in from virtually rabbit-free farmland.

In his 'Farmers' Ordinary' column in *Field* Robert Henriques referred to the 'astonishing' improvement of the hay crop, which on his farm was up by nearly 13 hundredweight (645 kilograms) per acre. This 'staggering' increase was not 'due to the weather, because for growing grass … last year was much the better of the two seasons. Nor was there any other factor, except the complete absence of rabbits.'[13] An editorial declared that 'the absence of rabbits has played an important part in the heavy crops of cereal and hay that have been produced in the last season.'[14] *Farmers Weekly* took the same line. Its editor wrote of 'enormous increases in grass and corn growth where myxomatosis has cleared the rabbits' and its regular columnist, A. G. Street observed:

> Unless something untoward happens soon 1955 will provide one of the best seasons for many years. Already it has given us one of the finest haymakings in living memory and, largely due to the lack of rabbits, one of the heaviest crops of greenstuff; while the same cheering abundance is generally to be found in roots and cereals.[15]

In the House of Lords Lord Listowel, who in 1950–51 had been a parliamentary secretary in MAF, observed that while it was impossible to quantify the financial benefits of the rabbit's demise to agriculture and forestry, they were 'very substantial', even to the point, as far as food and farming were concerned, of 'a minor agricultural revolution'.[16] Lord Dundee, who had been a member of the MAC until he resigned over the terms of the Pests Act in November 1954, was more definite. His enquiries indicated that rabbit-free medium quality mixed farmland in Scotland would yield an additional 35s (£1.75p) per acre. If this figure was 'anything like right' the potential gain for Britain as a whole promised to exceed £50 million per annum, 'which would be quite a useful help to any Chancellor of the Exchequer'.[17]

Not everyone was so certain. There was widespread agreement that the 1955 harvest was good, if not exceptional, but for Wentworth Day: 'A mild spring, a kindly summer, glorious harvest weather and an unprecedented increase in the use of combine harvesters are the main causes of the good harvest, not the disappearance of the rabbit.'[18] Others noted that bumper harvests were 'rare in our cycle of agricultural weather'. Consequently, 'we shall need several seasons of research and analysis before we can get an adequate and accurate estimate of what the effect has been.' In any case, some doubted the possibility of quantifying either the extent of pre-myxomatosis rabbit damage to agriculture or the boost rabbit depopulation gave the 1955 harvest.[19] Some of the figures presented by the MAC, it was alleged:

were based on an experiment carried out in Kent with an infestation of 20 rabbits to the acre. Anyone who knows a little about rabbits knows that a farm with 20 rabbits to the acre would be not just an infestation but a disaster. Why assess the overall damage throughout the country on surveys of this kind? It would appear that the whole method of estimating rabbit damage is based on if's, and but's and maybe's, and must be grossly exaggerated out of all reason.

Indeed, one letter to *Field* assessed annual crop damage as substantially less than £5 million per year and wondered 'if there ever was such a thing as rabbit menace'.[20]

Even though it sought the assistance of in-house and academic economists, the ministry found it difficult to quantify the benefits of MIRD to agriculture.[21] Two years to the day after myxomatosis was confirmed at Bough Beech, Amory held a press conference on the subject of 'myxomatosis and crop improvement'. The minister spoke of reports from all parts of England and Wales about 'remarkable improvements in crop yields which farmers claim are largely due to the virtual clearance of the rabbit pest following outbreaks of myxomatosis'. Though not able to differentiate between the influence of other factors such as weather and good husbandry, the one consistent feature in all reports from the shires was the absence of rabbits. The total gain could not be precisely calculated but Amory reported increased cereal yields of 'not far short of 2 cwt (approximately 102 kg) per acre (0.405 hectares)' and improved average crop yields of 25 per cent for the country as a whole. These figures were, moreover, conservative estimates. In short, a 'miracle' had occurred.[22]

Two weeks later Amory was rather more certain, not only about the statistics, but also their implications for farm incomes. Evidence that rabbit depopulation had increased the value of cereal production in England and Wales by £10–15 million prompted the minister to state that 'changes of this kind should be reflected in estimates of aggregate farming net income and thus taken into account at the Annual Price Review'.[23] The farming community was incensed. The executive of the NFU's Leicester branch called for Amory to substantiate his figures or resign. A Monmouthshire farmer wanted the NFU to tell the government

> in no uncertain manner that the losses inflicted by rabbits before the arrival of myxomatosis were never taken into consideration at price reviewing and there is no reason why any benefits derived now should be taken into account. Should the Government persist in so doing, then the control of the wild rabbit shall become the sole responsibility of the Government and any losses incurred by farmers through the Government's failure to carry out their obligations shall be recouped by farmers at Price Reviews.[24]

In an editorial headed 'Mr Amory cannot be serious', *Farmer & Stock-breeder* questioned whether cereal yields had improved to the extent suggested and argued that subsidies should remain unchanged until rabbits had been absent for 'a period of years'. One of its regular columnists dismissed as 'ridiculous' the idea that the bumper harvest of 1955 was caused entirely by the absence of rabbits. He thought the weather was without doubt 'the most important factor'. *Field* referred to the ministry's 'stupid propaganda'.[25]

Farmers' sense of grievance with Amory was heightened when the NUAW began to use MIRD as an argument to promote its wage claim. Any myxomatosis dividend for farmers, the union maintained, should mean higher pay for its members. As an editorial in the union's monthly magazine put it: 'farmers, who have often argued that they would pay more wages if they had the money, should remember that the £15 million which they have had handed to them "on a plate" would go a long way towards meeting the cost of our £7 [per week] wage demand.'[26]

Faced with widespread hostility from farmers, Amory was soon seeking to reassure a powerful interest group whose cooperation was vital if the Ministry's rabbit clearance campaign were to prosper:

> a statistical computation of the exact gain is extremely difficult to make and I have always said that I do not think it is worth

while to attempt to do so on present evidence. I have given estimates based on the best evidence available but I have pointed out when doing so that it is indeed a rough and ready estimate, and I have no means of checking the estimate made by the Myxomatosis Advisory Committee in 1954.[27]

The government would not simply assume that farmers' profits had risen by £10–15 million. For a while Amory continued to insist that the myxomatosis dividend would be a consideration in the annual price review but MAF soon stopped trumpeting the monetary gains to agriculture from the absence of rabbits.

Farmers were not entirely appeased. In 1959 *Farmer & Stock-breeder* continued to ponder the irony of farmers footing the bill for rabbit control only to find that the absence of rabbits provided an argument for reduced subsidies.[28] By this time, however, with rabbits coming back, albeit slowly and in small numbers, newspaper stories about higher farming incomes had been superseded by news that the government's extermination campaign was failing and predictions that agriculture stood to sustain losses as a result. As a *Farmers Weekly* editorial observed: 'If the estimate that, within five or ten years, rabbits may be doing £30,000,000 worth of damage on the farms of Britain is anything like correct, that means about 15s [75p] an acre – or £75 worth of damage every year on a 200-acre farm.'[29]

The 1956 harvest provided some support for those who thought weather, rather than MIRD, was chiefly responsible for the excellent crops of 1955. The early summer hay crop was patchy while the 'gales, floods, hail and incessant rain' of August prompted *Farmer & Stock-breeder* to run the headline: 'This May Be the Worst Harvest in 40 Years'. The next two years were little better. The 'wretched' summer of 1957 was 'depressing both for farmers and for holiday makers'. In 1958 a wet June 'demolished' the hay harvest; thereafter conditions remained poor until September.[30] So any advantages to agriculture brought about by myxomatosis were in some degree lost to bad weather. In contrast, the summer of 1959, with record-breaking heat and sunshine, was one of the best of the century thus far. Although some areas suffered from drought the harvest was generally excellent.

All of this is, of course, impressionistic. Any conclusions about the impact of rabbit depopulation on agriculture should be based on a statistical review of production and yield.

Table 8.1. UK Cereal Production and Yield, 1950–59

Year	UK cereal production (all cereals, million tonnes)	Area of cereal production in UK (million hectares)	Yield per hectare (tonnes)
1950	7.905	3.346	2.363
1951	7.846	3.149	2.492
1952	8.426	3.271	2.576
1953	9.060	3.300	2.745
1954	8.190	3.137	2.610
1955	8.913	2.958	3.013
1956	8.700	3.085	2.820
1957	8.264	3.013	2.742
1958	8.448	3.029	2.789
1959	9.409	2.914	3.228

Source: H. F. Marks and D. K. Britton, *A Hundred Years of British Food and Farming: A Statistical Survey* (London: Taylor & Francis, 1989) 162, 164.

UK cereal production figures provide the best indication of production and yield trends for crops known to be damaged by rabbits (Table 8.1). The key figures, in column four, show significant increase in cereal yields in the course of the 1950s, with peaks in the fine summers of 1955 and 1959. The increase predated the arrival of myxomatosis and, notwithstanding the (possibly weather-related) downturn of 1957 and 1958, continued afterwards. The first three years of the 1950s saw the lowest cereal yields of the whole decade. The yield of 1959 was 36.6 per cent higher than that of 1950; 29.5 per cent higher than 1951; and 25 per cent higher than 1952. The next worst yields of the 1950s occurred in 1954, the first full year of myxomatosis (when awful weather hit the growing and harvest seasons).

None of these figures, however, provides any indication of *why* yield figures performed as they did; none of them allows us to conclude that myxomatosis, as against several other possibilities, was responsible.

Agricultural historians have long pointed to the 'staggering' productivity gains of British farming between the 1930s and 1990s, a period that saw wheat yields, for example, rise from two tonnes per hectare to more than seven. The post-1947 years in particular have been identified as a period of agricultural transformation. Martin links the 'unprecedented increases' in yields to four causally-related factors: 'plant breeding which resulted in more productive varieties; fertilizers which raised the plant's photosynthetic capabilities; herbicides and pesticides which reduced competition and damage from weeds and insects; and improvements in mechanization which increased the efficiency of crop production'.[31] None of these, of course, has anything to do with rabbits or myxomatosis. Other historians of twentieth-century British agriculture, such as Holderness and Howkins, fail to mention rabbits or myxomatosis anywhere in their books. It appears, therefore, that MIRD is widely disregarded as an explanation for enhanced agricultural output. Only Martin accepts it as one of the factors that 'facilitated the expansion drive' in British agriculture. Indeed, he observes that reduced levels of rabbit damage 'were sufficient to account for the increase in British food production which took place between 1952 and 1956'.[32]

While Martin's point acknowledges nothing more than a theoretical and brief causal relationship, it does indicate that myxomatosis had a significant, if ultimately unquantifiable, impact on farm yields in the short term. Given that rabbit numbers have never returned to the levels of the early 1950s and that rabbit damage to cereals 'again become noticeable' only in the 1970s, it seems likely that longer-term benefits also ensued.[33] For how long is unclear; in 1982 Ross continued to refer to the 'great benefit' of myxomatosis to agriculture and forestry.[34] By the mid-1980s, however, MAF estimated that rabbit damage to food crops was at least £90 million per year and possibly as high as £120 million, with the potential to rise as high as £400 million. In 1998 the Mammal Society estimated the ongoing cost of damage at

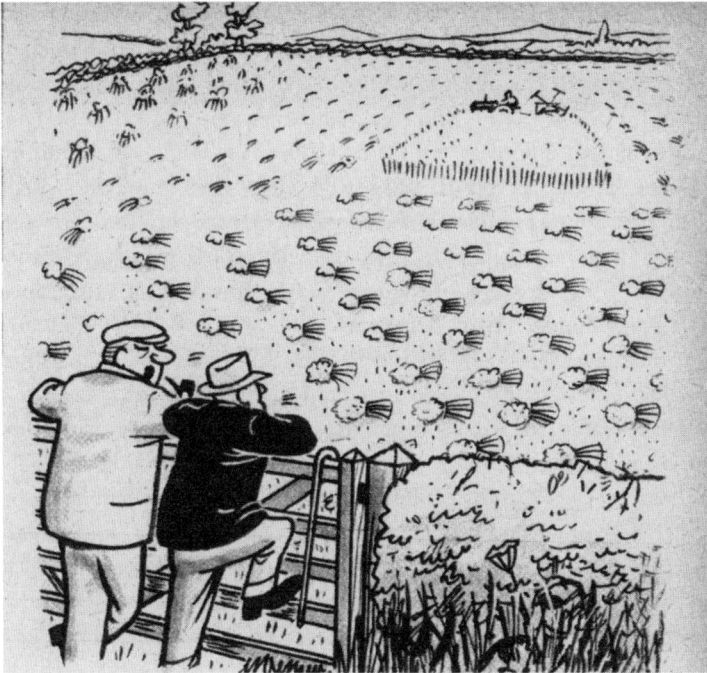

10. 'No excitement at harvest time since the rabbits went.'

£100 million a year. Large though such figures were, in real terms they were substantially lower than the £50 million widely suggested in the early 1950s. Things would have been worse without myxomatosis, for the number of wild rabbits probably stood at no more than 20 per cent of the pre-myxomatosis level in the 1980s and, notwithstanding viral attenuation, the disease was still inhibiting population recovery.[35] Mammal Society surveys in 1995 and 2004 indicated populations of 37.5 million and 40 million respectively, still far lower than even the most conservative estimate (60 million) for the early 1950s.[36] In any case, the state of British agriculture under the European Common Agriculture Policy in the 1980s was very different from what had prevailed three decades or so earlier. By this time the early-1950s' challenge of wringing every last ounce of food from the land had been transformed into one of controlling 'food mountains'.

Environment

The virtual elimination of rabbits had environmental consequences. By the twentieth century it was known that rabbits had an impact not only upon planted crops and tree plantations but also on flora, fauna and the natural environment. From 1900 'many studies' explored the influence of rabbits on Britain's wild vegetation.[37] In 1904 Wallis wrote that rabbits inflicted considerable damage on flora in some areas of Cambridgeshire.[38] In 1917 E. Pickworth Farrow, in 'the most important' English study of the effect of rabbits on vegetation, wrote about rabbit-induced plant degeneration and soil erosion on the *calluna* (ling) heaths of Breckland in East Anglia. He established experimentally that rabbit attack caused many wild plants, including species of campion, cranesbill, hawk's beard, lily, milfoil and trefoil, to become rare or disappear. Even a few rabbits could have a 'considerable cumulative effect'.[39] Subsequent research questioned whether rabbits 'determined Breckland vegetation quite so exclusively as Farrow supposed' or caused the erosion for which Farrow also blamed them. But the main conclusion, that the botany of the heath was created by 'the interaction of the overwhelming rabbit pressure on a small number of competing species', remained valid.[40]

Rabbits also had a 'very great effect upon vegetation elsewhere in the country'.[41] As the distinguished botanist and plant ecologist Arthur Tansley wrote in 1949, 'the aggregate damage they do is undoubtedly enormous'.[42] Almost anywhere, but especially on heaths and chalk grasslands where plant life was 'impoverished and the number of species diminished ... excessive rabbit pressure' degraded 'vegetation to a lower form'.[43] There was 'no proof that grazing by rabbits has eliminated any species from the flora of this country, but ... abundant evidence of local extermination'.[44] Military and monkey orchids were a case in point; botanists attributed their near disappearance from Berkshire and Oxfordshire to the explosion of the rabbit population since the second half of the nineteenth century.[45]

Rabbits could be blamed for much more than the scarcity of some attractive flowering plants. On hillsides their burrows and scrapes could initiate large-scale soil erosion and desertification. On heavily infested heaths and downs the invasion of rabbit-resistant plants such as bracken, ragwort, moss, elder, bramble, ground ivy, thistles, night-shade and nettles rendered land 'both agriculturally useless and aes-thetically depressing'. Tansley thought such areas 'ought to be taken in hand'. Securely fenced, they could support profitable warrens. Alter-natively, the rabbits they harboured could be exterminated and the land used for grazing or, where the soil was suitable, forestry.[46]

In woodland, where rabbits 'barked' saplings and ate the tips of seedlings, they restricted shrub and tree growth and inhibited regener-ation. They could also do serious damage to coastal vegetation. Perhaps, as Tansley suggested, voles and mice were more destructive of woodland and perhaps rabbits were not responsible for 'major changes either in sand-dune or salt-marsh vegetation'. But others were less forgiving. In 1913 Oliver observed that there was 'no end to the havoc they are capable of working' on dunes. Indeed, Davies thought that recent increases in the rabbit population had caused some dunes to break up. As Southern pointed out, 'the tale of the rabbit's mis-deeds is endless.'[47]

Little was written about rabbits having a beneficial effect on the environment, but certain annual plants that depended 'for their very existence upon constant and regular disturbance of the soil' flourished on heathland because the rabbit performed 'his ancient *rôle* of agriculturalist'.[48] As Farrow observed:

on Caversham Heath and elsewhere the rabbits very severely injure the grass-heath and keep it nibbled down very closely to the surface of the soil, and yet they enormously benefit it, since if it were not for the rabbits the grass-heath would not exist at all, but would become replaced by heather. The grass-heath owes its very existence to an extremely injurious influence which nevertheless greatly benefits it because it injures its com-petitor slightly more.[49]

Tansley noted that:

The crisp springy turf which covers much of the downs, and is so delightful to walk upon, owes its character to rabbit-nibbling, not where they are in enormous numbers that cause the devastation described, but where they are still fairly numerous. Under sheep-grazing alone, and in the complete absence of rabbits, down pasture supports a deeper herbage and the turf loses its resilience.[50]

On land not used for grazing:

a case can be made for temporarily preserving at any rate some of them [rabbits], in areas which are to be kept as pasture; this is particularly true if there is a local menace from upright brome, tor grass or the scrub which, if seed is available, invades pasture when it is left ungrazed or seriously undergrazed. Rabbits do keep these invaders at bay ... and they are more easily moved than scrub or tor grass.[51]

However, as Smith has noted, 'it is a very small step from attractive, close-cropped, simulated sheepwalk to the absolute destruction of the turf which is the mark of intensively populated rabbit territory.'[52]

Any judgement about whether rabbits exert an adverse or bene-ficial influence upon flora and the landscape depends in part on a subjective assessment about what is 'good' and what is 'bad' within a semi-natural or cultivated environment. Humans often dislike rabbit behaviour, especially their feeding and burrowing habits, for economic reasons (damaged plantations, lost and spoiled crops, competition for grazing with livestock, land rendered susceptible to erosion or inun-dation). But where income and assets are not threatened, subtler judgements, such as an aesthetic preference for one form of vege-tation or landscape over another, come into play. These preferences are subject to fashion. Many admire grassy chalk downland for its comparative rareness, open vistas and springy turf. But such land is not intrinsically 'better' or more beautiful than terrain covered with shrubs or trees. Most ecologists and naturalists stress the importance of environmental diversity whereby a rich mix of vegetation provides a variety of habitats capable of supporting a wide range of animal life from invertebrates to mammals. This may explain why, in 1944, a

British Ecological Society committee on nature conservation and nature reserves considered the wild rabbit a serious pest but also observed that 'most naturalists would be sorry to see rabbits disappear completely' and that 'there is a case for allowing the continued existence of a moderate rabbit population in some areas.'[53] The trouble with rabbits is that they do not restrict themselves to what humans consider reasonable numbers in selected areas.

As for the relationship between rabbits and fauna, since rabbits were 'in many parts of England ... one of the most important factors controlling the nature and direction of ecological succession in plant communities ... it is obvious that they have indirectly a very important influence upon other animals also'.[54] Hares, deer and voles competed with rabbits for grazing and could therefore suffer if rabbits were too numerous. Other animals benefited from their presence. For example, wheatears nested in rabbit holes; stone curlews, lapwings and sand lizards favoured either the short grass or bare ground created by rabbit grazing; large blue butterflies depended on short turf where thyme, a plant rabbits avoided, and a certain species of ant thrived; the larvae of the minotaur beetle fed on rabbit faeces.[55] Many animals eat rabbits. If, as is sometimes suggested, foxes and stoats relied on them for a substantial proportion of their diets (about 55 per cent in the case of foxes), a crash in the population could threaten predator numbers.[56] It also could force them to seek alternative food sources, either wild or domesticated. One *Field* contributor wondered

> from a game-preserving angle, what would vermin live on in a rabbit-less countryside? I suppose they are the main diet of buzzards, weasels, stoats, foxes and semi-wild cats. I see the probability of all these creatures turning their hungry looks towards the game. Another asked: 'if you rid a countryside of rabbits ... where will the fox go for his lunch, if not to our pheasants, partridges and hen runs?[57]

In the decades before Bough Beech when farmers and others deemed rabbit control vital, the potential consequences of a depleted rabbit population on flora and fauna was seldom discussed in print.

This virtual silence probably reflected an assumption that no such collapse was likely. In 1948, however, Max Nicholson, in arguing the case for 'the elimination of the rabbit over most agricultural and forest areas and its drastic reduction or, if possible, extermination in other areas', did reflect on the possible consequences for the natural environment. He acknowledged that there was 'always some risk in interfering with nature' and also that 'the rabbit is one of the biggest influences at work on the landscape at the present time.' But ecologists, including Tansley, had given

> no biological reason why the most practicable reduction of the numbers of rabbits should not be undertaken. Certain predators such as foxes, stoats and weasels, which live partly on rabbits, would possibly do increased damage in other directions during the process of adjustment, but this should not prove a serious offset.[58]

In other words, environmental considerations provided no valid reason for maintaining the wild rabbit. Plans for rabbit extermination proceeded although, as we have seen, little or nothing was achieved until myxomatosis struck.

Once myxomatosis had arrived, its implications for the balance of nature were recognized as a legitimate area of enquiry, if not concern.[59] Nicholson, by now director-general of the NC, was 'extremely interested' because 'it seems likely that if myxomatosis spreads it may become one of the biggest ecological events in Britain for some centuries.'[60] In consequence he pressed, unsuccessfully, for the appointment of a senior conservancy scientist to the MAC.[61] Notwithstanding Nicholson's appraisal, the MAC was unsure whether to take any account of ecological considerations. In November 1953 it remitted the question to its newly-established scientific subcommittee. The subcommittee judged that the possible impact of MIRD on the nation's flora and fauna was insufficiently important to influence any decisions.[62]

Although policy makers apparently regarded ecology as a peripheral issue, the NC was asked to explore 'the effect of extermination on the natural balance of fauna and flora'. A conservancy scientist, Dr

Norman Moore, drew up a tentative programme.[63] By coincidence, in October 1953 the NC had awarded Ronald Lockley a grant of £2000 over a two-year period to investigate 'the fundamental ecological populations and life history problems of the rabbit'. This project, which formally commenced on 1 December 1953, originally had nothing to do with myxomatosis, but following the Bough Beech outbreak, the impact of the disease, including on the balance of nature, became an important area of enquiry.[64]

Lockley had been researching rabbits and myxomatosis off and on since the 1930s when he collaborated with Charles Martin, but Charles Elton and Mick Southern of BAP and Charles Diver, first director of the NC, all had reservations about his capacity to undertake a project on rabbit ecology, let alone myxomatosis. Lockley certainly lacked formal qualifications. He was a gifted amateur naturalist and, as such, perhaps not the right person to make a meticulous scientific assessment of the ecological impact of myxomatosis. Ultimately, however, criticism, even from such eminent figures as Elton, Southern and Diver was inconsequential because Lockley had a friend and champion in Nicholson, whose support was probably the key factor in the award of a grant that ran not for two years but, in various guises, for almost six.[65] In the event, this support was well justified. Not only did Lockley prove 'a most reliable guide to the development of [myxomatosis] and its repercussions', his investigations also provided the basis for his classic study, *The Private Life of the Rabbit* (1965), in which the myxomatosis chapter is the longest.[66] This book, in turn, was an important source for the behavioural aspects of Richard Adams's bestselling novel, later a full-length cartoon film, *Watership Down* (1972).[67] Once Lockley had secured his grant even Elton and Southern proved cooperative, urging him in particular to investigate the consequences of rabbit depopulation on predators.[68]

Before Lockley began his work, he had certain expectations about the effects of a substantial fall in the wild rabbit population on Britain's flora and fauna. Far from predicting, as Nicholson had, 'one of the biggest ecological events in Britain for some centuries', he anticipated only short-term and limited impacts. He expected 'a very temporary increase' in predators while the supply of dead and dying rabbits was abundant. Then, as rabbits became scarce, he believed predators would rely more on the other creatures (hares, rats, mice and voles) that supplied a proportion of their diet anyway. Increased predation of these animals would check their tendency to increase as vegetation flourished in the rabbit's absence. Human culling of predators ought, therefore, to be avoided. If foxes attacked lambs, which sometimes they did even when rabbits were abundant, farmers should deal with them as the problem arose because foxes were 'easy to control'. Otherwise, stoats, which depended heavily on rabbits, might decrease while weasels, more dependent on small rodents, might increase with the disappearance of rabbits. The other main beneficiary might be hares, as competition for grazing was reduced. But Lockley cautioned that since fatal diseases seldom eliminated species, it was more likely that the myxomatosis virus would lose its virulence, the rabbit population would recover and 'the herbivorous fauna lately adjusted to rabbit-free (and rabbit-parasite-free) grazing' would suffer 'deleterious effects.'[69] Much of this proved remarkably prescient and underlines Lockley's standing, notwithstanding the jibes of professional ecologists, as an outstanding amateur naturalist.

Lockley's first report on the 'effects of myxomatosis on other species', in March 1955, noted that hares in France were 'healthy and thriving', despite a few isolated deaths from myxomatosis. Indeed, owing to the disappearance both of the rabbit as a food competitor and of rabbit-proof fences restricting their range, hare numbers appeared to be increasing. It was too soon to ascertain whether similar developments were occurring in England and Wales, though some reports were suggestive. Neither was it possible to determine the impact of myxomatosis on rabbit predators. In areas of west Wales, where rabbits and buzzards had been common, buzzards had 'glutted on dead and dying rabbits' throughout the summer and autumn. They also had assisted the government's mopping-up campaign by hunting rabbits, including perhaps some resistant individuals, more assiduously. But there was no evidence that the birds had begun leaving areas where rabbits had become rare. Lockley expressed scepticism

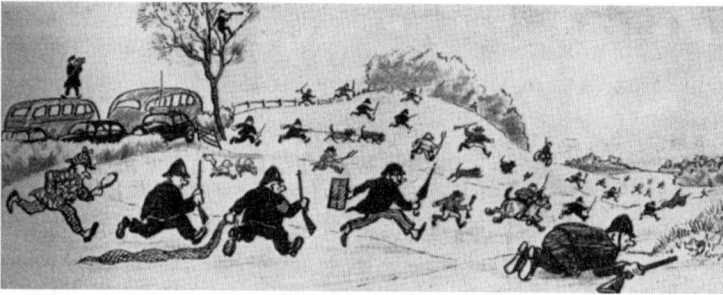

11. A rabbit has been seen in the district.

that starving ravens and foxes, denied the rabbits on which they normally fed, would soon be attacking ewes and lambs.[70]

Lockley paid some attention to the impact of rabbit depopulation on flora. The landscape might revert to its pre-Norman condition in which trees and shrubs were more abundant. Again, however, he thought it too soon to reach conclusions. In some locations the summer and autumn of 1954 had seen the growth of 'a tall thick sward' of grasses and other plants.

Winter weather had flattened this growth into 'a tough tussocky surface, the preliminary stages of change towards bush and woodland'. In existing woodland seedling trees and saplings had grown strongly. Reduced grazing by rabbits appeared to be a factor, but the wet weather of 1954 had been conducive to the growth of lush vegetation so the actual cause was unclear. The following year would reveal much. Unless farm stock grazed the heaths, downs and commons hitherto heavily populated by rabbits, the land could be expected to 'become thick with coarse grasses and plants of a woody nature'. In the longer term though, unless surviving rabbits were wiped out in the government's mopping-up campaign, population recovery might be dramatic in conditions of abundant food supply.[71]

In subsequent reports and elsewhere Lockley continued to suggest, apparently on the basis of personal observation or unattributed sources, that hares were becoming more numerous. Since they had 'hardly had time to multiply naturally to any unusual extent in the absence of their grazing competitor, the rabbit', he attributed their increased presence in areas where they were once scarce to the removal of rabbit proof fences on many farms and estates. As far as other animals were concerned, he found it difficult to determine any measurable impact, notwithstanding statements in the press and elsewhere to the contrary. No hard evidence was available, but rats were possibly scarcer; partly because of increased predation by foxes, buzzards, owls and other raptors in the absence of rabbits; and partly because of loss of underground cover as empty rabbit warrens silted up. Stoat numbers also might have declined. Foxes were preying more on poultry and, perhaps, on lambs and roe deer fawns, 'but not on any formidable scale'. Overall:

It is remarkable … how small the visible effects seem to be. Foxes are reliably reported to be taking more game than usual. Buzzards have had a less successful breeding season. There is no reliable statistical information available on the effects upon badgers, stoats and weasels, but stoats are said to be killing grey squirrels.

The effect on flora appeared 'more marked'. An end to over-grazing and soil erosion was bringing about the 'successful regeneration of palatable grasses, plants and trees, and the reduction of weeds and unpalatable species' to the benefit of both wild and domestic grazing animals. On ungrazed heaths spectacular change was evident. Skomer, previously a 'smooth-grazed lawn', had become a 'tussocky hayfield'.[72]

Lockley's post-1956 reports to the NC supplied little information about the relationship between rabbits (or the lack of them) and flora and fauna but in 1959, at the end of his project, Lockley concluded that the rabbit's 'four-footed enemies' had, 'contrary to expectation', become more numerous since myxomatosis first struck. Foxes, he thought, 'especially in the west country and Wales, have almost doubled their numbers'; stoats and weasels had also flourished. As a result, equilibrium between predator and prey was restored. These changes, however, he attributed less to myxomatosis or even to fluctu-ating rabbit numbers than to the abolition of the gin trap, which, until prohibited in 1958, had destroyed so many small carnivores.[73] Lockley made similar points in *The Private Life of the Rabbit*. As in centuries past, high numbers of predators were keeping rabbit and rat numbers low except where gamekeepers intervened. Lockley anticipated that this state of affairs would continue even if myxomatosis died out or persisted only in a non-lethal form. Rabbits were 'never likely again to become a general widespread plague'. Instead, something 'approaching a healthy equilibrium' between rabbits, less common than in the pre-myxomatosis past, and their natural predators had emerged.[74] What were the views of other naturalists and ecologists?

The fullest overview was written by two Cambridge biologists, Sumption and Flowerdew, in the mid-1980s. Their report, based on over 160 published sources covering the period up to 1983, comprehensively summarized the complex, multi-dimensional and 'dramatic' ecological effects of MIRD over a period of 30 years. These effects were far-ranging enough to include not only a shortage of food for many predators, but even the modification of bird nest construction caused by the unavailability of rabbit fur.[75] Subsequent appraisals, for example by Thompson and by Fenner and Fantini, have added little.[76] Except where alternative citations are provided, much of what follows on this issue is derived from Sumption and Flowerdew's paper.

Most observers agreed that MIRD produced short-term increases in the height, coverage and variety of grasses and other plants. It also allowed more flowering and seeding, thereby facilitating plant succession. Results were often striking. Cowslips, rockroses and other plants bloomed spectacularly on downland and elsewhere; *Pulsatilla vulgaris* (pasque flower), usually comparatively rare, transformed some areas into 'a sheet of purple'. Rare orchids also flourished locally. In Breckland many of the rabbit's 'favourite plants, such as the catchfly *Silene otites* and the curious fern *Botrychium lunaria*, which had survived for centuries in a bitten-down state, suddenly flourished'.[77] Another effect was woodland regeneration. Ash and oak saplings appeared where they were previously rare and woody plants such as ling and gorse spread on open ground. Less welcome was the blooming of toxic ragwort in unprecedented profusion in the summer of 1955. In some locations the extent of change was such that heath and downland began to revert to thicket. *Country Life* expressed fears that the chalk lion at Whipsnade was being lost to grass and weeds in the rabbit's absence.[78]

Longer-term consequences were often less clear. In general, however, the rich plant variety evident in the mid-1950s was soon lost as a small number of coarse grasses and woody shrubs became dominant. Sumption and Flowerdew listed 23 plants that had become less common since myxomatosis. One, ragwort, became comparatively scarce after a short period of abundance because an absence of rabbits meant loss of the bare ground necessary for reseeding. While this change was welcome, as were the long-term and 'widely spread … general benefits to woodland', other vegetational change was often regarded as degradation. For example, long coarse grass crowded out herbs; woody plants and scrub colonized chalk land, acidifying the soil and causing the permanent loss of some much admired and comparatively rare terrain. Rackham observed that the 'disappearance of rabbits has had disastrous consequences for the kinds of grassland and heath which they used to maintain'. It was, for example, a critical factor in destroying the last vestiges of Mousehold Heath in and around Norwich.[79] Accordingly, NC staff responsible for preserving heath or chalk downland welcomed the return of rabbits because their grazing prevented the spread of trees and coarse grasses.[80]

Fewer rabbits had an indirect but 'profound influence on animal life' from the meanest disease organism or parasite to the largest predator. The early profusion of flowering plants allowed bees to flourish even in the cool damp summer of 1956.[81] The longer grass probably led to a substantial increase of invertebrates, markedly assisting certain species, including snails and wood lice, along with Lulworth Skipper and Marbled White butterflies. Other butterflies suffered loss of habitat. It was argued that the longer grass produced by reduced grazing cut the numbers of Adonis Blue butterflies and, by causing a decline in the ant species that reared its caterpillars, led or contributed to the extinction of the Large Blue.[82]

Sand lizards lost breeding sites as bare areas of soil created by rabbits were grassed over. Rat numbers also may have declined, partly through loss of habitat and increased predation.[83] Mice and voles benefited from increased cover and food availability, even to the point of attaining 'plague' levels in the mid-1950s. One consequence was damage to forest nurseries, not unlike that inflicted by rabbits. Certain birds, including lapwings, stone curlews, wheatears, woodlarks, peregrine falcons and possibly the chough suffered decreases in their numbers through overgrowth of habitat. Others, such as skylarks, linnets, yellowhammers and meadow pipits may have benefited.

As far as predators were concerned, most studies of fox behaviour in the aftermath of myxomatosis demonstrated the animal's adaptability and catholicity of taste. In the absence of rabbits they turned to voles, rats, miscellaneous invertebrates, vegetable matter and even frog spawn. They also may have become more common as scavengers in towns and cities. Although more hunting effort may have been required than when rabbits were abundant, fox numbers did not decline over the longer term. Indeed, in the period to 1970 the population appears to have risen – partly, perhaps, because of the prohibition on trapping, though other factors such as more cover and a larger vole population may have contributed as well. Fears that hungry foxes would wreak havoc on poultry, lambs and game were largely unrealized. Such attacks had always occurred in some measure and, except 'in some localized areas', there was little evidence of much increase after myxomatosis.[84]

Rabbits comprised up to 80 per cent of the diet of stoats before the coming of myxomatosis. The stoat therefore was more threatened than any other predator by the loss of its staple prey. Although naturalists found that they changed their feeding habits, for example, by hunting squirrels in trees, the vermin books of large estates pointed to the animal's virtual disappearance. Only when the rabbit population began to grow substantially did stoat numbers follow them upwards. In contrast, weasels flourished until about 1970 because, much less dependent on rabbits than the stoat, they benefited from the prevalence of small rodents in the post-MIRD countryside. Thereafter, as things gradually returned to normal, weasel numbers declined.[85]

In common with stoats, buzzards depended heavily on rabbits for food. Moore found that 'myxomatosis had had a significant indirect effect' on reproduction. Whereas 1954 had been a good breeding season, with the result that buzzard numbers were thought to have reached a level unknown since the early nineteenth century, 1955 saw little successful breeding in areas cleared of rabbits. Although 1956 proved a better season, the buzzard population was in many areas much lower than in 1954. Tubbs subsequently took issue with some of Moore's findings. He thought Moore's suggestion of 20,000–30,000 buzzards prior to the myxomatosis outbreak was overstated by as much as 30 per cent. He also disputed the extent of post-myxomatosis buzzard decline, though he accepted that dramatic decline took place and that numbers had still not recovered by the 1970s. While food shortage was partly responsible, another factor may have changed human attitudes towards the buzzard; and this could also be linked to MIRD. Fearful that 'predators would become a great nuisance' in the rabbit-free countryside, 'nearly all farmers' embarked on a campaign of destruction. Poultry rearers and shooting men killed buzzards in large numbers. Directly or indirectly, therefore, myxomatosis 'caused a great reduction in breeding activities and a decline in the population of the buzzard'. It has been suggested that of all the predators, the buzzard was 'most severely affected by the loss of rabbits'.[86] In contrast, as Southern showed, tawny owl breeding suffered in the early years of MIRD, but the population apparently recovered speedily.[87]

In the early years of myxomatosis many ecologists and naturalists accepted, or at least suspected, that MIRD was having a significant impact on wildlife and the balance of nature. For example, Southern observed: 'The total effect [of myxomatosis on the web of British wild life] must be tremendous and far beyond our capacity to measure critically.'

Thompson agreed that the 'indirect effects of myxomatosis, and the reduction in rabbit numbers, upon other animals and upon plants have been considerable'. A few years later Thomas observed that rabbits had a 'great effect' upon vegetation and that myxomatosis was an 'event of major ecological importance'.[88] As we have seen, Lockley was less sure. Furthermore, Thomas's 1963 paper in the *Journal of Ecology* pointed out that returning rabbits were already reversing changes recorded between 1954 and 1957. He warned that 'generalizations based on short visits or even on the field work of others may produce misleading results through overlooking some important factor.' Compared with the influence of large-scale cultivation over a period of 4000 years, the 'increase and decrease of feral rabbits during the last 100 years is a minor incident in that long history of change'.[89] So were the environmental consequences of myxomatosis deep and permanent, slight and transient, good or bad? Was the balance of nature changed?

It is evident that MIRD affected different species of flora and fauna differently. While some prospered, either in the short or longer terms, others suffered, even to the point of eradication. The greatest effect was of course on the rabbit, which experienced a dramatic population crash. Yet the rabbit survived and eventually prospered, not perhaps to the extent that it did before the arrival of myxomatosis but certainly in its millions and even tens of millions. It seems to have done so as 'a tough and unsociable animal which lives on the surface and does not infect its colleagues', and hence as a somewhat different creature from its pre-myxomatosis forebears.[90]

Three decades after the arrival of myxomatosis, Sumption and Flowerdew referred to the 'wide-ranging effects' of myxomatosis on predator and herbivore populations and species that shared the rabbit's habitat. They considered 'reversal of many of the ecological effects of myxomatosis … unlikely'. Durrell also stressed the disease's profound and permanent impact: 'the effects of losing the majority of Britain's rabbits spread far beyond myxomatosis. It changed the balance of nature forever in Britain's countryside.'[91] A year later Moore took a more measured line; he thought 'the indirect effects of myxomatosis on vertebrates appear to have been relatively slight. Those on plants (and hence insects) were probably much greater, but they were masked by the much greater changes due to changes in grassland husbandry and forestry practice which were occurring at the same time.'[92]

As early as 1956 the minister of agriculture was asked for an opinion on the difficult question of whether myxomatosis was a blessing or curse in relation to fox, rat, weasel and buzzard numbers. He replied that buzzard numbers had fallen but since recovered, while 'rats and other small ground vermin' had declined owing to increased consumption by foxes. On balance, he thought 'the present evidence' pointed to myxomatosis as a blessing.[93]

It might be thought that this analysis reflected the understandable priority the minister placed on increased domestic food production in the immediate post-rationing era, as against the fate of a few species of wildlife. However, it seems likely that Amory had been briefed by the director general of the NC, for Nicholson accused rabbits of at least four 'ecological crimes'. These were over-grazing palatable and delicate plants, eroding banks and hillsides, preventing the natural regeneration of woodlands, and encouraging other species to become pests. Although they also had some beneficial effects, these were 'much less plain and undoubtedly far smaller'. Hence, from the ecological, as well as agricultural and forestry standpoints, there were 'quite decisive advantages of being without rabbits'.[94]

A quarter of a century later, in somewhat different circumstances, John Ross of MAF also reflected on whether myxomatosis was a blessing or curse. He concluded that aside from being 'a most unpleasant disease' it had 'caused great changes to our countryside', not all of them negative.[95] The sudden destruction of millions of rabbits undoubtedly changed the 'balance of nature' but as Harry Thompson consistently maintained, this balance is 'always in a state of fluctuation' and always in search of a new equilibrium.[96]

Chapter 9
Attitude and Opinion

Opinions expressed in parliamentary debates, magazine articles, sermons and press correspondence indicate that myxomatosis stirred strong emotions. Some regarded it as an efficient and humane way to deal with an intractable problem; those who spread it were benefactors to farmers, foresters and consumers. Others saw it as a hideous disease that caused unnecessary suffering; those who spread it were brutes akin to Nazi war criminals. Earlier chapters have discussed the attitudes of MPs and interest groups such as the NFU and RSPCA. In this chapter I examine a range of views aired in newspapers and periodicals. First, however, it is well to consider the attitudes of an institution not previously mentioned: the Anglican Church.

While the Church did not set out an official position on myxomatosis, several leading churchmen did express opinions. In the absence of any correction from the Archbishop of Canterbury, it is reasonable to take their observations as representative of the Church of England. In a sermon the Dean of Winchester drew attention to the 'appalling agony' and 'slow death' inflicted by the 'diabolical evil' of myxomatosis. He questioned whether rabbits cost agriculture the much trumpeted £50 million a year, lamented loss of the poor man's food and deplored damage to the balance of nature. His ire was particularly directed at those who engaged in deliberate transmission: 'methods of this kind are acts of sacrilege, of utter impiety, foreign to human decency, pointing not to man's triumph over nature, but to his enslavement by the powers of evil.'[1]

When the Archbishop of York, Cyril Garbett, was asked to state the Christian attitude towards myxomatosis, he responded in his diocesan letter. Although he described his opinions as personal, he believed many shared them. The archbishop accepted that rabbits did much damage to crops and gardens and that their numbers should be 'reduced ... painlessly and quickly as possible'. Also, any diseased rabbit should be humanely destroyed. But deliberate transmission of an agonizing disease was 'un-Christian and inhuman'. Furthermore, the wholesale extermination of rabbits through myxomatosis could have 'unexpected and undesirable results both on other animals and, possibly, on man himself'. The Bishop of Chester and Archdeacon of Chichester expressed similar views.[2] No doubt many parish vicars also voiced their opinions from the pulpit and in other ways. One, Reverend Oliver, vicar of Mayfield, Sussex, preached against the 'filthy disease', sent letters to the press and, in his capacity as chairman of Mayfield parish council, submitted a formal protest to MAF. Interviewed by a reporter from the *Kent and Sussex Courier*, he equated deliberate transmission of myxomatosis with 'germ warfare'.[3] No evidence has been found about the views of other churches.

What about public and media opinion? It is not difficult to find examples of newspaper and reader opinion. *The Times* digital archive allows the swift retrieval of editorials, feature articles and readers' letters. It is scarcely more troublesome to find such items in the *Glasgow Herald*, the one other indexed newspaper of the period. Thereafter the task becomes more difficult. Since most of the press accorded myxomatosis limited coverage, especially in correspondence columns and leading articles, it can be hard to determine either the range of reader opinion or a consistent editorial line. The difficulty is compounded by the tendency of newspaper editorials to express contradictory opinions within a short period for no apparent reason. Only by means of a time-consuming and impractical exercise involving page by page searches of the hundreds of general and specialist newspapers published in the 1950s would it be possible to access the sweep of attitudes to myxomatosis. Even then questions would arise about the selection process whereby certain letters were accepted for publication and others rejected, and the extent to which newspapers reflect the opinions even of their readers, let alone of society at large.

By the 1950s the British public was obtaining news and other information about current affairs not only from newspapers and magazines but also from radio and, to a lesser extent, television. Until September 1955, when independent television funded by advertising revenue first appeared, the BBC monopolized the broadcast media. In radio its monopoly continued much longer. BBC radio and television covered myxomatosis in 'Panorama', on 4 August 1954 and 17 October 1955, 'Farm Fare', 'Any Questions', 'Farming Today', 'On Your Farm', 'Woman's Hour' and a host of other programmes. With one exception, tapes of these transmissions have not survived. Extant film footage from 'Panorama' lacks a soundtrack. The one programme that survives intact, the BBC Home Service broadcast, *War on the Warren*, transmitted in September 1954, includes useful information but gives no hint either of the tenor of public opinion or of the corporation's editorial position on the disease.[4] Indeed, since the end of the war the BBC had adhered to earlier values in seeking to observe the strictest objectivity in its coverage of news and current affairs and never took an editorial position on any public issue.[5] As Reginald Pound wrote in the *Listener* following the first 'Panorama' programme:

> I was all attention when 'Panorama' put the arguments squarely on the screen, posing them with impeccable balance and summing up with judicial calm. Some of the pictures were indeed unpleasant, recruiting posters for a point of view which the programme was at pains to present while at the same time leaving the controversy unresolved.[6]

Hence, the loss of broadcast material, though regrettable, has probably not deprived us of insight into viewer, listener or official BBC opinion.

Britain's initial myxomatosis outbreak occurred in the relatively recent past. Many people still alive can recall the early 1950s. It is arguable, therefore, that attitudes towards myxomatosis are accessible through oral history. Although the present author considered the possibility of exploring public opinion towards the disease in the 1950s by means of structured interviews, the approach was rejected for two reasons. First, it was deemed impractical to locate and sample representative opinion among urban and rural residents in different parts of the country. Second, memory is faulty and, on an issue that affected most people only indirectly, reliable information would probably not be obtained by requesting the recollection of emotions and opinions across more than half a century. The passage of time, along with changed social attitudes towards animals, agriculture, scientific and political authority and the natural environment, will operate as distorting a mirror. Accordingly, in seeking to present and evaluate public opinion towards myxomatosis during the early period of its first occurrence, reliance has been placed on printed sources, which have the merit of capturing viewpoints at the time they were expressed. To sample a reasonable cross-section of opinion, a range of newspapers and periodicals has been consulted. Particular titles have been selected either because of their national prominence, because they carried a significant volume of material about myxomatosis and/or, in the case of periodicals such as *Shooting Times* or *Gamekeeper & Countryside*, because they represented the views of particular interest groups.

Local

A good starting point for establishing the view of a regional newspaper and its readers is *Southern Weekly News*, a long-established Brighton paper that, in the mid-1950s, had ten branch offices across Sussex and one in Tunbridge Wells, Kent.[7] On 30 October 1953, within a few weeks of MAF confirming the existence of myxomatosis at Bough Beech, a feature writer, Skim Coulter, covered the 'rabbit disease outbreak' as a front-page lead. Over the next two years or so Coulter and *SWN* raised the topic on many occasions, including as front-page headline stories and major feature articles on inside pages. Few newspapers accorded the disease any coverage at such an early date; seldom, if ever, did other newspapers accord myxomatosis so much space or prominence over such a lengthy period. *SWN*'s coverage culminated in a reader poll on the question: 'Would You Bring the Rabbit Back to England? ... Now Give Your View.' Readers were invited to return cut-out ballot papers to *SWN*'s editorial offices. Imperfect though the results of the poll may be as a guide to public opinion, they provide a rare guide to mass attitudes towards myxomatosis. Before considering the results of this poll let us explore *SWN*'s handling of the myxomatosis issue between October 1953 and

January 1956 (after which point the subject fell off the newspaper's 'radar').

On 30 October coverage was mainly factual, reviewing developments at Bough Beech over the preceding few weeks. However, the article also referred to the 'ghastly results' of myxomatosis and the 'terrible experience of dying rabbits in the last stages of the disease'. Furthermore, 'while farming interests have been pressing for the use of myxomatosis in this country, it is clear that many people would condemn its introduction on humane grounds, and there would also be a serious threat to the domestic rabbit industry.' *Southern Weekly News*, or at any rate Skim Coulter, evidently did not like myxomatosis.[8] As Coulter's next article made clear, he approved of the government's decision to try to contain the disease, questioned whether an outbreak offered the prospect of anything more than a brief respite from rabbit infestation and feared for the balance of nature.[9]

In June 1954 Coulter reported at length his visit to 'Sussex myxomatosis country' where he encountered 'a silent, deaf and sightless colony'. The experience was 'unbelievably shocking' and would 'have shaken anybody – except, perhaps, scientists seeing in it the fruition of long research'. Now Coulter had ethical as well as practical reasons to oppose the disease.[10] A subsequent news item reported that people walking on the Downs were 'appalled' by the sight of dying rabbits. Mrs Claydon, district officer of the Society of Sussex Downsmen, referred to the 'pathetic sight' of expiring rabbits: 'As for the dead ones it is revolting to go on to the Downs and you can't take a child there at all.'[11] In August an anonymous correspondent from Wimbledon observed that

an incalculable wrong is being practised in allowing so painful and cruel a disease to be thrust upon the unfortunate dumb animals who are incapable of helping themselves. Whoever thought of and contrived myxomatosis must have a background of Satanic cruelty and it is difficult to believe that an English government is responsible for so odious a remedy.

The writer praised the RSPCA for tackling the 'unhappy task' of destroying diseased rabbits and looked forward to the countryside becoming free of 'so disfiguring a blemish'.[12] Sixteen months later, the newspaper launched its poll with a full-page article by James Wentworth Day.

Day's piece, which was mainly about mopping-up, made it clear where his, and presumably *SWN*'s sympathies lay. Myxomatosis was 'the foulest disease since leprosy'; it had destroyed the trade in rabbit products and produced little if any benefit to agriculture:

> The truth is that myxomatosis has done more harm than good. It has knocked cheap meat sideways, half killed the hat trade, stolen 50 per cent of the profits out of the gunmakers' pockets, threatened the cheap fur trade and thereby the working girl, with a rise in prices, and finally, it has upset the balance of nature in a dozen different directions.[13]

A week later *SWN*'s main front-page story concerned the 'strong protest' of the NFU's Pulborough and Petworth branch against Day's 'save the rabbit' article. One member, J. Dallyn, complained about Day's 'falsehoods' and demanded that the branch send a letter of protest. Day, he thought, should stay in Essex and not 'come down poking about in our county' (Sussex). On its inside pages, however, *SWN* revealed that Day's article had elicited 'a host of [favourable] replies from readers'. Many of these correspondents emphasized the cruelty of myxomatosis; others bemoaned the loss of a cheap, plentiful, nutritious and tasty food source. On 3 February 1956 *SWN* announced the results of its poll, again as a front-page lead story. Of 348 votes cast, 339 opposed myxomatosis; only nine, several if not all of whom were farmers, 'considered that the disease was doing the countryside a service'.[14]

At least two other public opinion polls were conducted elsewhere. In 1955 727 people voted in an *Essex Chronicle* poll for the rabbit's continued existence in Essex; only 27 favoured extermination. A 'Save the Rabbit' poll at Felsted School, Essex produced a far closer result with 43 voters in favour of the animal and 38 against. Indeed, members of the school's Young Farmer Club voted 21–16 for the rabbit's destruction.[15] The *Chronicle*, which, like *SWN* accorded its poll result front-page headline prominence, had no doubt that the vote showed

MAF was 'completely out of touch with the wishes of the people in this matter'. This verdict was endorsed by the numerous letters it published over a three-week period; all favoured rabbits and many condemned myxomatosis out of hand.[16] While poll results, readers' letters and other coverage in two regional newspapers provide no definitive guide to public opinion, they may be taken as indicative. It is well to stress, however, that local newspapers were not unanimously opposed to myxomatosis.

In June 1954 the *Louth and North Lincolnshire Advertiser* noted the presence of myxomatosis just south of the Wash and observed that the disease 'read like the answer to a farmer's prayer'. It continued: 'Are we interested in Lincolnshire? Of course we are. If somebody would guarantee to get the rabbit plague going in this county and wanted £100 before he could do it, he could have the money in half an hour.'[17] The appraisals of other local newspapers such as the *Kent and Sussex Courier* and the *West Sussex Gazette* were more balanced. The *WSG* published readers' letters that described myxomatosis as a 'loathsome' and 'sickening' disease that involved wanton cruelty and slow death. As such, it was 'an affront to the Christian conscience'. But such opinions did not deter it from publishing thoughtful editorials that gave due emphasis to contrary positions.[18]

National

What views were expressed in the national press, starting with the most venerable and authoritative title, *The Times*? Though *The Times* published no leading articles on myxomatosis, its letters pages carried much correspondence on the subject. Roger Diplock, a Four Elms resident, was first to express an opinion. He thought MAF's efforts to contain the initial outbreak and protect a serious pest were absurd; even 'Lewis Carroll could hardly have imagined a more fantastic situation'. Sir Ronald Sperling, who had been writing to *The Times* about the depredations of rabbits since the 1930s, took much the same view: 'I see ... that attempts are being made to confine myxomatosis to certain areas where it has appeared. Why, and by whom, seeing that rabbits are our worst wasters of food and that myxomatosis has been tried with marked success in Australia?' Although

Arthur Harford, a farmer and forester from Hampshire, claimed to have mixed feelings about myxomatosis, his letter dealt entirely with the adverse effects of severe rabbit infestation and the difficulties of establishing effective controls. He concluded by asking whether 'the people of this over-populated island can afford the luxury of maintaining a rabbit population which may well equal them in numbers'. This too appears to have been a tacit vote for myxomatosis.

For Colin Baillieu of London, MAF's policy was 'symptomatic of the lack of understanding and singlemindedness in their planning of British farming'. Urban sentimentality should not be allowed to interfere with the rabbit's destruction. John Cherrington, another Hampshire farmer, 'plagued to distraction' by rabbits, appealed for 'a determined attempt to infect the whole rabbit population with myxomatosis'. Though motivated, like other *Times* correspondents, by economic considerations, Cherrington (and others) also defended myxomatosis as the humane option on the grounds that swift rabbit eradication would terminate the ongoing cruelty inflicted by other control methods. A correspondent from Pembrokeshire also took the view that myxomatosis was the only effective way to deal with rabbit infestation. He thought the suffering it caused was 'grossly overestimated. According to my own observations, I would say they suffer considerable discomfort but hardly intense pain.'[19]

Others expressed contrary views. Sylvia Assheton of Clitheroe was 'surprised and horrified' that some *Times* readers favoured the spread of a 'most unpleasant' disease. Even if rabbits were pests there was no 'justification for allowing the spread of a disease which is of a singularly painful and distressing type and far more cruel than any trap'. Brigid Longley, who farmed in Kent with her husband, wondered whether Cherrington had ever seen a rabbit with myxomatosis. Because their farm was overrun by rabbits, 'we thought to introduce the disease from our neighbours' infected animals':

However, before we had time to do so, we witnessed a wretched creature, sightless, nearly hairless, and half its entrails exposed, battering itself against the wall of the house.

As farmers we take an unsentimental view of destroying

animals, but we both felt that we could not be responsible for introducing this terrible disease on to our own land.[20]

It is difficult to generalize about these and other expressions of disgust and approval, beyond the obvious conclusion that readers of *The Times* held strong and conflicting opinions and that their newspaper strove to present a range of views. Some letters emphasized the immorality of myxomatosis, especially its deliberate transmission, regardless of economic considerations; others viewed rabbits as vermin that needed to be eradicated in the interest of food and timber production. While people often agreed about the need for rabbit control there were fundamental differences about acceptable means. Despite the lack of any objective criteria, opinions about the morality of biological control often rested on personal judgements about cruelty. Opponents of myxomatosis regarded the disease as cruel, perhaps crueller than other methods of control; others viewed it as no worse and perhaps more humane than the alternatives. All such evaluations reflected little more than sentiment or 'gut instinct'.

Insofar as *The Times* offered an editorial viewpoint, it did so in the occasional contributions of its agricultural and special correspondents. The first of these articles, published soon after the discovery of myxomatosis at Bough Beech, observed that MAF faced an unenviable task in dealing with the disease. On scientific and humanitarian grounds the writer approved the attempt to control it. At the same time, he noted that the rabbit was a serious pest and that farmers would 'look askance' at the containment exercise.[21] Within a fortnight its agricultural correspondent considered it natural that Britain's hard-pressed farmers should wonder why they were not 'allowed to make use of this weapon against waste which Nature has provided'. On the other hand, he urged farmers who favoured the use of myxomatosis to 'remember that Britain is a much more closely settled country than the sheep belts of Australia.' Furthermore,

Myxomatosis is a horrible disease, as those who visited France last summer know, and there would be a public outcry if our roads were littered with swollen rabbits in their death throes. It is impossible for man to know if this is a more painful death than trapping and gassing. It is certainly a lingering death painful to witness.

The loss of rabbit meat and the prospect of immune strains of rabbit in the future further complicated the issue. 'Lord Carrington's committee', the article concluded, 'has a teasing problem to solve.'[22]

These and other articles, along with the cross-section of opinion represented on its letters pages, indicate that *The Times* took a balanced view of the economic and humanitarian issues raised by the myxomatosis outbreak. In most respects it supported government policy, demurring only on the criminalization of deliberate transmission.

The *Manchester Guardian* published an editorial on myxomatosis in July 1954. It noted that many people were upset by the sight of infected rabbits and acknowledged that death from myxomatosis was unpleasant. At the same time, it cautioned against sentimentality:

> For all its pleasing furriness, the rabbit is no friend of man: it competes with man for food nearly as seriously as the rat, and its habits are appallingly destructive to agricultural land. City dwellers, looking to the countryside for food, must not be too squeamish about the methods used to counter the enemies of food production. Mankind is at war with the rabbit.

For all this, the newspaper drew the line at myxomatosis, for 'even in war all methods are not justified' and 'we recoil at the idea of bacterial warfare'. Paradoxically, the leader went on to support government action to eliminate the rabbit in the interests of humanity and economics, even by deliberate deployment of the disease.[23] Subsequent correspondence, though limited, showed a two to one majority in support of this proposal, with Wentworth Day the sole dissenter.[24]

The popular press took limited interest in myxomatosis. When it did address the issue, coverage ranged from the informative and dispassionate to the inaccurate, one-sided and emotional. Ritchie Calder (1906–82), the *News Chronicle*'s science editor (and chairman of the Association of British Science Writers) addressed 'The Strange Affair of the Vanishing Rabbits ... the Story of a Man-Made Plague' with a light but astute and non-judgemental touch.[25] In contrast, the *Daily Mail* and *Daily Mirror* provide examples of popular journalism at its worst. The *Mail*'s leading article, 'The Right to Life', appeared the day after the MAC published its second report. From first to last the editorial consisted of distortions and fabrications. As we have seen (Chapter 5), the MAC report discussed the possibility that it might be appropriate on humanitarian grounds deliberately to transmit a virulent strain of myxomatosis. Aware that the law would need changing before this could happen, it made no recommendations. The *Mail*, however, was aghast at the prospect of the rabbit becoming 'extinct as the result of an extraordinary proposal from' the MAC for deliberate transmission. It was even more upset that the committee should propose 'something illegal'. The committee's alleged attempt 'to show that infected rabbits are not really in agony' also roused the writer's anger. For the *Mail*, control of a destructive pest was acceptable and, from the farmer's perspective, 'an excellent thing'. But, for one species to 'abolish another, especially by the introduction of a fatal disease. That is a horrible thing. ... All living species, however, repellent we may think them, have a right to survive.'[26] While these were legitimate conclusions, few of the 'facts' supporting them passed muster.

The *Mirror*'s regular columnist, the outspoken 'Cassandra' (William Neil Connor), thought 'rabbits never did anything worse than knock the green stuff for six'. He therefore deplored the fact that man had attacked them with an 'unpronounceable, unspellable, unspeakable [and] revolting plague' that inflicted 'horrible torment'.[27] A staff writer followed up with an 'on-the-spot' report from Cranbrook, Kent, which possessed in melodrama what it lacked in authenticity:

On a dusty road outside this ancient town I met two weeping children. They stood staring at a small frenzied creature beating its wounded head against a gate-post. Then tear-stained and frightened they turned and ran back down the road ... and, while the wind grieved in the high trees, the little creature died beside the gate. It was then I began to sense the horror that myxomatosis is laying across the countryside.[28]

Soon the *Mirror* was reporting people's 'holidays of horror' as they encountered 'sick rabbits ... everywhere' on their summer vacations.[29]

The *People*, which boasted a circulation of 4.5 million, avoided the *Mail*'s inaccuracies but rivalled the *Mirror* for purple prose: 'There is death in the fields and spinneys of Britain – a slow, agonizing death. By tonight it will have claimed thousands more victims.'[30] Another tabloid, the *Daily Dispatch*, gave front-page prominence to a warning from the Animal Health Trust that the myxoma virus could mutate with awful consequences. On the same day a leading article condemned the 'horrible disease' that caused 'a lingering and painful death' and posed a potential threat to other farm animals and even humans. It roundly condemned the farmers who spread it deliberately.[31]

The most popular newspaper of all, the eight-million-circulation *News of the World*, first broached the subject on 1 November 1953 with an article by its agricultural correspondent headed: 'A Homely Little Creature Breaks into the News. Could You Get by Without that Rabbit Pie?' Accompanied by a line drawing of a smiling rabbit, the tone was sympathetic to 'Ole Brer Rabbit' and hostile to myxomatosis: 'For one thing, it's not a pretty fate – the stricken creatures, grossly malformed, leave their buries or woodland seats to wander blindly into the open and die a lingering death.' Yet, for all his journalistic flourish, the writer, who was optimistic that the rabbit would survive, compiled a fair and accurate account of developments in Australia, France and, more recently, Britain.[32] Ralph Wightman, the newspaper's country correspondent, addressed the issue in July 1954. Again, the approach, though opinionated, was balanced and accurate; rabbits did much damage and needed to be controlled but not by a 'ghastly' disease. 'The rabbit is a pest yet only the cold-blooded, perhaps, would wish for it the lingering agonizing death that the disease entails.'[33]

Scotland

The *Glasgow Herald* devoted considerable space to myxomatosis, and not only in its news columns. Months before William Milne introduced the disease to his Kincardineshire farm, the newspaper published a two-part article by a Glasgow University zoology lecturer entitled 'War against rabbits: the story of myxomatosis'.[34] Several months later, though still before the disease reached Scotland, the same author, S. A. Barnett, contributed another lengthy piece on 'myxomatosis and the balance of nature'.[35]

In August 1954, a few weeks after confirmation of Scotland's first outbreak, the *Herald* published its only leading article on myxomatosis. This piece, headed 'Pest and Pestilence', was perhaps the most robust defence of the disease ever to appear in a British newspaper editorial. The writer conceded that myxomatosis was 'disgusting, presumably painful and possibly prolonged', and also that it caused tumours, blindness and paralysis before death. Nevertheless, he dismissed those who protested against it as squeamish sentimentalists, for the common lot of the wild rabbit was starvation, predation and disease, against which its only defence was 'appalling breeding power'. Far from being the delightful creature of literary representation, the rabbit was actually an 'unpleasant pest', scarcely better than the rat. Since its demise would not threaten the balance of nature, which, 'if there is such a thing was effectively destroyed centuries ago', the only valid argument against deliberately spreading the virus was the possibility of mutation, with consequences for humans and other animals. On balance, the government's decision not to spread the disease deliberately was 'curious. ... The epidemic cannot be checked; the sooner it is finished with the better, and the less likelihood of a potentially dangerous virus becoming endemic. ... That myxomatosis is a distasteful ally should not be allowed to blind the country to the dictates of common sense.' The rabbit should be eliminated with all haste.[36]

The *Herald* published comparatively few letters on myxomatosis. Of those published several were from animal protection organizations wishing to outline their opinions.[37] On 24 July Captain Arthur McDougal wrote that the case for myxomatosis had not been stated because it appeared 'hard-hearted'. For him the salient points were that rabbits, most of which died violently either at the hands of man or in the jaws of a predator, were a plague that did 'untold damage'. They had to be controlled and all control methods involved animal suffering; better then to wipe out the animal than to have millions killed annually for ever more. Hence, myxomatosis was, for all its ugliness the most humane option. This opinion elicited some support, but also several responses that stressed that myxomatosis was a uniquely horrible death involving days, perhaps weeks, of prolonged suffering, that the rabbit had not long since helped eke out the meat ration, and that the disease would cause domestic breeders to lose their stock.[38]

The *Scotsman* devoted little space to myxomatosis, though its agricultural correspondent defended Milne who, in bringing myxomatosis to Scotland, was guilty merely of 'jumping the gun', since the disease would have arrived anyway. He also criticized the government for failing to provide proper leadership.[39] The (Aberdeen) *Press & Journal* provided much more coverage. It printed no editorial opinion, but did present a wide range of opinion about both the disease and Milne's behaviour in importing a diseased rabbit from England. It received a 'flood of letters on the myxomatosis controversy', and published a selection of them, including an acrostic poem headed 'The Weasel and the Bunny', which spelt out the phrase 'Myxomatosis is Death'. The *P&J* thought even farmers were divided, yet those it quoted were unanimous in their enthusiasm for the disease. Aside from the director of Aberdeen's Association for the Prevention of Cruelty to Animals, all the objectors quoted were landowners.[40] Letters printed subsequently contained much the same mix of opinion.[41]

Milne and his family took 'much abuse' for introducing myxomatosis. By early August they had received about 70 abusive anonymous letters, all of which 'went into the fire'. They also received newspaper cuttings addressed to 'Mr and Mrs Butcher Milne'. Their farm name plate attracted the attention of a graffiti artist who wrote: 'Diseased farm and farmer. Keep away or else'. Milne claimed that expressions of opposition or malice were outnumbered by letters of support and requests for advice. He also claimed to be unperturbed by his critics:

The criticism I have received from the point of view of inhumanity leaves me unmoved. The majority of those making such criticism have nothing to lose. They are not farmers and are not worried by rabbit damage.

To me and to most farmers rabbits are vermin, just like rats, and nobody has any scruples about how rats are exterminated.[42]

Countryside and Sport

Let us now turn to opinion within the rural community. *Gamekeeper &* *Countryside*, a monthly periodical first published in the 1890s, was quick to notice the appearance in England of 'the *most deadly disease known* to medical or veterinary science' (emphasis in original). Its 'Editorial Note Book' and L. R. James's article, 'This Disease is Dangerous', covered the outbreak in December 1953. Both pieces suggested that infected animals suffered distress, as did the humans who witnessed their suffering. To see 'blind and helpless rabbits crawling about in agony' was a 'pitiful sight'. James concluded:

> The writer does not wish to cause alarm, but apart from the obvious repercussions on sport, there is always the danger that a new strain of the virus may arise that might affect other animals beside the rabbit – with almost unthinkable consequences.
>
> This disease is dangerous, and we must do our utmost to stamp it out.[43]

Five months later, with the imminent prospect of the disease's resurgence following the winter lull, *G&C* hoped for no recurrence, partly because the symptoms of myxomatosis were 'particularly horrible', partly because the disappearance of rabbits would mean lost meat for the pot, lost sport for shooters, fox depredation in farms and gardens, and unpredictable environmental consequences: 'It would be the old story: remove one link in the chain, upset ever so slightly the balance of nature, and "things begin to happen" which had never been expected.'[44]

G&C's line remained consistent over the months and years and few letters from readers questioned its editorial position.[45] Dugald Macintyre of Oban deplored the use of 'germ warfare (which we dread if introduced among ourselves)' against 'innocent creatures, whose only crime is to dare to compete with us for the possession of the green leaf. What if rabbits do sixty-millions worth of damage annually to crops and trees?'[46] A reader from Launceston in Cornwall reported that myxomatosis was 'very bad' in his area; it was:

> a most sickening sight to see the poor creatures in such a state. I

am 86 years' old and I never thought that human beings could be so cruel as to introduce such suffering among innocent animals. We have enough disease in this country without introducing any more and we cannot estimate what damage we have done.[47]

'Gamekeeper' from Northumberland thought there was a case for spreading the disease 'in one big sweep, instead of it lingering here and there for probably years', if this would end it for good and thereby allow the rabbit trade to function again. But 'Gamekeeper' recognized myxomatosis was a 'dreaded disease' and that his opinion might be deemed 'callous'.[48] Another keeper offered a yet more robust defence. He regarded myxomatosis as 'one of the best things that ever happened'; with his boss's approval he had spread the disease all over his shoot and within six weeks was free of an animal that had caused him various difficulties (including complaints from farmers that he was not keeping them under control and the attentions of rabbit poachers). He suffered no additional trouble from foxes, stoats or weasels and was saved the trouble of fencing coverts; meanwhile, both farm crops and woodland benefited. He denied that the disease was as cruel as ferreting; the only disadvantage of myxomatosis being its 'unsightly' effects.[49] But this was the only published letter in *G&C* that expressed such views.

G&C's rival, *Gamekeepers' Gazette*, was the official organ of the Gamekeepers' Association of the United Kingdom. It did not carry leading articles, but its contributors, Dugald Macintyre prominent among them, and correspondents (including Wentworth Day) were overwhelmingly hostile towards the disease. 'WM' was typical: 'I am sure all experienced gamekeepers will be cursing this horrible disease and those who spread it, so will their wives when they are paying the butchers' bill.'[50]

Shooting Times, founded in 1882, was a weekly publication that appealed mainly to those who shot for sport. Of all the newspapers and magazines reviewed in this chapter it covered myxomatosis at the greatest length. It nailed its colours to the mast as early as 17 October 1953 when Leslie James reported on 'most disturbing' reports from France about the introduction of myxomatosis. By this time MAF had already confirmed the existence of the disease at Bough Beech, but

Shooting Times had evidently gone to press before this news broke and James wrote only of the possibility of a British outbreak. Most of his article discussed Australia's experience, both of the rabbit and myxomatosis. Such was the damage wrought by rabbits in Australia that James believed 'the Australian Department of Agriculture was probably justified' in introducing the disease:

> *But* Britain is *not* Australia, and our rabbit problem, severe though it may be in certain limited areas, is not so unbearable as to warrant the introduction of the horrors of biological control. Even the anti-sport fanatics will not condone the introduction of yet another new disease, and all of us will remember that it never pays mankind to take liberties with nature. Who knows whether a future mutation of the myxomatosis virus may not arise that may be as fatal to ourselves as it is to the rabbit ... it is the time for all sportsmen to register in advance their protest at any deliberate attempt to introduce biological control of any sort into this country [emphasis in original].

If food supplies were threatened, economic necessity might overide ethical considerations to the extent that chemical warfare against rabbits was justified: '*But* there *are* limits to the actions that a man is justified to take to protect himself, and the "biological control", even of vermin, is surely outside the limits of humane behaviour and one that arouses the same disgust as germ warfare, or atom bombing'[51] (emphasis in original).

Other *Shooting Times* columnists were also appalled by such a 'loathsome' disease.[52] In May 1954 a regular contributor, 'Tower-Bird', wrote a long article entitled 'A Scandal of Myxomatosis'. In this, the first of his many contributions on the subject, Tower-Bird accepted the need for rabbit control, but not by means of a 'foul, agonizing disease'. Its deliberate transmission 'shows that, at least in some quarters, the Englishman's nature is changing, and very much for the worse'. Come July he was ready 'to tie the body of a diseased rabbit round the neck of any farmer who deliberately introduced myxomatosis to his land, and allow the body to stay there until it fell off'. Other articles in the same vein followed, though he did accept that many farmers, especially younger ones, disapproved of the disease.[53] Some five months after myxomatosis arrived in Britain, Tower-Bird's opinions were unchanged: it was a 'foul, brutal disease' and the minds of those who introduced and spread it were also foul and brutal.[54]

Shooting Times' editorials were equally hostile. One referred to the 'sorry sight' of myxomatosis 'victims crawling about blind and helpless'. Another considered the 'outlook ... in this country is definitely disturbing'. Indeed, for 'shooting men of all kinds and to the gun and cartridge trade as a whole', the prospect of losing 90 per cent of Britain's rabbits was 'nothing less than tragic'. Most telling of all, *Shooting Times'* editor observed that: 'We ... find the whole business [of myxomatosis] utterly revolting, unsportsmanlike and un-British.'[55]

Almost without exception, readers' letters concurred with the sentiments expressed elsewhere in *Shooting Times*.[56] The author and illustrator 'BB' (D. J. Watkins-Pitchford) was one of many who endorsed Tower-Bird's words, not so much for the suffering myxomatosis inflicted on a dumb animal as for 'incalculable' loss to the rough shooter's sport. He blamed farmers and, to a lesser extent, large landowners and idle gamekeepers for the 'frightful tragedy' that had swept the land. The average farmer, he alleged, was concerned only with making money and did not care a 'fig' for the appearance of the countryside; myxomatosis had provided 'an easy way out'.[57] For most, however, the emphasis was on a disgusting disease and the un-English or un-British behaviour of those who spread it.

Not until mid-September 1954, when a Sussex farmer pleaded for more balanced judgements, did any correspondent point out the benefits of rabbit-free farming and the undesirability of excessive rabbit numbers. Even this writer conceded both the 'disgusting nature' of myxomatosis and the 'undesirability of artificial transmission'. He soon found himself roundly chastised for expressing such heresies and few others were prepared to offer any defence of the disease.[58] *Shooting Times*, in its feature articles, editorial comments and readers' letters, was utterly opposed to myxomatosis. Many contributors understood the need to control rabbits, but none thought that biological warfare was justified. Antipathy towards the disease was partly motivated by frustration that shooters lost an important prey, but also by genuine revulsion.[59] There was also concern about virus mutation, with its implications both for the health of humans and other animals and for adverse consequences to the balance of nature.

Field, founded in 1853, was the oldest of the country magazines considered in this chapter.[60] A weekly with high production standards, it sought readers interested in fishing, shooting, riding, hunting and non-field sports. It also covered farming, natural history and rural matters in general, styling itself, 'the country newspaper'. Its splendidly illustrated editorial content, including reports on public school sports plus reviews of luxury motorcars, along with its advertising pages full of high-quality goods, indicate that it targeted an affluent, well-educated audience. A fair proportion of this audience lived in urban areas. Whereas *Shooting Times* had a grudge against senior civil servants who, it thought, had the temerity to meddle in rural matters about which they knew little, *Field* readers probably included many senior-level Whitehall bureaucrats.

Field's first reference to myxomatosis in Britain appeared in an editorial on 11 November 1953. This short note observed that 'doubt exists as to whether myxomatosis would in the long run prove effective or desirable as a means of getting rid of [rabbits] in this country.'[61] Then, on the last day of 1953, C. M. Morrison's 'Diary of a Shoot' recorded the author's 'alarm' at the possible consequences of the disease:

> Ignorance breeds fear, and, perhaps, that is why I find it a little frightening to visualise this country without rabbits. ... A vast number of people would be deprived of sport, and a good many country folk would miss them from their larders. Possibly the dog and ferret will miss them most of all. Then again, from a game-preserving angle, what would vermin live on in a rabbit-less countryside? I suppose they are the main diet of buzzards, weasels, stoats, foxes, and semi-wild cats. I see the probability of all these creatures turning their hungry looks towards the game.[62]

Not until July 1954, by which time the disease had begun to take off, did any columnist offer further reflections. Then J. K. Stanford, who had yet to witness the disease, quoted with approval the views of a relative from Suffolk: 'if anyone wants to see something far more cruel than any gin, or even a pole trap, they can see it here. It's ghastly, and I would never wish even a rabbit a death like that.' Stanford remarked that although rabbits were very abundant in his home county (Wiltshire), 'I have no wish to see the pestilence in this neighbourhood.'[63]

Robert Henriques, in his regular 'Farmers' Ordinary' column, was the first contributor to assess the advantages and disadvantages of myxomatosis when he raised the question of whether farmers, himself included, should 'take advantage of myxomatosis to eliminate' rabbits. He thought complex issues of humanity and expediency were involved:

There is no doubt that the disease is ghastly to suffer and terrible to see. On the other hand, how do we measure suffering? In terms of the total pain inflicted on the whole species of rabbits, which of the two alternative courses is the more compassionate: to seek to eliminate all rabbits in one dreadful scourge, and to pursue relentlessly the few survivors; or to continue for countless generations our ineffective efforts to control them by means which, at their best, involve some degree of cruelty.

Expediency no longer seemed the overwhelming priority it had in the recent past when 'the zeal for higher agriculture output' was paramount. Farmers wished to see the back of rabbits whereas almost every sportsman and 'housewife' favoured their survival. If maximized, farm production came to 'be regarded as undesirable', as Henriques anticipated, 'the conflict between husbandry and sport' would be 'more evenly weighted'.[64]

This was a balanced and perceptive appraisal; if published in *Shooting Times* it would almost certainly have elicited furious reader reaction. *Field*, however, published no letters of criticism. The magazine's editorial position was set out in a leading article in August 1954. This was a measured, intelligent and dispassionate evaluation of the disease, the reactions of public and government and the future of the rabbit. It termed myxomatosis an 'evil' but found it 'difficult to blame a man trying to farm well for adopting this means of eradicating a pest which all too often frustrates his efforts to do so.' On balance, however:

it is equally difficult to view such operations with an entirely easy mind. Any form of major interference with the processes of Nature is apt to produce results that are not only unexpected but frequently unwelcome. Pestilence seldom benefits anybody and caution may yet obviate ultimate regret. Furthermore those who have seen what they were told to expect – the distressing and even alarming spectacle of rabbits suffering from myxomatosis – might well feel doubts as to the wisdom of helping it to spread, as well as to the ethics of deliberately exposing even a recognized pest to the suffering which myxomatosis brings.[65]

From all this it is fair to conclude that *Field*'s editorial position was antipathetic to myxomatosis. As later editorials observed, it was 'perfectly obvious' that myxomatosis was a 'disgusting disease' and 'a very bad thing' that inflicted prolonged stress and a cruel death. Furthermore, it 'would be a sad thing' if the 'loathsome pestilence' were entirely to 'denude the country of rabbits'.[66] Unlike *Shooting Times*, however, *Field* was willing to devote space to the contrary position.

The balance of opinion in readers' letters was against myxomatosis. One reader wrote that he had 'never seen anything so revolting and disgusting as this disease'; anyone who spread it deserved an anthrax injection. Another considered it 'almost incredible that "civilized" human beings have actually helped to spread this dreadful disease. Either they lack all imagination or their minds are as foul and corrupt as the scourge they have inflicted on thousands of helpless creatures.' Much more in a similar vein appeared.[67] But though most letters reviled myxomatosis and its consequences, a number of readers expressed different views. One wrote that 'the scare of this disease is being grossly over-played by those who are not farmers and think only of "dear little bunnies"'. Sir John Craster, who described himself as landowner, farmer, shooter and wild life enthusiast, even described myxomatosis as 'a heaven-sent boon'.[68]

Did views differ in Scotland? *Scottish Field*, a monthly, accorded rather less space to myxomatosis than its London-based counterpart. Its viewpoint is best indicated by a September 1954 editorial stating that the rabbit's ambiguous status (bane of farmers, darling of shooters) made 'any calm and reasoned assessment' of myxomatosis difficult. However, it then proceeded to provide just such an assessment: the disease was cruel, but the gin far crueller. Accordingly, if national opinion supported the rabbit's elimination and myxomatosis provided the means, then the disease would solve a problem. But myxomatosis would not wipe out rabbits. Since it was already present in Britain and was bound to spread regardless of human intervention, the condemnation of those involved in deliberate transmission was pointless:

> The main lesson to be drawn from the situation created by Myxomatosis is that no individual should be allowed to play around with virus disease, or to monkey with animal populations, without official approval, supervision and cooperation. We see what Dr Delille started in Europe. But, if we accept that ruling, we must see at once that we are allowing such playing around in this country every day of the week in the war against so-called vermin. Animal populations are too finely adjusted to be the sport of individuals. Our present methods of fox control are an object lesson in this respect. It seems to us that the time has come for a stated wildlife policy for this country.[69]

The magazine published few letters on myxomatosis. Only one, headed 'Spoiled Holiday', reflected on the morality of the virus:

> I have just returned from holidaying in Speyside, and it was considerably spoiled for us by seeing so many rabbits suffering from myxomatosis. It seems an extremely cruel way of ridding the country of this pest, and I cannot believe that they do not suffer intensely during the days before they die or are killed.[70]

The weekly 'glossy' *Country Life*, with its focus on fine art and stately homes, was more exclusive than either *Field* or *Scottish Field*. It was (and is) perhaps best known for its photographs of débutantes and advertisements for expensive property. It was, however, more than a mere adornment of domestic coffee tables and dentists' waiting rooms, for its contributors were often experts in their fields. H. N.

Southern of BAP was its main contributor on myxomatosis. *Country Life* was quick to pick up on myxomatosis. Major C. S. Jarvis, who wrote the regular feature, 'A Countryman's Notes', covered the French outbreak on 1 October 1953. Four weeks later he returned to the issue, this time in the British context:

> It is to be hoped that we escape a serious visitation, since, although in many parts of the country the rabbit is regarded as a destructive pest, the great majority of countrymen would not wish to see it exterminated altogether because of the dividend it pays as a foodstuff. Also, one gathers from the various accounts of it that myxomatosis is a most horrible disease, which causes intense suffering.[71]

An 'editorial note' endorsed these views, notwithstanding the acknowledged benefits that cheap and efficient rabbit extermination would bring to farming. The loss of rabbit meat, temporary nature of relief (as rabbits acquired immunity), and damage to the fur trade, rabbit breeders and pet keepers were major considerations. But above all 'there is the humanitarian aspect: even the rabbit's worst enemies could hardly wish to let loose a weapon of this nature.'[72] A later editorial reflected on the double-edged environmental impact of myxomatosis. On the one hand, woodland and forest would benefit from increased seed survival and improved natural regeneration; on the other, the rapid spread of scrub and trees would change the landscape and make some beauty spots inaccessible.[73]

Country Life published a number of letters on myxomatosis. These included an appeal from C. W. Hume (UFAW), which appeared in many publications, for people to join mercy squads, and a contribution from Wentworth Day.[74] Day's diatribe against 'pseudo-scientific-minded' farmers who, too lazy to control rabbits by conventional means, wanted a panacea for 'all the ills of nature', elicited an angry response from several readers. Aside from castigating Day for being 'ill-natured', several of them also offered justifications for myxomatosis. For example, a correspondent from Tenterden believed that the swift destruction of almost all wild rabbits would mean a reduction in overall suffering by rendering shooting, trapping, snaring and ferreting unnecessary.[75]

The *Countryman* was a quarterly that covered a wide range of rural topics. It first considered myxomatosis an 'ugly word' for a disease that was uglier still in spring 1954. An editorial comment observed that 'no one with a spark of humanity would knowingly have introduced it.' At the same time the *Countryman* recognized the disease as a wonderful opportunity to get rid of rabbits to the benefit of agriculture. Also, it was unconcerned about ecological consequences, believing that nature was highly resilient. Overall, therefore, the magazine took a relatively relaxed view of a disease that, for all its downside, also offered clear benefits and opportunities.[76]

Farming and Forestry

Farming opinion about myxomatosis is best gathered from *Farmers Weekly, Farmer & Stock-breeder* and, from a Scottish perspective, *Scottish Farmer*. *Farmers Weekly* dated from 1934 and covered all areas of British agriculture from high politics down. It was a paper for professionals and carried a diet of news items about parliamentary debates, ministerial speeches, NFU business, agricultural shows, new equipment and a host of other matters. There were also question and answer pages and regular columns by feature writers, one of whom, A. G. Street, was quite a national celebrity. *Farmers Weekly* also sought to appeal to the farmer's wife, by providing recipes, knitting patterns and so forth, and his children, through dedicated pages. It printed weekly editorials and carried thriving correspondence columns. The paper unfailingly stood up for farming interests, opposing, for example, the creation of the North Yorkshire National Park on the grounds that it would be a barrier to the reclamation of moorland for agricultural purposes.[77]

Before the advent of myxomatosis, *Farmers Weekly* carried occasional pieces about the damage rabbits (not to mention pigeons, rooks and other pests) did to agriculture. In correspondence columns, feature articles and elsewhere, the rabbit was almost always regarded as a pest in need of eradication. News of myxomatosis in France elicited a gleeful editorial response: 'We have often complained of the pests and diseases which reach us, willy-nilly, from across the Channel, but here is an "invisible export" for which I, for one, can hardly wait!'[78] Paradoxically, an item in the 'Editor's Diary' column in October 1953 approved MAF's decision to contain the Edenbridge outbreak: 'it is thoroughly sensible to defer the use of this method of control until the position can be thoroughly investigated.'[79] This cautious editorial approach was also evident subsequently with *Farmers Weekly* quickly accepting not only that myxomatosis was no panacea but an issue that posed humanitarian dilemmas, albeit that the gin trap was held to be crueller.[80]

The subject of myxomatosis seldom appeared in *Farmers Weekly's* opinion columns. There was no leading article on the issue until 1957 and this piece, headed 'Now or Never', dealt mainly with the need to take mopping-up seriously.[81] Only in 1959, when there was 'plenty of evidence that the rabbit [was] coming back', was myxomatosis again discussed with unadulterated approval: 'Providence, in the blessed shape of this wholesale killing disease, once almost cleared the countryside of the rabbit scourge.'[82] *Farmers Weekly* paid considerable attention to myxomatosis, but mainly in news and letters columns and feature articles rather than in its editorials. Its regular columnist, Arthur George Street (1892–1966), was a farmer, businessman, broadcaster and writer, well known for his many books (especially *Farmer's Glory* 1932), newspaper and magazine articles, and appearances on radio programmes such as 'Any Questions' (in one of which he spoke up for myxomatosis).[83] He also contributed in various capacities to Ministry of Information films on wartime agriculture. He is probably 'best remembered' for his weekly contributions to *Farmers Weekly* over a period of 30 years in which he expressed his forthright, common-sense views on a range of farming and countryside issues.[84]

Street did not have a good word for the wild rabbit; in fact, he 'loath[ed] the little beast'. It was 'a noxious, expensive pest' and 'a much bigger menace than the rat'. Street was, consequently, 'tremendously' attracted to 'anything that would exterminate it'. Scarcely better than the rabbit were the bunny-loving sentimentalists of Britain who stood in the way of extermination.[85] Though initially cautious about the introduction of a highly infectious disease that could wipe out domestic rabbit stocks and create other difficulties, Street was much impressed by the reported gains in Australian agricultural production once myxomatosis had struck. Before long he cast caution aside and called upon MAF to help 'British agriculture to spread myxomatosis throughout the country'. When he heard that the disease had been discovered near his farm in Wiltshire, he 'rejoiced'. Subsequently, he ran through further emotions, fuming at Wentworth Day's defence of the rabbit and ultimately rueing the animal's comeback.[86]

If Street were *Farmers Weekly*'s standard bearer for anti-rabbit and pro-myxomatosis opinion, as he was, the newspaper's letters pages provided the main forum for an exchange of views. The process began in September 1953 when a Graham Boatfield asked 'if anyone, official or otherwise, has considered "importing" into this country the disease which is apparently exterminating the rabbits of France and other countries. Judging by reports, this method seems both simple and cheap.'[87] Following the disease's arrival several readers, including 'Bewildered' of Pembrokeshire, reacted with amazement to the news that MAF was attempting to prevent its spread.[88] Once this attempt had failed, advocates of deliberate transmission stepped forward: 'No one wants to see animals suffering, and the logical and realistic reaction would be to encourage the spread of the disease all over the country.'[89]

In the opinion of a Kent correspondent, such action need not be eschewed on grounds of inhumanity for he thought rabbits suffered less than some people thought: 'in my opinion, if the affected rabbits were capable of feeling they would surely make more attempt to get away … instead of sitting in a state of coma.' He thought the ghastly appearance of infected rabbits gave the false impression that the creatures were in pain; in reality, the 'pain' was felt by their distressed observers. The gin trap was far more painful.[90] A medical doctor from Cornwall defended farmers against accusations that they were 'callous and inhuman brutes, fiends, devils incarnate, bracketed with the originators of the Nazi concentration camps and other extravagant and wholly unjustifiable epithets'. He reminded readers that: 'Diseases are caused by bacteria and viruses, which, after all, were created by the Almighty, and all man has done in this case is to encourage their spread.'[91] As for opposition to myxomatosis and those who spread it, the correspondence pages of *Farmers Weekly* were largely silent. Only one issue carried such letters and one of these came from the chief secretary of the RSPCA.[92]

On one occasion a reader congratulated *Farmers Weekly* for being virtually the only British newspaper to take an unsentimental approach towards the rabbit and myxomatosis.[93] Certainly, the pages of *Farmer & Stock-breeder*, Britain's other main farming weekly, carried much less material supportive of the disease. Though its news columns covered the progress of the British outbreak at length, comparatively few readers' letters either praised myxomatosis or berated the 'bleeding hearts' who deplored its presence. In contrast, those who reviled it, including Wentworth Day and C. W. Hume, were accorded considerable space in which to express their views.[94] No leading articles or contributions by regular columnists made the case for the disease as Street did in *Farmers Weekly*. To be sure, in October 1953 *Farmer & Stock-breeder*'s weekly commentator, 'Blythe', wondered: 'Why so much fuss in official circles because myxomatosis … has made its appearance here?' Like many others, he could see no good reason why MAF wished to prevent its spread.[95] Although Hume was quick to disagree, a Ripon reader was equally bemused.[96] But thereafter debate about the ethics and practicalities of myxomatosis did not develop as it did elsewhere.

One other farming weekly merits consideration: the Glasgow-based *Scottish Farmer*. As noted above, the Scottish NFU, in its evidence to the MAC, was the one organization that favoured deliberate transmission of myxomatosis. Did *Scottish Farmer* take a similar view? In fact, it took little interest in the subject while the disease was confined to England. Not until late July 1954, following the Kincardineshire outbreak did its 'Current Topics' column raise the issue of whether it was crueller to have introduced the disease deliberately or to have awaited the inevitable natural outbreak. In addition, the writer expressed regret that rabbit infestation should have been allowed to become so bad that a farmer was forced to take the step of spreading a virus. In other words, there was no suggestion that Milne or anyone else had behaved badly in bringing myxomatosis to Scotland.[97]

A week later *Scottish Farmer* published its first letters on the issue. Aside from airing UFAW's standard line, as represented in a letter from Hume, it published Arthur McDougal's four point defence of deliberate transmission. It was, McDougal concluded, 'reasonable to say that on the long view it is more humane to spread the disease to the benefit of farming, forestry, food production and of the untold millions of rabbits that will never be born to suffer the eternal persecution they get now.'[98] Some correspondents took issue with this analysis. 'Ex-Shepherd' foresaw such large-scale fox depredation of lambs and sheep following the disappearance of rabbits that 'farmers will require to sleep by their sheep'. 'AJW' of Kilmarnock attributed large-scale rabbit infestation to a lack of traditional control methods. As for myxomatosis, 'such a despicable and uncivilized method of exterminating any pest is to be despised and completely thrust aside.'[99] So *Scottish Farmer*'s correspondence columns display a mix of opinion.

The journal's first leading article on the subject appeared in March 1955. Mainly concerned with the question of mopping-up, it portrayed the rabbit as an unmitigated pest that inflicted great damage on British agriculture and forestry. By implication, myxomatosis was a good thing because it provided an opportunity to eliminate the animal. Also by implication, it was no crueller than control methods already in use.[100] Yet, when a later editorial revisited the issue, *Scottish Farmer* reached rather different conclusions. Questions were raised, for example, about the failure of some farmers to tackle rabbit infestation in an effective way before the arrival of the epizootic. It also questioned the desirability of the disease. One concern was the impact on Scottish tourism of vast numbers of dead and dying rabbits throughout the countryside; another was the consequences of rabbit depopulation on the diet of the poor, the millinery business and the incomes of impoverished farmers. The writer pointed out that while traps, snares and gas involved cruelty, use of such controls was a matter for individual consciences. In contrast, myxomatosis could be 'thrust upon those who strongly disapprove of its use'. Above all, the editorial was concerned that the deliberate introduction of a devastating disease constituted a huge gamble for no good purpose if a race of resistant rabbits should result. 'For, of course, we are far from being able at this stage to assess the outcome of the disease or even its potential dangers.' It regarded interference with the balance of nature as a 'risky business'. Increased fox raids on poultry and other farm stock might be one consequence, but what if animals other than the occasional hare proved susceptible to the disease? In short: 'Have we leaped before we really looked and is not more research on the disease overdue?'[101] In sum, the columns of *Scottish Farmer* presented a somewhat ambivalent view of myxomatosis and lend some support to the notion that farmers initially approved of myxomatosis but later, as they came to see the consequences, were less sure.[102]

The *Quarterly Journal of Forestry*, published by the Royal Forestry Society, had been championing strict rabbit control for years before the arrival of myxomatosis.[103] In early 1953 its 'Notes' section discussed with enthusiasm the prospect of 'a new weapon against the rabbit'; viral 'assault' offered 'the best possible answer' to trappers, felt manufacturers and farmers who had an economic interest in protecting rabbits. The authorities were urged to launch 'large-scale tests'. The piece carried no suggestion that biological control might be unethical.[104] An editorial note observed that the ministry's attempt to contain the initial outbreak, though 'rather puzzling' at first sight, was justified. So too was the appointment of the MAC, provided a report was produced swiftly. It recognized myxomatosis as a 'horrible disease' that caused great suffering and a 'lingering death', but also wondered whether myxomatosis was crueller than other means of killing rabbits apart from being more apparent to the public. More than anything the *QJF* welcomed the disease for providing a 'unique opportunity of ridding this country of one of its greatest pests'. Aware that myxomatosis would not achieve this outcome by itself, it also championed mopping-up operations.[105]

Veterinary
Veterinary opinion about myxomatosis is best gauged from the pages of the *British Veterinary Journal* and *Veterinary Record*. Although the *BVJ* mainly published scientific papers, including a report by Shanks et al. on their experiments with myxomatosis in the Hebrides, a 1954 editorial set out its considered view about myxomatosis a year or so after the disease reached the UK.[106] This editorial recognized the deep disquiet the disease had caused among the animal-loving British public. But compassion, though laudable, could warp judgements:

The present [myxomatosis] epidemic has given rise to many such cases. The lurid accounts of the terminal stages of the disease have been the cause of great sorrow and anxiety in spite of the fact that the period of suffering is relatively short, that a few hours before death the animals are eating and gambolling as usual, and what animal eats and plays if he be in pain, and also that the sensation and apprehension in the apparent rather ghastly end are soothed and dulled by a gradually increasing coma.

Although rabbits were attractive, gentle and, in reasonable numbers, desirable to have around, they needed to be controlled when their numbers got out of hand. All controls involved some cruelty and it 'is debatable and even doubtful if myxomatosis occasions more pain and suffering than some of the alternative methods'. In any case, rabbit suffering should not be judged by human standards and the *BVJ* thought 'this simple fact may bring some degree of comfort to those whose hearts are sorely troubled.'[107]

The *Veterinary Record*, founded in 1888, was published by the British Veterinary Association. It was therefore the organ of the professional body in the same way that the *British Medical Journal* was and is the organ of the British Medical Association. Like the *BMJ* the *Record* published research reports, readers' letters, book reviews, news items and obituaries. Unlike the *BMJ*, it did not publish leading articles. So, while it covered myxomatosis with some regularity and carried papers by the likes of Bull, Ratcliffe, Ritchie, Thompson and Lockley, it did not adopt an editorial stance. Also, the topic was not raised in correspondence until, in 1955, F. B. Edwards, a vet practising in mid-Wales, wrote to bemoan the spread of the disease:

The tragedy of myxomatosis has swept through this country during the dismal summer and now the lonely hills are lonelier for the lack of the cheerful, scurrying forms of the rabbits. We must look back with shame at the times when we begrudged these fellow beings their quota of food. Did they really do so much harm that a Government edict of total extermination had to be promulgated? Surely such an inhuman decree is wrong, and all our instincts prompt us to resist its application at all times.

Before closing with a quotation from Robbie Burns, he blamed recent cases of black tongue in farm dogs on the disease.[108]

These comments elicited several responses, including one from Alastair Worden, who later co-authored a book, *The Rabbit*, with Harry Thompson. Worden rejected Edwards's views about black tongue and commended his humanitarianism:

> but as one who has had the privilege of undertaking research both on the effects of gin-trapping and, to a limited extent, on the transference of myxomatosis, I find it difficult to escape the conclusion that considerably more pain and suffering are caused to the rabbits themselves by trapping than by the disease. If willingness to eat and to mate are any criterion of freedom from suffering, then many rabbits must be relatively unaffected in this respect until the late stages of myxomatosis. The suffering caused by the gin trap; however, is unquestionable.

At the same time, Worden emphasized the serious damage rabbits did to agriculture and the likelihood that the balance of nature would cope with fluctuating rabbit numbers.[109] R. H. Smythe agreed that the rabbit's long-term survival was assured, for 'the rabbit is no ecologic nitwit'.[110]

Conclusion

What scope is there to generalize about public and media opinion? Tentative judgements can be offered, albeit with the reservation that evidence can be found to contradict them all. There was widespread agreement in the early 1950s that rabbits were too numerous and that culling was required in the interests of food production during a period of austerity. However, widespread acceptance of the need for controls did not necessarily mean a willingness to contemplate extermination, especially by biological means. Self interest led most farmers to regard rabbits as vermin. They needed to be killed and any effective method was acceptable. Consequently, many farmers welcomed myxomatosis and regarded its deliberate transmission as either a good thing or, at least, not the callous activity that many suggested. The chairman of the NFU's Cornwall branch went so far as to describe myxomatosis as 'a beautiful disease. ... There are no disadvantages, it is something worth having. We have had it and should be very grateful.'[111] Shooters, on the other hand, liked rabbits for their sporting and culinary qualities and equated them not with 'vermin' but with pheasants, partridges and hares, that is as noble prey undeserving of death by disease.

For the non-farming, non-hunting public who formed the mass of the population, attitudes were determined more by a mix of moral and emotional than by economic considerations, though loss of a source of cheap meat was a concern. The morality of extermination was one issue but more important was the belief that myxomatosis was cruel.[112] Public attitudes towards myxomatosis as a disease so loathsome that there could be no justification for visiting it on one of God's creatures no doubt reflected 'a lot of very pleasant sentimentality'.[113] Probably they also indicated a deeper distrust of science and government created by recent history and the international climate of the time. Nazi genocide and the experiments of Nazi doctors were recent memories in the early 1950s and references to such horrors often occurred in newspaper discussion of myxomatosis. Similarly, public concern about the cold war, atomic weapons and germ warfare also figured in public debate. As Sheila Wheble wrote to the *Illustrated London News*, 'isn't modern life hideous enough without inflicting this ghastly suffering on defenceless creatures?'[114] For some, perceptions of national identity and self worth were important; biological warfare against a sentient mammal was repeatedly described as un-English (or British) and un-Christian. Farmers who spread myxomatosis were engaging in 'a form of beastliness altogether foreign to the ideas of any decent Britisher'.[115]

It is likely that public opinion was also influenced by the portrayal of rabbits in popular fiction and film.[116] As the Scott Henderson committee observed in 1951: 'Until about 1850 ... few books had been published which had animals as their central characters, but since then, and especially since the end of the 1914–18 war, such books have been written and published in ever increasing numbers.'[117] Rabbits have featured in children's literature at least since 1865 when Alice followed Lewis Carroll's White Rabbit down the burrow that led to Wonderland. Indeed, the online encyclopaedia, *Wikipedia* lists as many as 66 fictional rabbits. Neither does this list include the White Rabbit, Thumper (who appeared in Walt Disney's 1942 film and Felix Salten's 1923 book, *Bambi*), or the eponymous anti-hero of Aardman Aniation's 2005 film, *Wallace and Gromit and the Curse of the Were-Rabbit*.[118] Some of those on the list, including Carroll's March Hare, are actually not rabbits at all. Others, such as the Duracell/Energizer pink bunnies are less fictional characters, more advertising icons. But for all the list's shortcomings, 66 is an impressive number, beaten by cats and dogs alone.

A good many fictional rabbits, especially in cartoons and film, postdate the early 1950s. *Watership Down*, for example, was first published in 1972. Roger Rabbit, who featured first in a novel, then in the partially animated Hollywood film, *Who Framed Roger Rabbit?* dates from the 1980s. Nevertheless, when myxomatosis reached Britain in 1953 most people would have been familiar with at least some fictional rabbits. Thumper and the White Rabbit aside, characters such as Brer Rabbit (in books and Disney's 1946 film *Song of the South*), Beatrix Potter's Peter Rabbit (and his extended family); A. A. Milne's Rabbit (friend of Winnie the Pooh) and Bugs Bunny were all well established in the public consciousness in the early 1950s. All of these rabbits possess human characteristics and are portrayed in a flattering light. Several may be rogues, but they are decidedly lovable rogues whose misdeeds, as they toy with such witless adversaries as Elmer Fudd, Mr McGregor and Brer Fox, are endearing rather than appalling. The White Rabbit and Rabbit, far from being scallywags, are vulnerable neurotics, and no less sympathetic for that. It is not surprising that a public reared on such fare reacted with disgust to a viral disease that disfigured and killed such lovable creatures. Who could view with equanimity the prospect of Potter's Flopsy Bunnies riddled with myxomatosis?[119] Not Philip Larkin apparently who, for all his misanthropic reputation, wrote a sensitive poem about the disease in 1955:

'Myxomatosis'
Caught in the centre of a soundless field
While hot inexplicable hours go by
What trap is this? Where were its teeth concealed?
You seem to ask.
I make a sharp reply,
Then clean my stick. I'm glad I can't explain
Just in what jaws you were to suppurate:
You may have thought things would come right again
If you could only keep quite still and wait.

(italics in original)

Did public and newspaper opinion influence political decision making? It is clear that government departments and agencies monitored the press and received unsolicited correspondence from representatives of concerned organizations and members of the public.[120] It is difficult to believe that public clamour had no influence on MAF, the MAC and politicians. On the one hand the ministry acted upon requests 'to do what they could by educational means to correct the Flopsy, Mopsy, and Cottontail attitude', by producing educational booklets.[121] On the other, public opinion played a part in the government's acceptance of the King amendment to the 1954 Pests Bill.

Robert Henriques ridiculed the 'absurdity [of] those gay inspired little books where creatures, dressed in human clothes and living in human habitations, suffer the same feelings, and act from the same motives, as human beings'. But he had no doubt that their influence and that of 'their offspring such as Walt Disney films – persists into adult legislation'. No politician, he maintained, would dare even to consider making a case for myxomatosis.[122] While this was not entirely true; some politicians, at least in the House of Lords, did express favourable views about the disease; Lord Carrington has confirmed to the author that official perceptions of public sentiment did influence the MAC's deliberations and recommendations.

Chapter 10

Conclusion

In this chapter I discuss some general issues relating to myxomatosis in Britain. I consider whether the epizootic marked a turning point in attitudes towards the natural environment and animal cruelty. I also compare and contrast the first myxomatosis epizootic of the mid-1950s with animal disease crises of recent decades: foot and mouth disease (FMD), bovine spongiform encephalopathy (BSE) and the H5N1 strain of avian influenza (AI).

Environment
In 1987 Norman Moore, a retired NC officer, wrote that 1954 marked 'the beginning of the present conservation era, in which conservation was seen to be a matter both of site protection and of the general protection of the environment from disease and pollution', because of the arrival in Britain of the myxoma virus and 'the first recognition that pesticides could affect wildlife significantly'.[1] He went on to argue that myxomatosis 'made many biologists even more aware of the potential danger of introducing non-native species to this country' and 'forced conservationists to take a wider view of their profession'. He detected little evidence that the epizootic altered public attitudes:

> when, a few years later, biological control was extolled as a sub-
> stitute for the use of pesticides few people were restrained by
> their experience of myxomatosis. The public's main concern
> was for the rabbit and for themselves. They were outraged by
> the horrible appearance of the disease, and worried that cir-
> cumstances might arise in which they could be poisoned by
> eating diseased rabbits or in which they could get the disease.[2]

Are Moore's claims justified?

The origins of environmentalism and conservation have attracted considerable scholarly attention. Many authors have shown that concern about degradation of the natural environment has a history that long predates the 1950s. David Evans stated in 1992 that the 'nature conservation movement as we know it in Britain today is 100 years old'.[3] Philip Lowe goes back still further when he identifies 1830 as the beginning of the first of four overlapping stages of nature conservation in Britain.[4] They are:

1. Natural history and humanitarian period, 1830–90.
2. Preservationist period, 1870–1940.
3. Scientific period, 1910–70.
4. Popular/political period, 1960–present.[5]

Brian Clapp argues that Thomas Malthus (1766–1834) 'has some claims to be regarded as the first conscious and celebrated conservationist'.[6] Keith Thomas takes an even longer view, drawing numerous examples of changing attitudes towards the natural world from the sixteenth and seventeenth centuries.[7]

Moore claimed, however, to identify a development involving something other than a generalized concern about nature and wildlife. He detected the beginning of a new era in which specialists became concerned about site protection, pollution and disease control. But even in this restricted sense Moore's claim is dubious. Measures to address river and air pollution can be traced over several centuries; similarly, concern about links between bad air (miasma) and disease, and attempts to clean up the natural environment in the interests of health, have a pedigree at least as long.[8] Furthermore, in Lowe's analysis the 1950s barely feature.

Insofar as environmentalism flourished in the second half of the twentieth century, the 1960s, 1970s and later years were more important than the 1950s. Sheail cites a host of international and domestic developments during the 1960s and early 1970s, including Adlai Stevenson's speeches at the United Nations in 1965, Harold Wilson's address to the Labour Party conference four years later and the Stockholm conference on the human environment in 1972.[9] In Britain the destruction of the oil tanker *Torrey Canyon*, which hit a reef between the Scilly Isles and Land's End in 1967 and leaked 31 million gallons of crude oil, is often regarded as a critical incident. Rachel Carson's book, *Silent Spring*, published in Britain in 1963, and Dennis Meadows's *Limits to Growth* (1972) were influential texts, along with the government's White Paper, *The Protection of the Environment, The Fight against Pollution* (1970) and the *Ecologist*'s 'Blueprint for Survival' (1972). Innovative political developments include the appointment of a standing Royal Commission on Environmental Pollution in 1969, the declaration of European Conservation Year in 1970 and the formation of Britain's Green Party in 1973.

Moore alone identifies the 1950s as a pivotal decade. More often, and not without reason, the 1950s are cast as years of inertia.[10] Some legislation was enacted, but with little significant environmental impact. For example, the 'Great Smog' of 1952 resulted in the passage of the Clean Air Act, 1956, though with a noteworthy lack of governmental enthusiasm. The measure was far from radical and anyway was more concerned with protecting the health of human city dwellers than preserving the natural environment.[11] Concern about human health was also behind the Agriculture (Poisonous Substances) Act, 1952. This act notwithstanding, the 1950s was something of a golden age for the agricultural use of chemicals. Both aldrin and dieldrin were widely used to control fungal and insect pests; officialdom usually shrugged off the simultaneous rise in deaths among small birds as a price worth paying for elevated farm production.[12] As Moore notes, 'in the 1950s studies on the side effects of pesticides were largely incidental and anecdotal, and the need for international cooperation between the scientists concerned was hardly recognized.'[13] Only in the mid-1960s was use of aldrin and dieldrin restricted.[14] Even so, Burchardt argues that in Britain it was not until 'the 1980s that concern about the total impact of modern farming practices on the countryside became widespread'.[15]

Moore's claim that myxomatosis heightened biologists' awareness of risks associated with the introduction of non-native species to the UK is also unconvincing. First, the rabbit was so well established in mid-twentieth century Britain that it could hardly be regarded as non-native. When, in 2005, the Royal Geographical Society debated the issue of invasive plants and animals, rabbits went unmentioned. An audience voted that the zebra mussel was the worst offender, causing more damage than the American mink, *rhododendrum ponticum*, Reeves's muntjac deer, ruddy duck, grey squirrel, signal crayfish, Oxford ragwort, Spanish bluebell, harlequin ladybird and Australasian flatworm. Neither were rabbits judged beneficial imports (as the roe deer and pheasant were); they were apparently viewed either as benign or an integral part of the country's ecological furniture.[16] Second, it was not decimation through disease that raised questions about the presence of the species but the vast expansion of rabbit numbers before myxomatosis arrived. It was the rabbit's virtual elimination, rather than its presence, that posed environmental problems.

Moore's claim that Britain's myxomatosis epizootic of the mid-1950s changed the outlook of conservationists and biologists is also questionable. Insofar as attitudes changed, it was more at a popular level than in the 'corridors of power'. Public and newspaper debate about the disease focused on greedy and idle farmers, meddling scientists and the demise of traditional British values. In contrast, official literature, especially the MAC reports, was technocratic. It was not the expert who was sounding the alarm but the person in the street.

James Wentworth Day's views about myxomatosis probably coincided with mass public opinion. As we have seen, Day took much interest in myxomatosis, publishing numerous letters and articles in newspapers and magazines, as well as devoting lengthy sections of his 1957 book, *Poison on the Land* to the issue. Among other things, he was the moving force behind the *Southern Weekly News* poll on the rabbit in 1956. It was Day, rather than any bureaucrat or politician, who warned that: 'Wild life in Britain today is at the crossroads. Birds, animals, fish, insects, wild flowers and even trees are menaced by the mechanization of farming, the increasing use of dangerous crop sprays and other poisons, and the appalling pollution of rivers and streams.' He went on to berate 'the man who "flogs" his land with chemicals, [and] denies it natural living'.[17] The extent of Day's influence is debatable but the important point here is that he was a popular author, not a professional biologist or conservationist.

Cruelty

Concerns about cruelty loomed large during the early years of myxomatosis. Unlike Australia, no government department or agency in Britain deployed the virus. Consequently, except for those who believed that the disease was developed by government scientists and spread by bureaucrats, the cruelty question really centred on the issue of deliberate transmission. Although C. W. Hume of UFAW said myxomatosis was 'a cruel death' regardless of how it was transmitted, the Country Landowners' Association rightly drew a distinction between 'deliberate cruelty arising out of human machinations' and suffering due to natural causes:

> It is appreciated that public opinion may well deprecate the effects of myxomatosis, but insofar as these arise from a natural source such opinion cannot affect the issue. It is only in regard to the question of taking positive measures to stimulate the spread of the disease that consideration need be given.[18]

In other words, while there is suffering in nature, there can be no cruelty without human intervention.

Even when deliberately spread, can myxomatosis legitimately be regarded as cruel – as it regularly was by members of the public? Dictionary definitions of the word 'cruelty' emphasize intent to inflict suffering, lack of compassion and indifference to or delight in the pain and misery of other people or animals. Cruelty can be mental or physical.[19] In the early 1950s English and Scottish law defined animal cruelty as the infliction of 'unnecessary suffering'. The legislation then in force, however, mainly applied to domestic animals. As the Scott Henderson Committee pointed out in 1951, wild animals 'in their wild state ... have no legal protection at all'.[20] Myxomatosis cannot therefore be regarded as cruel in strictly legal terms, even if it did impose severe and unnecessary pain and suffering.

The moral position is more complex. Opinion varied over whether and to what extent myxomatosis inflicted pain, distress, misery or suffering, all words that tended to be used interchangeably and rather loosely in contemporary debate. Lord Carrington informed the House of Lords that the disease caused 'acute suffering'; Lockley wrote that it was 'decidedly painful'.[21] However, A. S. Thomas of the NC, referred to French evidence indicating that little suffering was involved since rabbits continued to feed until they died.[22] At least two members of the MAC, Lord Dundee and R. B. Verney, were greatly impressed by such evidence. Their colleagues, Lord Merthyr and Harold Collison were prepared to support deliberate transmission of myxomatosis if infected rabbits did not suffer. The MAC concluded that it was impossible 'to assess the extent of pain felt by animals'. The committee also agreed, however, that myxomatosis was unsightly and that infected rabbits were 'clearly distressed'. As a result, the committee doubted whether the 'general public could be convinced that the disease was not painful to the rabbit'. In the absence of consensus about the extent to which myxomatosis caused suffering, public perception was a prime consideration.[23]

This brings us back to the 'fluffy bunny' issue. Shortly before the onset of myxomatosis the Scott Henderson Committee referred to the 'marked tendency in recent years for public concern about animals to be based more on sentiment than on … real understanding'. Much of this sentimentality focused on deer, foxes and rabbits. In contrast, rats were regarded with revulsion: 'Yet the rat is an intelligent and highly sensitive creature and probably suffers far more than some of the animals which attract a great deal of sentimental interest.' Although both rats and rabbits were serious pests, the committee received many representations about cruelty to rabbits but 'practically no evidence' about cruelty to rats.[24]

During the myxomatosis epizootic some observers drew attention to the different attitudes towards rabbits and other pests. As Lord Rennell enquired: 'If it is not humane to kill rabbits by a disease, is it not equally inhumane to kill rats with phosphorus?'[25] Presumably the rat's links with human disease made it fair game for attack by any means, humane or not. But what of 'the simple, delicate, pale green, translucent greenfly [a] lovely member of God's community of creatures, whose only crime is that it preys upon … roses?' In this case status on the evolutionary scale was a consideration.[26] Rabbits were widely viewed as sentient, sporting and cuddly creatures with culinary merit. They therefore won sympathy that rats, greenfly and some other creatures were denied.

The first MAC report, eschews the word 'pain' and makes no reference to cruelty, but describes myxoma rabbits as 'unsightly' and 'plainly in distress'. The committee opposed deliberate transmission partly because of 'clear and obvious objections on humanitarian grounds to infecting an animal deliberately with an unpleasant disease in order to reduce its numbers'.[27] A committee member later wrote that humanitarianism was a 'major reason' behind the official decision to reject and deprecate deliberate transmission:

> Infected rabbits are a revolting aspect; their eyelids are so swollen that their eyes are closed; their faces, the bases of their ears and often their genitalia are swollen. When they are ill they come into the open and sit about, breathing slowly and often with difficulty, for several days before they die. Letters to newspapers reporting that they are 'in agony' and attempting suicide need not be literally believed; nevertheless there is a very powerful and vocal humanitarian argument against spreading the infection in order to obtain economic rewards.[28]

Notwithstanding its humanitarian concerns about myxomatosis, the MAC welcomed the demise of the rabbit and recommended that those not killed by the disease should be eliminated by other means. Thereafter, extermination became government policy. Even the RSPCA and UFAW approved.[29] Yet, a decision to exterminate rabbits necessitated choices about killing methods, which, in turn, involved judgements about cruelty, cost, effectiveness and public safety. Environmental and agricultural considerations, however, were not relevant to any debate about the *means* of extermination. Neither, since all killing methods were utilized for economic reasons, was Andrewes's reference to the unacceptability of deploying a biological control in the interests of financial gain pertinent. Morally, killing animals for pleasure by hunting or, in the case of rabbits, shooting, was more dubious than their destruction in the interests of higher food production.

Only if myxomatosis were crueller than other killing methods could it legitimately be regarded as unacceptable on humanitarian grounds. A senior RSPCA inspector referred to the 'intense agony and misery' inflicted by myxomatosis over a prolonged period.[30] But all other control methods were also subject to criticism and objection from one quarter or another. The Scott Henderson Committee regarded gin traps as 'diabolical'; it also stated that shooting and snaring could inflict 'a great deal of suffering'. Ferreting, which anyway was not a practicable control method on a large scale, also involved suffering. The committee enthused about cyanide gas but Wentworth Day was in no doubt that this was extremely cruel.[31] In humanitarian terms the only clear distinction between myxomatosis and other ways of killing rabbits *en masse* was the length of time between infection and death, and this difference hardly mattered if rabbits suffered little during the killing period. Otherwise it was the unpleasant appearance of myxomatosis, the ingrained sympathy for the rabbit on the part of those who suffered no direct loss from its depredations and the infected animal's tendency to die in vast numbers on open ground accessible to the public that marked the disease as different. Alternative controls were less efficient and often did their work underground or on private land removed from the public gaze.

No alternative method could compete with myxomatosis in terms of cost, effectiveness and safety. Not only did the most virulent form of the disease kill 99 per cent of all rabbits afflicted, it did so at virtually no cost to the public purse and without posing any direct threat to humans or other animals (aside from a few hares). The main hazard to human health came from millions of dead and decaying rabbits that provided a breeding ground for flies, especially during the summers of 1954 and 1955. In the early 1950s, when infectious diseases remained a matter of public concern and postwar poliomyelitis epidemics were fresh in the mind, public health hazards could not be overlooked. But the potential public health threat of myxomatosis, though sometimes raised in the press, was not a serious concern for bureaucrats once it was established, as it was before the disease reached Britain, that the virus was highly specific.[32]

Those who engaged in the deliberate transmission of myxomatosis were probably not motivated by a desire to inflict suffering. They may have lacked compassion but they merely accelerated a natural process and it is hard to avoid the conclusion that myxomatosis was widely regarded as cruel less because of the length of time between infection and death, more because it was novel. As such it was reviled in the same way that poison gas was during the First World War, notwithstanding that death or disablement by high explosive is, objectively, no less appalling than death or disablement by chemical inhalation.[33]

As we have seen, members of the public often condemned those who engaged in deliberate transmission. The Pests Act, 1954 made deliberate transmission illegal on humanitarian grounds. Accordingly, questions arise whether myxomatosis generated new attitudes towards animal suffering and ushered in a new era of concern about the mistreatment and exploitation of animals.

It is not easy to chart fluctuation in the level of public interest about animal welfare but Robert Garner argues that the creation of animal protection organizations provides a useful guide to the strength of concern about animals. He identifies 35 'major groups' with a national focus, significant concern for the protection of animals and 'either a large membership or considerable wealth or a high public profile'. Unfortunately, he fails to define the terms 'major', 'large', 'considerable' and 'high'. But leaving this point on one side, his 35 organizations range chronologically from the RSPCA, founded in 1824, to SHAC (Stop Huntingdon Animal Cruelty), dating from 1999. Eight of these bodies were established in the nineteenth century, eight in the period 1902–44 and eighteen between 1961 and 1999. Only one, the Captive Animals Protection Society (1957) dates from the years 1945–60.[34]

Membership of bodies concerned with animal protection appears also to have boomed in the final four decades of the twentieth century. The emergence of local animal protection groups, often with radical agendas, was another feature of these years. From 1961 support for animal protection and animal rights surged. In contrast, the decade and a half following the Second World War, whether gauged by the creation of new organizations, growth in membership or radicalism, were years of quiescence.[35] For a variety of reasons, therefore, it is hard to see myxomatosis, which received maximum publicity in

1954–55, as a significant factor in stimulating concern about animal cruelty.

Insofar as cruelty to wild animals was of concern in the 1950s, this concern predated the advent of myxomatosis. In 1949, following the presentation of parliamentary bills on hunting and hare coursing, the Home Office appointed a committee to investigate cruelty to wild animals. Chaired by John Scott Henderson, who later served on the MAC, it enquired into cruelty to British wild mammals, whether at large or in captivity, and included extensive discussion of rabbits. It focused on the pursuit or capture of animals for sport or food and on other methods of control or destruction; rabbits loomed large in its report.[36]

Comparisons and Contrasts

Britain's myxomatosis outbreak of the mid-1950s can be viewed as an animal disease crisis. It prompted parliamentary questions and debates, the appointment of an official committee of inquiry, interventions at the highest level of government, legislation, mass concern among the general public and special interest groups, extensive coverage on BBC radio and television, reams of newsprint in the national, regional and specialist press, and a nationwide campaign to exterminate a mammalian species. Most fundamentally, of course, it resulted in the deaths of tens of millions of sentient animals that, at least in some quarters, were well loved.

Myxomatosis was neither the first nor last animal disease crisis in the United Kingdom. Before and since the 1950s there have been serious outbreaks or concerns about foot and mouth disease (FMD) cattle plague, anthrax, fowl pest, BSE, H5N1 avian influenza (AI) and other diseases. In terms of animals killed, myxomatosis dwarfs any other epizootic. Britain's FMD outbreak of 2000–1 resulted in the deaths of more than ten million farm animals (perhaps one-ninth of the number of rabbits killed by myxomatosis in the mid-1950s), but most of them were healthy cattle slaughtered in an effort to prevent disease transmission. The more serious FMD epizootics (in terms of number of outbreaks) of 1923–24 and 1967–68 produced much lower death tolls in the region of 300,000 and 442,000 respectively.[37]

Following its discovery at the end of 1986 the number of bovine spongiform encephalopathy (BSE) cases grew rapidly over the next few years. A statistical peak was attained in 1992 when more than 36,000 cases were diagnosed. Numbers have since declined steadily.[38]

Aside from the number of animals affected, the most fundamental difference between myxomatosis and the other three animal diseases considered here concerns their negative impact on human interests. FMD, BSE and H5N1 AI, all affect animals reared for the food market and have exerted, or at least threatened, serious economic consequences. Abigail Woods points out that for much of the nineteenth century FMD was regarded as little more than a minor inconvenience to farmers and meat traders, as against the major catastrophe it came to be regarded during the twentieth century. She argues that the slaughter policies used to control FMD since the end of the nineteenth century have 'manufactured' a plague from a non-fatal and comparatively mild ailment.[39] These policies, along with those implemented to eradicate BSE, have imposed vast expense on the rural economy and taxpayers. As well as lost markets (the EU ban on the export of British beef remained in place until May 2006) and damaged livelihoods, the consequences have included shattered dreams, broken families and premature deaths, including by suicide.

In February 2007 H5N1 finally reached Britain after several previous false alarms (the dead swan discovered on the east coast of Scotland in April 2006 was transformed from a harbinger of doom to a non-event in a matter of days) when an outbreak was discovered at Bernard Matthews's turkey 'farm' in Holton, Suffolk.[40] Though only a small proportion of the birds was infected, a mass cull of 160,000 was carried out in a matter of days. Local poulterers and bird keepers were required to prevent their stock from coming into contact with wild birds – initially assumed to be the source of the infection. In addition, various steps were introduced to prevent further outbreaks. These included the establishment of *cordon sanitaires*, which imposed restrictions of varying severity on the movement of poultry according to distance from Holton. Many countries, Japan, Russia, South Africa and Norway among them, quickly banned British poultry imports. At the time of writing it is too early to speculate about the possible impact on public consumption of chickens, turkeys and other domestic fowl. It is also too early to determine the impact on either Bernard Matthews, a business that had already suffered an *annus horribilis* in 2006 because of media and public concerns about the dietary qualities of some of its fast-food brands, or on the British poultry industry more generally. Precedent suggests short or medium term difficulties but a return to normality over the longer period.[41]

The main economic impact of myxomatosis was beneficial in that it boosted agriculture yields and forestry, at least in the short to medium terms.[42] Britain's farm animals were economic assets; in the eyes of MAF and most farmers and foresters the country's wild rabbits were pests. Myxomatosis did impose emotional costs. Principally, these involved upset (trauma may be too strong a word) associated with the loss of pets and the sight of millions of distressed, dead and dying rabbits strewn across the countryside. But such costs were modest compared with those associated with FMD and BSE.

FMD, BSE, H5N1 and myxomatosis also vary in terms of feared or actual human susceptibility. FMD is a highly contagious viral disease that affects cloven hoofed animals. It has never been regarded as a serious threat to human health even though people have very occasionally contracted it. Woods does not mention the occurrence of human cases but in 1966 Bob Brewis, a 34-year-old Northumberland salesman who lived on a farm, was confirmed as having the disease. His symptoms were mild and he suffered no long-term ill effects. Public health officials, infectious disease specialists and politicians sought to reassure the public, insisting that FMD carried no significant threat to human health. Even so, for a while there was a media scare that people were at risk.[43]

The issue of human susceptibility to FMD resurfaced in 2001 with reports that Paul Stamper, a Cumbrian contract worker employed by MAF to assist in culling animals, had become only the second person in Britain to contract FMD. Stamper, who was in frequent contact with infected animals, was at some point 'accidentally sprayed with some material from a cow'. A fortnight later he developed mouth ulcers along with sore and itchy hands. A Department of Health official accepted that the worker exhibited 'all the symptoms' of FMD and an official investigation was mounted. Before this had concluded, various experts had dismissed the possibility of a human case of FMD. Angus Nichol, director of the Communicable Disease Surveillance Unit at the Public Health Laboratory Service (PHLS) described FMD as an animal disease caused by a virus that 'doesn't like human beings'. Professor Tony Hart of Liverpool University concurred. A PHLS spokesperson told BBC News Online that the laboratory had been informed of several cases of human FMD since the beginning of the 2000–1 outbreak, none of which were confirmed. Far from it being 'a big public health issue', FMD in humans was 'vanishingly rare'. Within a week 13 people tested by the laboratory for the disease were given the all clear. Although Stamper alleged a government cover-up, there is no reason to doubt that FMD is for all practical purposes an animal disease to which humans are not susceptible.[44]

In the 1990s, when BSE was a major issue for government, media and the public, a prime concern was the possibility of a link between the consumption of infected meat or meat products and the onset of new variant Creutzfeldt-Jakob disease (vCJD). BSE (mad cow disease) affects the brain and central nervous system of adult cattle. It is one of a number of transmissible spongiform encephalopathies (TSEs) or prion diseases caused by an accumulation of prion proteins. It was first observed in 1986 and has been linked with the practice, banned in the UK since 1988, of feeding cattle infected meat and bone meal. CJD has been known as a rare form of dementia affecting older people since the 1920s. In 1996, however, a new strain of the disease (vCJD) began to be seen in younger people. By the end of 2005 153 deaths had been attributed to the disease in the UK. Since the prion protein found in the brains of sufferers was similar to that found in the brains of BSE-infected cattle, a link between the fatal diseases of BSE and vCJD was established: 'the most likely origin of this new disease was human exposure to the BSE agent.'[45]

At the time of writing there are concerns that the H5N1 virus, responsible for the deaths of large numbers of birds, especially in the Far East, and a small number of human beings worldwide (164), could mutate to become a threat to human health on the scale of the 1918 influenza pandemic ('the most devastating plague in history') which affected about one billion people and caused vastly more deaths than the First World War. Although news media repeatedly carry reassurances that the risk to human health is miniscule, these same media also reiterate the possibility that bird flu could affect people to a catastrophic degree. Furthermore, John Oxford, professor of virology at Queen Mary's College, London, is reported to rate the chances of a pandemic as 'high'.[46] In February 2007 Gordon Young, a government veterinarian involved in investigating the H5N1 outbreak in Holton was taken ill and removed to an isolation ward in a Nottingham hospital. Despite having no previous exposure to H5N1 and having been dressed in 'full protective clothing', including breathing apparatus, throughout his time at Bernard Matthews, Young was tested for AI. These tests proved negative.[47]

In the case of myxomatosis, Charles Martin found in the 1930s that the virus was 'highly specific', affecting only the European wild rabbit and its domesticated relatives.[48] Later experience showed that while this conclusion was not entirely true in that hares were occasionally affected, myxomatosis was almost exclusively a disease of the European wild rabbit. In the early 1950s Australian scientists (Frank Fenner, Macfarlane Burnet and Ian Clunies Ross) inoculated themselves, to no ill effect, with myxomatosis virus to reassure their compatriots that the disease posed no threat to humans.[49] Nevertheless, in Britain C. P. Quick, assistant secretary (namely head) of MAF's animal health division, warned that while there was

> no evidence that myxomatosis *in its present form* is communicable or otherwise dangerous to man or, indeed, to any animals other than rabbits and hares. Virus diseases can, and do, change their character in course of time and it would be unwise to assume that a form of myxomatosis may not ultimately appear that would constitute a danger to other animals or possibly to man.[50] (emphasis in original)

Doctors and the government's chief veterinary officer assured the public that people were not at risk, as did the MAC.[51]

No case of myxomatosis in humans has ever occurred. Initially, however, the British press and public were not convinced that the disease could not, or even was not, affecting humans and other animals, including domestic pets. In November 1953, the *Daily Telegraph* reported the case of William Cass, assistant pest officer for Kent, who developed a skin complaint after helping with the Edenbridge outbreak. He was absent from work for several weeks with an inflamed eye and swelling under the chin. He believed he had contracted his ailment from diseased rabbits. However, his doctor diagnosed impetigo, a highly-contagious bacterial skin infection caused by staphylococci or streptococci.[52] In December 1953, under the heading, 'This Disease is Dangerous', L. R. James raised the prospect of a new strain of myxomatosis emerging 'that might affect other animals beside the rabbit – with almost unthinkable consequences'. James did 'not wish to cause alarm' but since he characterized myxomatosis as 'the *most deadly disease known* to medical or veterinary science' (emphasis in original), it is hard to see how his words could do otherwise. Indeed, a later *Gamekeeper & Countryside* editorial noted that 'learned opinion' recognized the propensity of viruses to change 'character in a mysterious fashion, and no one can be quite certain where the thing will end'. This 'sobering thought' had been given 'insufficient publicity'.[53] This was to change, however, when the *Daily Dispatch* ran a front-page article and an editorial informing its readers of a warning from the scientific director of the Animal Health Trust (AHT), W. R. Wooldridge, that myxomatosis could mutate and become a threat to humans.[54]

Wentworth Day picked up the issue and used it to promote his 'save the rabbit' campaign. With Wooldridge as his authority, Day warned that there was 'no guarantee' myxomatosis would not mutate into a form capable of infecting humans and animals other than rabbits: 'I hear, already, of a farm worker who developed severe swellings after handling a dead rabbit and was only cured by penicillin. Is this the first of many cases? Further, what of the risks of pus from dead rabbits being sprayed on corn by combine harvesters?' He went on to refer to a cat that had died 'with all the symptoms of myxomatosis' and to request information from members of the public about the occurrence of the infection in any animals other than rabbits.[55] The implication was that the AHT was seriously concerned about myxomatosis affecting animals other than wild rabbits and the occasional hare.[56] Before long, Wooldridge clarified the trust's position. He accused Day of selective quotation and other distortions that gave 'an import to my quotations far more unusual than is warranted'. Nevertheless, the dermatologist who examined Britain's first alleged case of human myxomatosis judged it possible that 'human cases of myxomatosis will occur, particularly as the virus seems to be unstable.'[57] Suggestions in the press that 'mystery illnesses' among dogs and other animals continued to crop up from time to time but gradually the public panic about human myxomatosis subsided.[58] In all this there are parallels with subsequent scares over FMD, BSE and H5N1.

There are resonances between the myxomatosis outbreak of the 1950s and other animal disease crises of recent years. At least in the public mind BSE was linked with animal exploitation and greed: feeding animal products to herbivores in order to bulk them up for the market. Farmers' deliberate transmission of myxomatosis in order to increase agricultural production was also seen as caused by greed. The 2000–1 FMD outbreak gave rise to concern about a public health hazard associated with the release of carcinogenic dioxins from animal pyres. Indeed, a government minister, Malcolm Meacher, admitted that these pyres did constitute a health risk.[59] In 1954–55 fears centred on the prospect of infected rabbits entering the food chain or polluting public water supplies. In addition, 'flies which had been feeding on the diseased carcasses often went straight to other animals or to food exposed for sale.'[60]

These similarities should not be overstated. The notion that meddling scientists were implicated in the myxomatosis outbreak is little evident in the case of the other diseases. And nobody has suggested that these diseases were deliberately created or spread (though such allegations have been made in relation to HIV/AIDS). For all that, myxomatosis was the almost perfect killing disease; with few exceptions its main consequences for humans were either neutral or beneficial. It did damage the interests of hatters, furriers and trappers, worry some ecologists and upset members of the public. But, overwhelmingly, it killed 'only' wild rabbits, an animal widely viewed as one of the most serious agricultural pests. Had it been otherwise and killed almost all the nation's dogs, cats, horses, cattle or sheep, myxomatosis would have loomed far larger in the national consciousness. Furthermore, if the epizootic had arrived 40 or 50 years later it would surely have roused the anger of animal rights groups and raised much bigger questions about 'germ' warfare and the threat to natural environment. As it was, myxomatosis in 1950s Britain was 'merely' a disease of wild rabbits. As such, it was a catastrophe for the rabbits, though one from which they recovered impressively, but not for humans. To paraphrase Kipling, a rabbit is only a rabbit but a good dog is a pet (and a good cow an economic asset).

Notes

Chapter 1. Before Bough Beech

1. See NA. MAF 131/132. Myxomatosis: outbreak at Edenbridge, undated and unsigned notes; MAF 255/216. Third report of C. P. Quick, 13 October 1953.
2. P. W. Brown et al., 'Rabbits and myxomatosis in the north east of Scotland', *Scottish Agriculture*, 35 (1956) 205; NA MAF 131/113. Paper on experimentally induced outbreaks of myxomatosis – programme of research on Scottish islands; MAF 105/311. Minutes of meetings of Research Group of MAC Scientific Sub-Committee, 22 December 1953 and 12 January 1954; *Press & Journal*, 4 November 1954.
3. F. M. Burnet, *Viruses and Man* (London: Penguin, 1953) 10.
4. H. V. Thompson, 'Myxomatosis for rabbit destruction', *Quarterly Review of the Royal Agricultural Society of England* (1953) 15–16.
5. www.cs.cf.ac.uk/Rabbits/intervet.html; E. Boden (ed.) *Black's Veterinary Dictionary* 20th edn (London: A&C Black, 2001) 350; F. M. Burnet, *Mosquito-Borne Myxomatosis* (Melbourne: CSIRO, 1951); NA MAF 131/115. Research report of MAC Scientific Sub-Committee, December 1953–December 1955.
6. H. Kean, *Animal Rights: Political and Social Change in Britain since 1800* (London: Reaktion Books, 1998) 199.
7. C. J. Martin, 'Observations and experiments with *myxomatosis cuniculi* (Sanarelli) to ascertain the suitability of the virus to control the rabbit population', *Fourth Report of the University of Cambridge Institute* (1934–5) 16–38.
8. P. Ambrosioni, 'Giuseppe Sanarelli', in C. C. Gillispie (ed. in chief) *Dictionary of Scientific Biography* (New York: Charles Scribner's Sons, 1980 edn) vol. 12, 96–7; J. M. Morton (ed.) *Morton's Medical Bibliography* (Aldershot: Scolar, 1991 edn) 403.
9. G. M. Findlay, 'Notes on infectious myxomatosis of rabbits', *British Journal of Experimental Pathology*, 10 (1929) 214–19; Martin, 'Observations and experiments', 17.
10. L. B. Bull and C. G. Dickinson, 'The specificity of the virus of rabbit myxomatosis', *Journal of the Council for Scientific and Industrial Research*, 10 (1937) 291–4; J. F. Kessel et al., 'Occurrence of infectious myxomatosis in southern California', *Proceedings of the Society for Experimental Biology and Medicine* 28 (1930–31) 413–14.
11. T. M. Rivers, 'Infectious myxomatosis of rabbits: observations on the pathological changes induced by virus myxomatosum (Sanarelli)', *Journal of Experimental Medicine*, 51 (1930) 965–76.

12. See J. R. Hobbs, 'Studies on nature of infectious myoma virus of rabbits', *American Journal of Hygiene*, 8 (1928) 800–39; T. M. Rivers, 'Changes observed in epidermal cells covering myxomatous masses induced by virus myxomatosum (Sanarelli)', *Proceedings of the Society for Experimental Biology and Medicine*, 24 (1926–27) 435–7; T. M. Rivers, 'Some general aspects of pathological conditions caused by filterable viruses', *American Journal of Pathology*, 4 (1928) 91–124.

13. Martin, 'Observations and experiments', 18; Rivers, 'Changes observed', 435–7; Rivers, 'Infectious myxomatosis', 966; F. W. Stewart, 'The fundamental pathology of infectious myxomatosis', *American Journal of Cancer*, 15 (1931) 2013–28. Stewart referred to 13 published papers on myxomatosis since Sanarelli's original report 33 years earlier.

14. F. Fenner and B. Fantini, *Biological Control of Vertebrate Pests: The History of Myxomatosis in Australia* (Wallingford: CABI, 1999) 72, 117.

15. E. C. Rolls, *They All Ran Wild* (Sydney: Angus & Robertson, 1969) 6–25; J. Sheail, *Rabbits and their History* (Newton Abbot: David & Charles, 1971) 210–12; *The Times*, 27 August 1936. Sheail questions whether the impact of the rabbit was as extreme as has sometimes been alleged. He speculates that bad husbandry and over-grazing by sheep may have accounted for much of the damage for which the rabbit was a convenient scapegoat.

16. W. E. Abbott, *The Rabbit Pest and the Balance of Nature* (n.p.: Wingen, NSW, 1913) i.

17. D. G. Stead, *The Rabbit Menace in Australia in 1933 and the Way Out* (Sydney: F. E. Moore, 1932) 5.

18. F. Fenner and F. N. Ratcliffe, *Myxomatosis* (Cambridge: Cambridge University Press, 1965) 272; Sheail, *Rabbits and their History*, 178–9.

19. Fenner and Fantini, *Biological Control*, 116–18.

20. Ibid., 118; Rolls, *They All Ran Wild*, 170–1.

21. Fenner and Fantini, *Biological Control*, 119–21; Rolls, *They All Ran Wild*, 171–2.

22. Anon., 'Control of rabbit infestation by the use of a virus', *Nature*, 138 (1936) 396–7; H. Chick, 'Sir Charles James Martin' http://www.oxforddnb.com.; Fenner and Fantini, *Biological Control*, 123.

23. Martin, 'Observations and experiments', 16.

24. Ibid., 20; Findlay, 'Notes on infectious myxomatosis', 215.

25. Martin, 'Observations and experiments', 28–9.

26. Ibid., 32–3.

27. Ibid., 36–7.

28. D. Lush, 'The virus of infectious myxomatosis of rabbits on the chorioallantoic membrane of the developing egg', *Australian Journal of Experimental Biology and Medical Science*, 15 (1937) 131; C. J. Martin, 'Observations on *myxomatosis cuniculi* (Sanarelli) made with a view to the use of the virus in the control of rabbit plague', *Commonwealth of Australia Council for Scientific and Industrial Research, Bulletin no. 96* (Melbourne, 1936) 24; F. C. Minett, 'Diseases of animals: prevention and treatment', *Journal of the Royal Agricultural Society of England*, 98 (1937) 246–72; *The Times*, 27 August and 26 October 1936. The prickly pear, which became a nuisance following its introduction to Australia was successfully controlled by means of a moth (*cactoblastis cactorum*) brought

from South America. See H. V. Thompson, 'Myxomatosis of rabbits', *Agriculture*, 60 (1954) 503–8.

29. Fenner and Fantini, *Biological Control*, 118–19; R. M. Lockley, 'My island and our life there. 19. An experiment in the extermination of rabbits – our boat beaten back', *Countryman* (July 1939) 557–71; R. M. Lockley, 'Some experiments in rabbit control', *Nature*, 145 (1940) 767–9; R. M. Lockley, 'Myxomatosis: a factual survey', *Field*, 9 December 1954, 1174–5; R. M. Lockley, 'The observed effects of myxomatosis on rabbit populations and behaviour and on wild life generally', *La Terre et La Vie. Revue d'Histoire Naturelle*, 3 (4) 1956–57, 211–19, 260–2; R. M. Lockley, *The Island* (London: Andre Deutsch, 1969) Chap. 8; R. M. Lockley, *The Private Life of the Rabbit* (London: Book Club Associates, 1980 edn) 116–17; NA MAF 112/181. Rabbit destruction campaign, paper no. 6, 20 July 1950.

30. *Report of the Select Committee of the House of Lords on Agriculture (Damage by Rabbits) together with the proceedings of the committee and minutes of evidence* (London: HMSO, 1937). Evidence of Sir Ronald Sperling, 70, 72.

31. *La Terre et La Vie. Revue d'Histoire Naturelle*, 3–4 (1956–57) 261.

32. Bull and Dickinson, 'The specificity', 293.

33. Fenner and Fantini, *Biological Control*, 125.

34. Ibid., 126; J. A. Button, 'The insect vector in relation to myxomatosis in Australia', *Journal of Agriculture. West Australia*, 3rd ser. 1 (1952) 819–21, 823, 825, 827–9.

35. Fenner and Fantini, *Biological Control*, 126–8.

36. L. B. Bull and M. W. Mules, 'An investigation of *myxomatosis cuniculi* with special reference to the possible use of the disease to control rabbit populations in Australia', *Journal of the Council for Scientific and Industrial Research*, 17 (1944) 1–15. See also Anon., 'Rabbit control by virus infestation', *Nature*, 144 (1939) 145.

37. Fenner and Fantini, *Biological Control*, 128.

38. F. M Burnet, 'Myxomatosis as a method of biological control against the Australian rabbit', *American Journal of Public Health*, 42 (1952) 1522–6; J. E. Nichols, 'Rabbit control in Australia: problems and possibilities', *Nature*, 168 (1951) 932–4; F. N. Ratcliffe, *The Rabbit Problem: A Survey of Research Needs and Possibilities* (Melbourne: CSIRO, 1951) 1.

39. Fenner and Fantini, *Biological Control*, 132–4; Rolls, *They All Ran Wild*, 176–8.

40. Fenner and Fantini, *Biological Control*, 137; Ratcliffe, *The Rabbit Problem*, 5; Rolls, *They All Ran Wild*, 179–80.

41. Burnet, 'Myxomatosis as a method', 1523; Burnet, *Mosquito-Borne Myxomatosis*.

42. Burnet, 'Myxomatosis as a method', 1524.

43. Fenner and Fantini, *Biological Control*, 137. See Anon., 'Information for the press, for release to morning papers published on Thursday 1 March 1951', Oxford University Zoology (Elton) Library. BAP Reprint Collection.

44. Burnet, 'Myxomatosis as a method', 1524.

45. Fenner and Fantini, *Biological Control*, 143.

46. Ibid., 145; Rolls, *They All Ran Wild*, 179–80, 185; *The Times*, 18 October 1951.

47. Lockley, 'Myxomatosis: a factual survey', 1174–5; Lockley, *Private Life of the*

Rabbit, 118; P. A. Reid, 'Some economic results of myxomatosis', *Quarterly Review of Agricultural Economics*, 6 (1953) 93–4; Rolls, *They All Ran Wild*, 184; *The Times*, 10 February, 16 November 1953.
48. *The Times*, 2, 4, 7, 10 November 1953.
49. F. N. Ratcliffe et al., 'Myxomatosis in Australia: a step towards the biological control of the rabbit', *Nature*, 170 (1952) 9.
50. Bull and Mules, 'An investigation', 15.
51. Fenner and Ratcliffe, *Myxomatosis*, 273.
52. Ratcliffe et al., 'Myxomatosis in Australia', 7–11.
53. K. Myers, 'Studies in the epidemiology of infectious myxomatosis of rabbits II: field experiments, August–November 1950, and the first epizootic of myxomatosis in the riverine plain of south-eastern Australia', *Journal of Hygiene*, 52 (1954) 47.
54. *Report of the Advisory Committee on Myxomatosis* (London: HMSO, 1954) 2.
55. Fenner and Fantini, *Biological Control*, 134, 138.
56. *The Times*, 26 July 1951.
57. Myers, 'Studies in the epidemiology', 47–8.
58. In a personal communication to the author (1 January 2005), Frank Fenner confirmed that Ratcliffe released the virus at Gunbower in May 1950 and later at four sites on either side of the Murray River 'as a final deliberate attempt to introduce the virus into the wild rabbit population'. Professor Fenner expressed regret that he and Fantini had used the word 'escape' in their book.
59. See, for example, *The Times*, 31 January, 26 July, 15 September, 18 October 1951.
60. Fenner and Fantini, *Biological Control*, 212.
61. NA. CAB 124/2884. R. M. Lockley, 'Report on myxomatosis in France: a survey for the Nature Conservancy', undated.
62. NA. MAF 191/145. Rabbit myxomatosis in France. J. W. Evans's Report of inquiry, 22–25 September 1953; Fenner and Fantini, *Biological Control*, 213–14; CAB 124/2884. Lockley, 'Report on myxomatosis in France'.
63. NA. MAF191/145. Evans's report of inquiry; CAB 124/2884. Fenner and Fantini, *Biological Control*, 213; Lockley, 'Report on myxomatosis in France'; *The Times*, 5 November 1953.
64. *The Times*, 5 November 1953.
65. NA. MAF191/145. Evans's report of inquiry; NA. CAB 124/2884. Lockley, 'Report on myxomatosis in France'; MAF 131/37. Reports of the situation in France. Legal proceedings against Dr Armand Delille; Fenner and Fantini, *Biological Control*, 213; *The Times*, 5 November 1953, 27 September 1954, 12 January and 2 December 1955, 26 January and 8 August 1956.
66. Lockley, *Private Life of the Rabbit*, 118.
67. NA. MAF191/145. Evans's report of inquiry; *The Times*, 5 November 1953.
68. NA. MAF191/145. Evans's report of inquiry.
69. H. V. Thompson and A. N. Worden, *The Rabbit* (London: Collins, 1956) 149.
70. *Report of the Advisory Committee on Myxomatosis*, 2; *The Times*, 26 January, 8 April, 28 May, 8 September 1956.

Chapter 2. The War on the Rabbit

1. L. D. Stamp, *Man and the Land* (London: Collins, 1973 edn) 211; H. V. Thompson, 'The rabbit in Britain', in H. V. Thompson and C. King (eds) *The European Rabbit: The History and Biology of a Successful Colonizer* (Oxford: Oxford University Press, 1994) 64–107.

2. G. E. H. Barrett-Hamilton, *A History of British Mammals* (London: Gurney & Jackson, 1913) vol. 2, 184; Lockley, *Private Life of the Rabbit*, 14; *PP* 1950–1 viii (Cmd. 8266) Report of the Committee on Cruelty to Wild Animals, 518; Sheail, *Rabbits and their History*, 9; Stamp, *Man and the Land*, 212; Thompson, 'The rabbit in Britain', 62; Thompson and Worden, *The Rabbit*, viii; E. Veale, 'The rabbit in England', *Agricultural History Review*, 5 (1957) 85–90.

3. See for example J. E. Harting, *The Rabbit* (London: Longmans, Green & Co., 1898) 1.

4. J. Drakeford, *Rabbit Control* (Wykey, Shrewsbury: Swan Hill Press, 2002) 9.

5. E. P. Farrow, 'On the ecology of the vegetation of Breckland. III. General effects of rabbits on the vegetation', *Journal of Ecology*, 5 (1917) 5–6; J. Marchington, *Pugs and Drummers: Ferrets and Rabbits in Britain* (London: Faber & Faber, 1978) 31–40.

6. E. Ayrton, *The Cookery of England* (London: Penguin, 1974) 105; Drakeford, *Rabbit Control*, 9; M. Lorwin, *Dining with William Shakespeare* (New York: Atheneum, 1976) 172; Thompson, 'The rabbit in Britain', 64; Veale, 'The rabbit in England', 89.

7. J. Simpson, *The Wild Rabbit in a New Aspect* (Edinburgh: Blackwood & Sons, 1893) 23.

8. C. Arscott, 'Sentimentality in Victorian paintings', in G. Waterfield (ed.) *Art for the People* (Dulwich: Dulwich Picture Gallery, 1994) 78; Harting, *The Rabbit*, 222–4, 233.

9. N. Fletcher, *500 Sixpenny Recipes* (London: Harrap, 1934) 7.

10. J. Grigson, *English Food* (London: Penguin, 1993 edn) 234.

11. H. Glasse, 'First Catch Your Hare': *The Art of Cookery Made Plain and Easy* (Totnes: Prospect Books, 1995 edn) 7–8, 14; M. McKendry, *The Seven Centuries Cookbook* (New York: McGraw-Hill, 1973) 39, 178.

12. I. Beeton, *Mrs Beeton's Book of Household Management* (London: Ward Lock, 1888 edn) 181, 593, 629–34, 657–8, 665.

13. I. Beeton, *Mrs Beeton's All-About Cookery: With over 2000 Practical Recipes* (London: Ward Lock, 1923) 635.

14. Fletcher, *500 Sixpenny Recipes*, 109–14.

15. I. Beeton, *Mrs Beeton's Book of Household Management: A Complete Cookery Book* (London: Ward Lock, 1950) 144, 177–8 633–4, 1077. See also D. Hartley, *Food in England* (London: Macdonald, 1954); C. Spry and R. Hume, *The Constance Spry Cookery Book* (London: J&M Dent, 1956). Both books include several rabbit dishes.

16. See for example J. Burnett, *Plenty and Want: A Social History of Diet in England, 1815 to the Present Day* (London: Scolar, 1979 edn); J. C. Drummond and A. Wilbraham, *The Englishman's Food: A History of Five Centuries of English Diet*

(London: Cape, 1957 edn); D. J. Oddy, *From Plain Fare to Fusion Food: British Diet from the 1890s to the 1990s* (Woodbridge: Boydell, 2003).

17. P. Munsche, *Gentlemen and Poachers: The English Game Laws, 1671–1831* (Cambridge: Cambridge University Press, 1981) 5–7, 11.

18. Sheail, *Rabbits and their History*, 132.

19. Ibid., 109–11.

20. Ibid., 136–7.

21. Ibid., 10; Barrett-Hamilton, *A History of British Mammals*, vol. 2, 188; British Ecological Society, 'Nature conservation and nature reserves', *Journal of Ecology*, 32 (1944) 62; Simpson, *The Wild Rabbit*, 15–16; A. G. Tansley, *The British Islands and their Vegetation* (Cambridge: Cambridge University Press, 1949) 133, 185.

22. Gathorne-Hardy says there were no rabbits in Argyll until 1845. A. E. Gathorne-Hardy, *Autumns in Argyleshire with Rod and Gun* (London: Longmans Green, 1900) 12–13. See also *Field*, 4 August 1955, 215; *Gamekeepers' Gazette*, 281 (1954) 4232–3; D. Macintyre, *Nature Notes of a Highland Gamekeeper* (London: Seeley, Service & Co. Ltd, 1960) 159; Sheail, *Rabbits and their History*, 132.

23. *The Times*, 7 September 1963.

24. Farrow, 'On the ecology', 6.

25. A. G. Tansley and R. S. Adamson, 'Studies of the vegetation of the English chalk. III. The chalk grasslands of the Hampshire–Sussex border', *Journal of Ecology*, 13 (1925) 211.

26. *PP* 1846 ix (2) Select Committee on Game Laws, report, 16, 23; see A. S. Thomas, 'Changes in vegetation since the advent of myxomatosis', *Journal of Ecology*, 48 (1960) 287–306.

27. *PP* 1872 x Select Committee on Game Laws, evidence, 272, 368.

28. Ibid., evidence of Hon. Adolphus Liddell QC, 35.

29. *PP* 1873 xii Select Committee on Game Laws, report, 5.

30. Ibid., 6.

31. 3 *Hansard*, 252 (27 May 1880) 599–602. See M. Stenton and S. Lees, *Who's Who of British MPs* (Hassocks: Harvester, 1976–81) vol. 1, 201, 306.

32. A. D. Middleton, *The Control and Extermination of Wild Rabbits* (Oxford: Bureau of Animal Population, 1940). BAP was an Oxford University research institute between 1932 and 1967. Its director throughout this period was the pioneering ecologist, Charles Elton. In 1939 Elton submitted a plan to the ARC proposing that in the event of war BAP staff should engage in applied biological research on rodent control. In practice, staff devoted their attention to rats, house mice and rabbits. Doug Middleton, on secondment from ICI after an earlier spell with the Bureau (1932–37), and H. N. (Mick) Southern, on the BAP staff from 1938 to 1967, were mainly concerned with the rabbit. H. V. Thompson, who later joined MAF's Infestation Control Division and was closely involved with Britain's first myxomatosis outbreak, was a BAP researcher between 1942 and 1946. See P. Crowcroft, *Elton's Ecologists: A History of the Bureau of Animal Population* (Chicago: University of Chicago Press, 1991); C. Elton, 'Research on rodent control by the Bureau of Animal Population', in D. Chitty and H. N. Southern (eds) *Control of Rats and Mice* (Oxford: Clarendon Press, 1954) vol. 1, 1–24.

33. Ground Game Act, 1880, 43 & 44 Vict. c. 47.

34. Harting, *The Rabbit*, 173.

35. Sheail, *Rabbits and their History*, 195–7.

36. *Select Committee of the House of Lords on Agriculture*, evidence, 66.

37. Ibid., evidence, 30–1. The Ministry of Agriculture and Fisheries was created, in succession to the Board of Agriculture and Fisheries by act of parliament (9 & 10 Geo. V c.91) in 1919. See E. H. Whetham, *The Agrarian History of England and Wales vol. viii 1914–1918* (Cambridge: Cambridge University Press, 1978) 122.

38. Order of 30 March 1917. S R & O no. 208, 1917 (London: HMSO, 1917) 279. In 1917 WAECs were established throughout England and Wales. They were responsible for carrying out agricultural and food production policy in every county and, through district subcommittees, every parish and farm. Members included farmers, estate agents landowners and trades unionists drawn from county agricultural subcommittees appointed by the board. In 1919 WAECs were replaced by county agricultural committees that exercised various powers, including over the control of pests. See Whetham, *Agrarian History*, 97–102, 122–3.

39. 7 & 8 Geo. V c.58 s.10.

40. Sheail, *Rabbits and their History*, 197.

41. Whetham, *Agrarian History*, 98–9.

42. *The Times*, 29 December 1917.

43. *Select Committee of the House of Lords on Agriculture*, evidence, 30–1.

44. Forestry Act, 1919, 5 & 10 Geo V c. 58. The commission, appointed in the aftermath of a war that had demonstrated Britain's dangerous dependence on imported timber, was responsible for promoting forestry and afforestation and increasing domestic timber production.

45. *Select Committee of the House of Lords on Agriculture*, report, iv, evidence, 8–10. In 1954 it was suggested that the commission was spending £500,000 per annum to protect plantations against rabbits. British Library. National Sound Archive. *War on the Warren*, BBC Home Service Broadcast on Myxomatosis, 14 September 1954.

46. *PP* xii 1921 (Cmd. 1401) (Edinburgh: HMSO, 1921).

47. *Select Committee of the House of Lords on Agriculture*, evidence, 30–1. Councils of agriculture, one for England and one for Wales, were set up under the terms of the Ministry of Agriculture and Fisheries Act, 1919. They comprised two members of each county agricultural committee plus representatives from other bodies such as the NFU and agricultural workers' unions. They were charged with providing assistance to the ministry and were obliged to meet, in public, at least twice a year to discuss matters of public interest connected with agriculture and rural industries. See Whetham, *Agrarian History*, 123.

48. *Select Committee of the House of Lords on Agriculture*, evidence, 30–1.

49. 5 *Hansard* (Lords) 67 (3 May 1927) 31–2. Lord Atholl supported the rabbit-control objectives of the 1928 bill but was concerned about investing authority in the Scottish Board of Agriculture. He considered that the board was opposed to field sports and, under a Labour government 'likely to be swayed

by Socialism'. He was far more sympathetic to control by county councils on which landowners and farmers were heavily represented. See NAS GD 325/1/182. Atholl to Erskine Jackson (Secretary of the Scottish Land and Property Federation) 7 July 1928.

50. 5 *Hansard* (Lords) 67 (3 May 1927) 39.

51. *Select Committee appointed to consider the Rabbits and Rooks Bill [H.L.]* (London: HMSO, 1927) report, 2–4.

52. 5 *Hansard* 231 (1 November 1929) 477–8; 236 (7 March 1930) 843–76; 239 (29 May 1930) 1487; 240 (30 June 1930) 1746; 244 (31 October 1930) 341; 244 (7 November 1930) 1227–60; *PP* 1929–30 IV, 1–4; *PP* 1930–31 iv, 193–6, Bill to make provision for the prevention of damage by rabbits; *The Times*, 8 March, 8 November 1930.

53. 5 *Hansard* (Lords) 67 (3 May 1927) 31–2. David Cannadine has written about the 'revolution in landholding between 1910 and 1922'. The sale of great estates in this period, he argues, 'amounted to a transfer of property on a scale rivalled in Britain this millennium only by the Norman Conquest and the Dissolution of the Monasteries'. D. Cannadine, *The Decline and Fall of the British Aristocracy* (New Haven: Yale University Press, 1990) 704–5.

54. *The Times*, 23 September 1935.

55. Cited in P. Lewis, *The People's War* (London: Thames Methuen, 1986) 162–3.

56 *The Times*, 13 April 1936.

57. Ibid., 20 April 1936. See also letters of 20 and 27 April.

58. 5 *Hansard* (Lords) 103 (4 November 1936) 42.

59. *Select Committee of the House of Lords on Agriculture*, evidence, 11, 41, 67, 88, 91, 96, 99–100, 102, 111–13. For a fuller indication of the views of the Scottish Land and Property Federation, see NAS AF 43/200. Rabbits Bill, 1938, 'Notes for Members' (December 1936).

60. *Select Committee of the House of Lords on Agriculture*, report, iii–v.

61. *The Times*, 1 July 1937.

62. NAS AF 43/200. Rabbits Bill 1938.

63. R. G. Stapledon, *The Plough-up Policy and Ley Farming* (London: Faber & Faber, 1939) 159.

64. 2 & 3 Geo. VI c.43.

65. *The Times*, 26 July 1939.

66. Ibid., 29 July 1939. In 1926 Captain (later Major) C. W. Hume founded the University of London Animal Welfare Society (ULAWS). In 1938, following its spread to several other universities, it became the Universities Federation for Animal Welfare (UFAW). See C. Hume, *Man and Beast* (London: UFAW, 1962) 8, 12.

67. E. W. Fenton, 'The influence of rabbits on the vegetation of certain hill-grazing districts of Scotland', *Journal of Ecology*, 28 (1940) 438–9; Ministry of Information, *Land at War: The Official Story of British Farming, 1939–1944* (London: HMSO, 1945) 50; Sheail, *Rabbits and their History*, 202.

68. S R & O no. 927 (1939) 772.

69. S R & O no. 1493 (1939) 909–10; S R & O. no. 431 (1940) 295–6. As in the First World War, WAECs (in England and Wales) were responsible for

ensuring that government policy was implemented at local level. See J. Martin, *The Development of Modern Agriculture. British Farming since 1931* (Basingstoke: Macmillan, 1931) 43–7; H. Newby, *Country Life: A Social History of Rural England* (London: Weidenfeld & Nicholson, 1987) 183–4. For Scotland see S R & O nos.1465/S.105 and 1654/S.121 (1939) 805–6, 911.

70. See NA MAF 170/11. Ministry of Agriculture policy on the destruction of rabbits and pests.

71. *The Times*, 27 December 1941.

72. Ibid., 16 January 1943. See Ministry of Information, *Land at War*, 50.

73. *The Times*, 31 May 1945.

74. Martin, *The Development of Modern Agriculture*, 70.

75. 10 & 11 Geo. VI c.48 ss.98, 100. CAECs were required 'to promote agricultural development and efficiency' and ensure 'minimum standards of husbandry and estate management'. They lacked the 'draconian powers' of the WAECs they replaced, but until they were rendered toothless in 1957 they could, and did, take action that led to the dispossession of farmers. Martin, *The Development of Modern Agriculture*, 72, 75–6.

76. 11 & 12 Geo. VI c.45 s.39. Scotland had regional, rather than county, AECs.

77. NA FT1/1. E. H. Havelock to C. Driver, 19 October 1948; R. Davis to C. Driver, December 1948; R. Franklin to C. Driver, 2 January 1950; MAF 131/136. Rabbit Policy Group. Memorandum on the development of organized rabbit control in England and Wales, 9 January 1957.

78. *The Times*, 14 February 1950. See also 5 *Hansard* (Lords) 185 (26 January 1954) 422.

79. NA MAF 131/136. Rabbit Policy Group. Memorandum on the development of organized rabbit control in England and Wales, 9 January 1957; MAF 191/143. H. C. Gough to I. Thomas, 2 January 1950; Memo of H. V. Thompson, 30 July 1950; I. Thomas to W. Davies, 8 August 1950; 5 *Hansard* 481 (23 November 1950) 503–4; *Quarterly Journal of Forestry*, 44 (1950) 181–2; *The Times*, 31 July 1950. Similar developments occurred in Scotland. See MAF 131/5.

80. Report of the Committee on Cruelty, 525.

81. 5 *Hansard* (Lords) 185 (26 January 1954) 423.

82. *Field*, 9 July 1953, 91.

83. 5 *Hansard* (Lords) 176 (8 April 1952) 34–5.

84. NA MAF 131/136. Rabbit Policy Group. Memorandum.

85. 5 *Hansard* 531 (22 October 1954) 1510–11. See also (Lords) 185 (26 January 1954) 417; NA MAF 131/122. Rabbits in the Dukeries, undated.

86. 5 *Hansard* (Lords) 185 (26 January 1954) 422.

87. *Farmers Weekly*, 26 April 1957, 41; C. S. Jarvis, 'A countryman's notes', *Country Life* 114 (1953) 1031; *La Terre et La Vie*, 3–4 (1956–57) 255; *Report of the Advisory Committee on Myxomatosis*, 4; Sheail, *Rabbits and their History*, 202. In December 1953 *Land Worker* (9) estimated the number at 250 million.

88. Sheail, *Rabbits and their History*, 181–2, also mentions use of alcohol and poisons. The Scott Henderson committee considered that man and disease exerted the greatest check on rabbit numbers. See Report of the Committee on Cruelty, 519.

89. Kean, *Animal Rights*, 170.

90. NA HO 45/21811, 'Control of wild rabbits', 16; *Select Committee of the House of Lords on Agriculture*, evidence, 35.

91. Sheail, *Rabbits and their History*, 182. See Arscott, 'Sentimentality', 65–81, especially 77–81. Chlorine gas was first used on the Western Front in April 1915. July 1917 saw the first deployment of mustard gas. D. Winter, *Death's Men: Soldiers of the Great War* (London: Penguin, 1979) 121.

92. *Select Committee of the House of Lords on Agriculture*, evidence, 35–8.

93. The Protection of Animals Act, 1911 as amended by the Protection of Animals (Amendment) Act, 1927 made it an offence to place poison on land or in buildings except, and provided reasonable precautions were taken to protect other animals, to destroy invertebrates, rats, mice and small ground vermin. In 1936 the Home Office's legal adviser stated that it 'would seem doubtful whether rabbits can properly be regarded as small ground vermin'. *Select Committee of the House of Lords on Agriculture*, evidence, 3.

94. Stead, *The Rabbit Menace in Australia*, 12–13; *The Times*, 22 March 1932.

95. NA MAF 131/10. Supplies of cyanide gassing powder. New subsidy scheme. See NAS AF74/24. 'Pests Control Branch. Rabbits. Gassing'; *Select Committee of the House of Lords on Agriculture*, evidence, 35–6, 121–5; *The Times*, 28 May 1935.

96. W. H. Buckley, 'Report on a solution of the rabbit problem: cyanide gassing', *Veterinary Journal*, 91 (1935) 210–15; W. H. Buckley, 'One man's war against the rabbit', *Field*, 24 October 1957, 724–5; NA MAF 131/124. W. H. Buckley, 'The Wild Rabbit in West Wales' (unpublished paper, dated January 1957); *The Times*, 31 May 1935. An article in *The Times* (16 March 1936) stated that a badly infested farm of 200 acres could be cleared of rabbits by means of Cymag for about £5 (excluding the cost of the rotary fan blower).

97. Lockley, 'My island and our life there', 557–71; Lockley, *The Island*, 129–31.

98. NAS AF74/24. Draft undated and unsigned letter to J. Macleod; *Select Committee of the House of Lords on Agriculture*, evidence, 36, 121–7; *The Times*, 28 May 1935.

99. *Select Committee of the House of Lords on Agriculture*, report, vii.

100. 2 & 3 Geo. VI c.43 s.4. As previously stated, this measure applied only to England and Wales. The Agriculture Act, 1947 (for England and Wales) and the Agriculture (Scotland) Act, 1948 confirmed the legality of gas in the control of wild rabbits.

101. Report of the Committee on Cruelty, 463. See also MAF 112/181. Rabbit destruction campaign, paper no. 9, 20 July 1950; Ministry of Information, *Land at War*, 50; NA MAF 131/10. Supplies of cyanide gassing powder. New subsidy scheme; NAS AF74/24. P. Gold to G. Anderson, 3 December 1955. In the mid-1950s the government subsidy ran to 4s 8d (23p approximately) per 7lb tin, which meant a retail price of about 15s (75p).

102. J. Wentworth Day, *Poison on the Land: The War on Wildlife and some Remedies* (London: Eyre & Spottiswood, 1957) 61. See also *Manchester Guardian*, 23 July 1955.

103. 'Gas that rabbit', *Farming News*, 15 February 1958; 5 *Hansard* 481 (23 November 1950) 504; NAS AF74/24. Undated (1955?) pamphlet, 'Gassing of

rabbits' issued by DAS. Towards the end of the 1950s concerns arose about cyanide leaching into rivers and drinking water supplies. In addition, growing evidence linked cumulative exposure to health problems in humans. See NAS AF74/24, *passim*. Relevant documents include R. Bell to Secretary of DAS, 4 August 1959; Memorandum of F. Cann, 13 August 1959; H. David to Mr Whimster, 5 November 1959.

104. A. H. B. Kirkman, *Man versus Rabbit* (London: ULAWS, 1934) 2; Sheail, *Rabbits and their History*, 144–51.

105. Middleton, *The Control*, 12. Middleton states that a single trapper could keep 70–100 traps, and in favourable circumstances many more, working efficiently.

106. *Select Committee of the House of Lords on Agriculture*, evidence, 35.

107. Kirkman, *Man versus Rabbit*, 15–25; *Select Committee of the House of Lords on Agriculture*, report, vi–vii, evidence, 13–15.

108. K. Thomas, *Man and the Natural World* (London: Allen Lane, 1983) 23, 109–10, Chapter 4, 279, 290–1. See also E. S. Turner, *All Heaven in a Rage* (London: Michael Joseph, 1964).

109. 3 Geo IV c.71. Act to prevent the cruel and improper treatment of cattle. Notwithstanding its title, the act also applied to horses and sheep. 5 & 6 Will. IV c.59. Act to consolidate and amend the law relating to the cruel and improper treatment of animals.

110. Kean, *Animal Rights*, 69, 111, 185–7; *The Times*, 13 July 1934.

111. Turner, *All Heaven in a Rage*, 230.

112. Ground Game Act, 1880, 43 & 44 Vict. c.47, s.6. Subsequent court decisions established that section 6 applied to occupiers only and not to landowners or the owners of sporting rights. As a result, such people were entitled to set gin traps in the open. In evidence to a select committee in the 1930s O. F. Dowson, legal adviser to the Home Office, stated that this entitlement 'appears to have been not quite in accordance with the original intention of Parliament'. See *Select Committee of the House of Lords on Agriculture*, evidence, 2.

113. Report of the Committee on Cruelty, 449–50, 456–7.

114. 5 *Hansard* (Lords) 97 (28 May 1935) 8–46; Hume, *Man and Beast*, 34; PP (Lords) I (1934–5). There had been similar bills previously. See for example 5 *Hansard* 245 (20 November 1930) 637.

115. *Select Committee of the House of Lords on Agriculture*, report, vi–vii.

116. 2 & 3 Geo. VI c.43.

117. Conference on humane methods of rodent control held in Oxford, 10 May 1945. Oxford University, Zoology Library, Bureau of Animal Population Reprint Collection; S R & O II (1941) 8. Order in Council no. 50 (1941) adding to and amending the Defence (General) Regulations, 1939.

118. Report of the Committee on Cruelty, 454.

119. Hartley, *Food in England*, 173. See also 60–1.

120. Report of the Committee on Cruelty, 449.

121. Ibid., 436.

122. 2 & 3 Eliz. II c. 68. Pests act, 1954.

Chapter 3. Narrative of a Disease

1. MAF 131/12. F. Winch to H. Ashton et al., 19 August 1953. RPOs possessed the status of higher executive officers in the civil service. In 1953 they were paid between £715 and £865 per annum. See *British Imperial Calendar and Civil Service List* (London: HMSO, 1954).

2. In the 1950s the MAF, with its network of scientific, educational, advisory, statistical and other divisions, plus research stations dotted around the country, was one of the largest government departments. It directly employed hundreds of veterinarians. See *British Imperial Calendar and Civil Service List* (London: HMSO, 1953).

3. NA MAF 131/113. Circular No. 53/36 to all veterinary officers. Myxomatosis in rabbits, 15 September 1953.

4. MAF 131/12. Minute of L. Hughes, 10 October 1953; NA MAF 131/113. Myxomatosis Advisory Committee (MAC). Minutes of meetings and related papers; MAF 255/216. Third report of C. P. Quick, 13 October 1953; J. N. Ritchie et al., 'Myxomatosis', *Veterinary Record*, 66 (1954) 796–802. See also H. V. Thompson, 'The origin and spread of myxomatosis with particular reference to Great Britain', *La Terre et La Vie. Revue D'Histoire Naturelle*, 3–4 (1956–7) 142. Thompson and Worden suggest that the outbreak may have started as early as August 1953. See Thompson and Worden, *The Rabbit*, 149.

5. British Library. National Sound Archive. *War on the Warren*, BBC Home Service Broadcast on Myxomatosis, 14 September 1954.

6. Rabbit syphilis was widespread in 1953 as was coccidiosis, another fatal disease of rabbits. *The Times*, 9 November 1953.

7. C. J. Armour and H. V. Thompson, 'Spread of myxomatosis in the first outbreak in Great Britain', *Annals of Applied Biology*, 43 (1955) 511–18; MAF 131/12. Minute of L. Hughes, 9 October 1953; MAF 131/14. Minute of R. H. Franklin, 16 October 1953; MAF 131/12. Sankey's note on myxomatosis in Kent and East Sussex. Action taken by Infestation Control Division, 18 November 1953; NA MAF 131/132. Timetable of myxomatosis outbreak at Edenbridge, Kent; *War on the Warren*.

8. NA MAF 131/12. A. V. Neal to W. D. Baylis, 24 October 1953. For an early unofficial account of developments at Bough Beech see *Southern Weekly News*, 30 October 1953.

9. NA MAF 255/216. First report of C. P. Quick, 10 October 1953.

10. MAF 131/113. MAC Paper no. 5, undated; NA MAF 131/12. Suspected myxomatosis outbreaks in Kent. Resumé of the events since the first reports, 20 October 1953, Minute of L. Hughes, 9 October 1953; NA. MAF 255/216. Second report of C. P. Quick, 10 October 1953.

11. NA. MAF 255/216. Third report of C. P. Quick, 13 October 1953; NA MAF 131/12. W. D. Baylis's Report to date on rabbit clearance scheme (myx) at Bough Beech, 15 October 1953.

12. MAF 131/113. L. R. Sankey to H. N. White, 10 October 1953 (*sic*), unsigned and undated note no. 5 to H. N. White, L. R. Sankey to H. Gardner, 14

October 1953, L. R. Sankey to H. N. White, 16 October 1953, L. R. Sankey to
H. N. White, 28 October 1953, L. R. Sankey to H. N. White, 3 November
1953; MAF 131/132. Myxomatosis–situation report by Major C. J. Armour, 5
February 1954. Leslie Thompson, head of the Bough Beech shooting
syndicate, applauded MAF's containment efforts; NA MAF 131/12. Minute of
J. N. Ritchie, 13 October 1953. See *The Times*, 13 November 1953.

13. Ritchie et al., 'Myxomatosis', 799.
14. MAF 131/132. Myxomatosis–situation report by Major C. J. Armour, 5 February
    1954; NA MAF 131/113. L. R. Sankey to H. Gardner, 14 October 1953, L. R.
    Sankey to H. N. White, 16 October 1953, L. R. Sankey to H. N. White, 10
    October 1953 (sic), unsigned and undated note no. 5 to H. N. White; Sankey
    to White, 28 October 1953, L. R. Sankey to H. N. White, 3 November 1953.
15. NA. MAF 255/216. Press notice of 19 October 1953. According to Lord
    Carrington in 2005, the government was keen to create the impression that 'we
    were in control'. Author's recorded interview with Lord Carrington, 23 May 2005.
16. NA. MAF 191/145. Rabbit myxomatosis in France. J. W. Evans's report of
    inquiry, 22–25 September 1953.
17. MAF 131/113. L. R. Sankey to H. N. White, 28 October 1953; NA MAF
    131/13. Minute of H. Gardner, 27 October 1953, Report of Major A. Franklin
    (DVO), 28 October 1953.
18. NA MAF 131/13. Minutes of L. Hughes, 26 and 27 October 1953, minute of
    J. N. Ritchie, 27 October 1953, report of Major A. Franklin (DVO), 28
    October 1953.
19. NA MAF 131/13. Minute of H. Gardner, 27 October 1953. In fact, late 1953
    saw exceptionally mild weather. The temperature in London on 2 December
    reached 63° Fahrenheit (17°C). See I. S. Macadam (ed.) *Annual Register of World
    Events, 1953* (London: Longmans, Green & Co., 1954) 64.
20. NA. MAF 255/216. Lord Carrington to R. H. Franklin, 27 October 1953.
21. MAF 131/113. L. R. Sankey to H. N. White, 31 October 1953; NA MAF
    131/13. Minutes of L. R. Sankey, 28 and 31 October 1953, press notice of 30
    October 1953.
22. NA MAF 131/13. H. Gardner to R. H. Franklin, 29 October 1953; MAF
    131/113. L. R. Sankey to H. N. White, 31 October 1953, L. R. Sankey to H. N.
    White, 3 November 1953.
23. NA MAF 131/113. L. R. Sankey to H. N. White, 31 October 1953.
24. NA. MAF 255/216. R. H. Franklin to H. Gardner, 2 November 1953, notes
    for chairman's opening statement (prepared by L. R. Sankey) to the first
    meeting of the MAC on 4 November 1953. Sankey was the second most
    senior official in MAF's infestation control division.
25. NA MAF 131/113. L. R. Sankey to H. N White, 3 November 1953; MAF
    131/13. L. R. Sankey to H. J. Gill (East Sussex AEC) 9 November 1953.
26. NA MAF 131/113. L. R. Sankey's note on present outbreaks for the period 4–
    6 November, L. R. Sankey to H. N. White, 13 November 1953, L. R. Sankey's
    notes on action by Infestation Control Division, 14–17 November and 3–6
    December 1953, L. R. Sankey's note on present outbreaks for the period 18–
    24 November.

27. *Gamekeeper & Countryside*, May 1954, 135.
28. NA MAF 131/113. Minutes of fifth meeting of MAC, 23 February 1954; minutes of sixth meeting of MAC, 15 March 1954.
29. 5 *Hansard* 531 (21 October 1954) 1370, (22 October 1954) 1505, 1555; (Lords) 189 (22 November 1954) 1755; NA MAF 131/94. Minutes of joint meeting of MAC and LPAC, 26 July 1954; *Press & Journal*, 14 July 1954. This dramatic spread occurred even though the summer of 1954 was 'dreadful' and, therefore, not necessarily propitious for the insects that served as virus vectors. After a brief heat wave in May 'the weather broke and never, in England, at any rate recovered. ... A dreary series of rain storms followed one another in endless succession.' Autumn saw successive floods and gales. I. S. Macadam (ed.) *Annual Register of World Events, 1954* (London: Longmans, Green & Co., 1955) 47, 65.
30. *Farmer & Stock-breeder*, 13–14 July 1954, 51; *La Terre et La Vie. Revue d'Histoire Naturelle* 3–4 (1956–7) 263; *Shooting Times*, 30 July 1954, 501.
31. R. Page, *The Decline of an English Village* (London: Denis-Poynter, 1974) 117.
32. Lockley, 'Myxomatosis: a factual survey', 1174; Lockley, *Private Life of the Rabbit*, 123–4; NA FT 4/26. R. M. Lockley, Rabbit investigation, note 6.
33. NA MAF 131/31. Summary of replies to rabbit questionnaire, July 1955.
34. NA MAF 131/115. Appendix to MAC paper no. 17.
35. *Press & Journal*, 30 May 1955.
36. *Farmer & Stock-breeder*, 29–30 March 1955, 43; *Farmers Weekly*, 26 April 1957, 41; *Field*, 5 February 1959, 223; NA MAF 131/136. Minutes of first meeting of Rabbit Policy Group, 6 March 1957; *PP* 1956–7 xvii. Annual Report of Nature Conservancy, 1955–6, 472; *PP* 1957–8 xvi, Annual Report of Nature Conservancy, 1956–7, 452–5; K. J. Sumption and J. R. Flowerdew, 'The ecological effects of the decline in rabbits (*oryctolagus cuniculus* L.) due to myxomatosis', *Mammal Review*, 15 (1985) 151–3; *The Times*, 3 January 1955, 22 July and 29 November 1957, 5 May 1958, 13 January 1960.

Chapter 4. Accident or Design?

1. British Library. National Sound Archive. *War on the Warren*, BBC Home Service Broadcast on Myxomatosis, 14 September 1954.
2. *Report of the Advisory Committee on Myxomatosis*, 2, 3. As we have seen, the disease had been introduced on the Welsh island of Skokholm in the 1930s. In 1952 and 1953 North of Scotland College of Agriculture staff attempted to exterminate the rabbit population of the Heisker islands in the Hebrides using myxomatosis. See for example P. L. Shanks et al., 'Experiments with myxomatosis in the Hebrides', *British Veterinary Journal*, 111 (1955) 25–30.
3. P. Carrington, *Reflect on Things Past: The Memoirs of Lord Carrington* (London: Collins, 1988) 90.
4. H. V. Thompson, 'The rabbit disease: myxomatosis', *Annals of Applied Biology*, 41 (1954) 362.
5. Thompson, 'The rabbit in Britain', 73.
6. Fenner and Ratcliffe, *Myxomatosis*, 322.

7. BBC Television, *Rabbits Wanted: Dead or Alive* (30 January 1977); *British Imperial Calendar and Civil Service List* (London: HMSO, 1955).

8. Thompson, 'The rabbit disease', 358.

9. Thompson and Worden, *The Rabbit*, 135. See also H. V. Thompson, 'The origin and spread of myxomatosis with particular reference to Great Britain', *La Terre et La Vie. Revue D'Histoire Naturelle*, 3–4 (1956–7) 142.

10. BBC Television, *Rabbits Wanted: Dead or Alive*.

11. Thompson, 'The rabbit in Britain', 73.

12. BBC Television, *Rabbits Wanted: Dead or Alive*.

13. Thompson, 'The Rabbit disease', 359. In another paper he wrote that once the disease was established in France and elsewhere in Europe 'it became evident that suitable vectors were present in the area and probably that the disease would eventually cross the Channel.' See Thompson, 'The Origin and Spread', 142. In *The Rabbit*, 135–6, he and Worden considered it 'highly probable', rather than 'inevitable' that myxomatosis would cross the Channel. When myxomatosis appeared on an island 200 miles from the Australian mainland the authorities were 'quite satisfied that the disease had not been introduced by man'. See NA MAF 131/115. Minutes of tenth meeting of MAC, 18 June 1956.

14. Thompson, 'The origin and spread', 142; Thompson, 'The rabbit disease', 362; Thompson and Worden, *The Rabbit* 149. Some thought the 1951–52 foot and mouth epizootic reached Britain via birds migrating from Europe. A. Woods, *A Manufactured Plague: The History of Foot and Mouth Disease in Britain* (London: Earthscan, 2004) 92.

15. E. J. Moynahan, 'Myxomatosis', *Practitioner*, 174 (1955) 709–14.

16. Brown, P. W. et al. 'Rabbits and myxomatosis in the north east of Scotland', *Scottish Agriculture*, 35 (1956) 204–7; R. M. Lockley, 'Has the rabbit a future?' *Countryman*, 53 (1956) 658–60.

17. C. H. Andrewes, 'Myxomatosis in Britain', *Nature*, 174 (1954) 529–30; C. H. Andrewes, *The Natural History of Viruses* (London: Weidenfeld & Nicholson, 1967) 156.

18. Stamp, *Man and the Land*, 213.

19. Day, *Poison on the Land*, 43; Marchington, *Pugs and Drummers*, 109.

20. BBC Television, *Rabbits Wanted: Dead or Alive*; N. W. Moore, *The Bird of Time: The Science and Politics of Nature Conservation* (Cambridge: Cambridge University Press, 1987) 123; C. J. Smith, *Ecology of the English Chalk* (London: Academic Press, 1980) 261. See also D. Evans, *A History of Nature Conservation in Britain* (London: Routledge, 1992) 108. Smith supports his point by citing Lockley's *Private Life of the Rabbit*. However, nothing in Lockley's book indicates that myxomatosis was brought into the UK intentionally.

21. J. Sheail, 'The management of an animal population: changing attitudes towards the wild rabbit in Britain', *Journal of Environmental Management*, 33 (1991) 196.

22. NA. MAF 255/216. Third report of C. P. Quick, 13 October 1953; see MAF 131/12. I. Thomas to B. Engholm, 23 June 1958.

23. Thompson, 'The rabbit in Britain', 73.

24. J. N. Ritchie et al., 'Myxomatosis', *Veterinary Record*, 66 (1954) 797–8; Thompson, 'The rabbit disease', 358–66.
25. F. Fenner and J. Ross, 'Myxomatosis', in H. V. Thompson and C. King (eds) *The European Rabbit: The History and Biology of a Successful Colonizer* (Oxford: Oxford University Press, 1994) 208.
26. Fenner and Ratcliffe, *Myxomatosis*, 322.
27. C. J. Armour and H. V. Thompson, 'Spread of myxomatosis in the first outbreak in Great Britain', *Annals of Applied Biology*, 43 (1955) 511–18.
28. Fenner and Ratcliffe, *Myxomatosis*, 322.
29. Fenner and Fantini, *Biological Control*, 225. Fenner and Fantini quote without comment Thompson's observation that a local man brought the disease to Britain by importing a myxomatous rabbit. In 2005 Frank Fenner informed the author by email that his opinion about the deliberate introduction of the disease into the UK originated with Harry Thompson. He also insisted that he did not change his opinion between 1994 and 1999; in other words, he continued to believe that the British outbreak was started deliberately. The fact remains, however, that Fenner and Fantini did express uncertainty about how the disease crossed the Channel and that this uncertainty was absent when Fenner and Ross addressed the issue in 1994.
30. Drakeford, *Rabbit Control*, 16; O. Rackham, *The History of the Countryside* (London: J&M Dent, 1986) 48.
31. National Sound Archive C900/11062C1. Millennium Memory Bank.
32. *Shooting Times*, 28 November 1953, 764.
33. *Field*, 3 November 1955, 812; *Gamekeeper's Gazette*, 275 (1953) 4092; *Shooting Times*, 23 July 1954, 482, 485.
34. *Southern Weekly News*, 20 January 1956. In fact, the presence of myxomatosis in Britain was confirmed more than eight months before the derationing of meat.
35. NA MAF 131/14. M. Lane to R. Franklin, 20 October 1953.
36. S. Mills, 'Rabbits breed a growing controversy', *New Scientist*, 109 (1986) 50–4.
37. *Gamekeeper's Gazette*, 275 (1953) 4092.
38. R. F. Sellers, 'Possible windborne spread of myxomatosis to England in 1953', *Epidemiology and Infection*, 98 (1987) 119–25.
39. M. W. Service, 'A reappraisal of the role of mosquitoes in the transmission of myxomatosis in Britain', *Journal of Hygiene*, 69 (1971) 105.
40. NA MAF 131/114. Minutes of joint meeting of MAC and LPAC, 26 July 1954.
41. R. C. Muirhead-Thompson, 'Field studies of the role of *anopheles atroparvus* in the transmission of myxomatosis in England', *Journal of Hygiene*, 54 (1956) 477; R. C. Muirhead-Thompson, 'The part played by woodland mosquitoes of the genus aëdes in the transmission of myxomatosis in England', *Journal of Hygiene*, 54 (1956) 471.
42. Service, 'A reappraisal', 105.
43. NA MAF 131/12. B. Engholm to J. Hensley, 24 June 1958.
44. *The Times*, 5 June and 10 July 1953.
45. NA FT 1/1. J. W. Evans, The Rabbit Problem, 6 November 1952; MAF 131/153. J. W. Evans to C. B. Williams, 20 October 1950.
46. On the experiments of Martin and Lockley, see Chapter 1.

47. NA MAF 131/2. Note by J. Scott Watson, 27 July 1948.
48. NA MAF 131/2. Control of rabbits in Australia, undated.
49. NA MAF 131/2. W. M. Gracie's paper, 'Control of wild rabbits', 16 December 1949.
50. NA FT 1/2. Lord Rothschild to E. M. Nicholson, 8 June 1953.
51. NA HO 45/21811.
52. NA MAF 131/152. Draft interim report of working party on control of wild rabbits, undated.
53. NA MAF 112/181. Rabbit destruction campaign, paper no. 6, 20 July 1950.
54. NA FT 1/1. J. W. Evans, 'The rabbit problem', 6 November 1952. In conversation with the author Lord Carrington unequivocally dismissed the suggestion that government introduced the disease and thought it 'quite unlikely' that farmers were responsible. Author's recorded interview with Lord Carrington, 23 May 2005.
55. MAF 112/181. Rabbit destruction campaign, paper no.6, 20 July 1950.
56. NA FT 1/2. R. M. Lockley to E. M. Nicholson, 17 October 1953.
57. NA MAF 105/311. Summary of minutes of first and second meetings of research group of MAC Scientific Sub-Committee, 22 December 1953, 12 January 1954. Though it might seem remarkable that in 1952 a virulent disease organism could be deployed, even offshore, without official sanction, civil service and legal opinion indicated that infected rabbit carcasses and laboratory samples of virus could be imported and used to spread myxomatosis with impunity. MAF 131/113. Opinion of Bazil Wingate-Saul, 7 December 1953; legal aspects, further note, 11 March 1954; MAF 131/22. C. P. Quick to H. White, 13 November 1953. The North of Scotland College of Agriculture obtained the virus from ICI and acknowledged the assistance of various parties but not of any government department or civil servant. The Heisker experiments failed because of the scarcity of suitable insect vectors. On the Scottish mainland rabbits were heavily infested with fleas. See R. M. Allan, 'A study of the populations of the rabbit flea, *spilopsyllus cuniculi* (Dale) on the wild rabbit *oryctolagus cuniculus* in the north-east of Scotland', *Proceedings of the Royal Entomological Society of London. Series A. General Entomology*, 31 (1956) 145–52; Brown et al., 'Rabbits and myxomatosis', 204–7; NA MAF 131/113. Minutes of second meeting of research group of MAC Scientific Sub-Committee, 12 January 1954, Paper on experimentally induced outbreaks of myxomatosis–programme of research on Scottish islands; NAS AF 70/128, AF70/722, AF70/784. Annual reports of the North of Scotland College of Agriculture, 1951–2, 1952–3, 1953–4; Shanks et al., 'Experiments with myxomatosis'; P. L. Shanks et al., 'Myxomatosis in rabbits with special reference to the north of Scotland', *Transactions of the Royal Highland and Agricultural Society of Scotland*, 68 (1957) 4.
58. NA FT 1/1. J. W. Evans, 'The rabbit problem', 6 November 1952.
59. NA MAF 131/100. T. J. Marjoram to H. Ashton (Cheshire CAEC) 29 December 1952, F. Winch to E. R. Morgan, 5 February 1953.
60. NA MAF 131/100. T. J. Marjoram to C. R. C. Jeffery, 27 March. 1953.
61. NA MAF 131/100. L. R. Sankey to J. Williams, 28 July 1953.

62. See Muirhead-Thompson, 'Field studies', 472; Muirhead-Thompson, 'The part played', 461.
63. NA MAF 131/100. J. W. Evans to J. A. Boycott, 30 July 1953. See also MAF 113/367. Memorandum of J. Scott Watson, 23 March 1953; MAF 131/94. Minutes of first meeting of LPAC, 2 March 1953.
64. 5 *Hansard*, 517 (14 July 1953) 152.
65. NA MAF 131/100. 'The use of myxomatosis for rabbit destruction', 12 August 1953.
66. NA MAF 131/100. J. W. Evans to H. N. White, 13 August 1953.
67. NA MAF 113/367. J. W. Evans, 'Pest Control – Research Aspects', 3 April 1953.
68. NA MAF 131/19. Memorandum to CAECs. Animal and bird pests control campaign 1953/54, 20 August 1953. See MAF 113/367. Agricultural Improvement Council for England and Wales. Extract from minutes of sixty-third meeting (23 September 1953). Notes on LPAC.
69. NA MAF 131/100. Sir Thomas Dugdale to Sir Arnold Gridley, 7 September 1953.
70. NA MAF 131/100. J. W. Evans to H. N. White, 13 August 1953.
71. NA MAF 131/100. J. D. Westlake to L. R. Sankey, 21, 25 August 1953.
72. NA FT 1/1. J. W. Evans, 'The rabbit problem', 6 November 1952.
73. NA MAF 131/94. Minutes of second meeting of LPAC, 20 April 1953.
74. See, for example, 5 *Hansard* (Lords) 185 (26 January 1954) 422; *The Times*, 14 February 1950.
75. NA MAF 113/367. Memorandum of J. Scott Watson, 23 March 1953.
76. H. Thompson, 'Myxomatosis for rabbit destruction', *Quarterly Review of the Royal Agricultural Society of England* (September 1953) 15–16. See also NA MAF 131/12. Minute of C. Quick, 10 November 1953.
77. NA FT 1/2. H. V. Thompson to R. M. Lockley, 17 October 1953.
78. NA MAF 131/14. R. Franklin to M. Lane, 22 October 1953; J. Ross, 'Myxomatosis: the natural evolution of the disease', *Symposia of the Zoological Society of London*, 50 (1982) 94.
79. Ritchie et al., 'Myxomatosis', 799–800.
80. NA. MAF 255/216. Third report of C. P. Quick, 13 October 1953.
81. NA MAF 131/115. Minutes of tenth meeting of MAC, 18 June 1956.
82. NA MAF 131/12. I. Thomas to B. Engholm, 23 June 1958. From 18 October 1954 there was a single Minister of Agriculture, Fisheries and Food. The ministries were formally amalgamated in the following April. D. Butler and G. Butler, *British Political Facts 1900–1994* (Basingstoke: Macmillan, 1994 edn) 24, 50; National Archives Guide, 504/1/1. The designation Ministry of Agriculture, Fisheries and Food (MAFF) should therefore be used in any reference to the Ministry subsequent to this date.
83. NA MAF 131/12. I. Thomas to B. Engholm, 23 June 1958.
84. NA. MAF 255/216. Third report of C. P. Quick, 13 October 1953.
85. *Southern Weekly News*, 30 October 1953.
86. Williams died on 5 August 1954, aged 82, following an operation. *The Times*, 7 August 1954.
87. Author's recorded interview with Georgina Coleby, 18 July 2005.

88. Author's recorded interview with Cyril Skinner, 14 December 2005.
89. Ibid; BBC Television, *Rabbits Wanted: Dead or Alive*.
90. *Farmers Weekly*, 29 October 1954, 85; *Press & Journal*, 5 August 1954; *Scotsman*, 21 July 1954.
91. Author's recorded interview with Stuart Wicks, 29 May 2006.

Chapter 5. The Myxomatosis Advisory Committee

1. NA. MAF 255/216. R. H. Franklin to H. Gardner, 14 October 1953; *Report of the Advisory Committee on Myxomatosis*, 1.
2. MAF 131/132. Myxomatosis–situation report by Major C. J. Armour, 5 February 1954; NA MAF 131/113. L. R. Sankey to H. Gardner, 14 October 1953.
3. NA. MAF 255/216. R. H. Franklin to H. Gardner, 14 October 1953. Lord Carrington informed the author that he was required to take on the chairmanship: 'It wasn't a question of agreeing. I was the parliamentary secretary; I did what I was told.' Author's recorded interview with Lord Carrington, 23 May 2005.
4. Carrington, *Reflect on Things Past*, 89.
5. Ibid., 90; NA. MAF 255/216. R. H. Franklin to H. Gardner, 14 October 1954; *Quarterly Journal of Forestry*, 48 (1954) 3.
6. NA MAF 131/113. Minute of appointment of advisory committee, 6 November 1953; MAF 255/216. Press Notice of 4 November 1953. Members served in a personal capacity, not as representatives of particular organizations. Carrington who pressed for Woolley's inclusion, was told that his attendance as a member of the Gowers committee on foot and mouth disease had been 'most irregular.' See MAF 255/216. R. H. Franklin to H. Gardner, 14 October 1953; MAF 131/14. Minute of W. C. Tame, 15 October 1953. In the event Woolley attended only one of the six MAC meetings held prior to publication of its first report. On every other occasion J. F. Phillips of the NFU substituted for him.
7. Carrington, *Reflect on Things Past*, 90.
8. T. J. Cartwright, *Royal Commissions and Departmental Committees in Britain* (London: Hodder & Stoughton, 1975) 84. See G. Rhodes, *Committees of Inquiry* (London: Allen & Unwin, 1975).
9. NA MAF 131/101. Minute of L. R. Sankey, 16 March 1954.
10. NA MAF 255/216. First meeting of MAC, 4 November 1953. Undated and unsigned notes for the chairman's opening statement; See also 5 *Hansard* (Lords) 184 (11 November 1953) 285–6 for Carrington's response to Rennell, which took very much the same line as Sankey.
11. NA MAF 147/73. Minutes of district CAEC, Swaffham, Norfolk, 6 November 1953; *The Times*, 2 and 4 November 1953 (letters of R. Diplock and R. Sperling).
12. 5 *Hansard* (Lords) 184 (11 November 1953) 257, 286. 'Gilbertian', namely ludicrous or paradoxical, as in the situations created by W. S. Gilbert in his operatic collaborations with Arthur Sullivan. See www.oed-online.

13. L. Harrison Matthews, *Mammals in the British Isles* (London: Collins, 1982) 191–2; L. Harrison Matthews, *Man and Wildlife* (London: Croom Helm, 1975) 25.

14. NA MAF 255/216. First meeting of MAC, 4 November 1953. Undated and unsigned notes for the chairman's opening statement.

15. NA MAF 255/216. R. Franklin to H. Gardner, 2 November 1954, H. Gardner to A.C. McCarthy, 3 November 1953; author's recorded interview with Lord Carrington, 23 May 2005.

16. NA MAF 255/216. R. Franklin to H. Gardner, 2 November 1954, H. Gardner to A. C. McCarthy, 3 November 1953.

17. NA MAF 255/216. Press notice of 4 November 1953.

18. NA MAF 131/113. Minutes of first meeting of MAC, 4 November 1953. Fear of an 'outcry' from 'old ladies in Bournemouth' or 'the Peter Rabbit people' horrified by the sight of masses of dead and dying rabbits was a concern for the committee. As a farmer Carrington welcomed the disease; as a politician he worried about it becoming an issue that could damage the government. Author's recorded interview with Lord Carrington, 23 May 2005.

19. NA MAF 131/13. L. R. Sankey to H. N White, 6 November 1953.

20. NA MAF 131/113. Minutes of second meeting of MAC, 10 November 1953. The minister rejected a ban on the importation of live rabbits on the grounds that it was impractical, unnecessary and unreasonable. In particular, 'to prohibit the importation of live rabbits would have little effect compared with the risk of spread of the disease that exists from infected rabbits already in this country.' MAF 131/20. Undated and unsigned memorandum headed importation of live rabbits.

21. NA MAF 131/113. Minutes of second meeting of MAC, 10 November 1953, Preliminary meeting of the Scientific Sub-Committee.

22. NA MAF 131/113. Minutes of second meeting of MAC Scientific Sub-Committee, 3 December 1953; MAC paper no. 7, 8 December 1953.

23. NA MAF 131/113. L. R. Sankey's notes on action by Infestation Control Division, 3–6 December 1953; MAF 131/113. Minutes of third meeting of MAC, 10 December 1953.

24. Ibid.

25. Ibid.; NA MAF 131/113. Press Notice of 11 December 1953; undated and unsigned notes for the information of those giving evidence before the MAC.

26. NA MAF 131/113. Paper MAC (evidence) no. 2.

27. NA MAF 131/113. Undated general note by the Earl of Dundee; Minutes of fourth meeting of MAC, 20 January 1954. For the views of the RSPCA see its Annual Report 1954, 19–20 and the society's monthly publication, *Animal World*, January and September 1954, October and December 1955.

28. NA MAF 131/113. MAC (evidence) no. 9.

29. NA MAF 131/113. MAC (evidence) no. 1 and no. 7.

30. NA MAF 131/113. MAC (evidence) no. 6.

31. NA MAF 131/113. L. N. Messing and W. S. Smith to C. T. Plumb, 2 December 1953; L. G. Fein and K. Hollebone, 'Report to the Board of Trade by the Fur Trade Export Group, including regarding the value of wild rabbit skins in the United Kingdom', undated; A. J. Jackson et al., to C. T. Plumb, 16

December 1953, including appendix A on the use of wild rabbits for food and their skins as raw material for fur felt and hats and Appendix B on the annual crop of wild rabbits in the United Kingdom.

32. NA MAF 131/113. MAC Note by the Board of Trade, January 1954.

33. NA MAF 131/113. MAC paper 11; minutes of fifth meeting of MAC, 23 February 1954.

34. NA MAF 131/113. MAC (evidence) no. 4.

35. NA MAF 131/113. MAC (evidence) no. 5.

36. NA MAF 131/113. MAC (evidence) no. 11.

37. NA MAF 131/113. Opinion of Bazil Wingate-Saul, 7 December 1953; MAC Paper no. 12.

38. NA MAF 131/113. Minutes of fourth meeting of MAC, 20 January 1954.

39. NA MAF 131/113. MAC Paper 11; Minutes of fifth meeting of MAC, 23 February 1954.

40. It is not known who wrote the report. In 2005 Lord Carrington could not remember who was responsible, but denied it was him. A MAF civil servant, probably Sankey, is the most likely candidate. Author's recorded interview with Lord Carrington, 23 May 2005.

41. NA MAF 131/113. Minutes of fifth meeting of MAC, 23 February 1954.

42. NA MAF 131/113. Minutes of sixth meeting of MAC, 15 March 1954.

43. *Report of the Advisory Committee on Myxomatosis*, 9.

44. NA MAF 131/101. Minute of H. Gardner, 22 March 1954.

45. NA MAF 131/101. Minute of R. H. Franklin, 24 March 1954.

46. 5 *Hansard* 526 (9 April 1954) 83.

47. NA MAF 131/101. Minute of H. Gardner, 22 March 1954.

48. NA MAF 131/101. Minutes of L. R. Sankey, 16, 31 March 1954.

49. NA MAF 131/101. Minute of H. N. White, 31 March 1954; Minute of R. H. Franklin, 5 April 1954.

50. NA MAF 131/114. Press notice of 9 April 1954.

51. NA MAF 131/101. Minute of L. R. Sankey, 31 March 1954.

52. *The Times*, 10, 19 April 1954.

53. 5 *Hansard* 526 (15 April 1954) 1319. In its first references to the disease, in 1953, *Hansard* consistently misspelt the word (myxamatosis). See for example 5 *Hansard* 514 (29 April 1953) 107–8; 517 (14 July 1953) 152.

54. NA MAF 131/101. Minute of H. Gardner, 22 March 1954; Minute of R. H. Franklin, 29 March 1954; Minute of L. R. Sankey, 31 March 1954.

55. NA MAF 131/101. Minute of H. Gardner, 30 March 1954.

56. NA MAF 131/101. Minute of E.A. Hitchman, 25 March 1954; Minute of R. H. Franklin, 29 March 1954.

57. NA MAF 131/101. Minute of H. Gardner, 30 March 1954.

58. NA MAF 131/114. Memorandum to CAECs. Myxomatosis in rabbits, 9 April 1954.

59. SI 1954 no. 927. Non-indigenous rabbits (prohibition of importation and keeping) order, 1954, 122; NA MAF 131/114. Press notice of 29 July 1954. See also *Farmer & Stock-breeder*, 6–7 July 1954, 34; NA MAF 131/23. The order was issued under the terms of the destructive imported animals act, 1932 (22

&23 Geo. V c.12). Although the act dealt with musk rats, section 10 gave the minister power to extend its provisions to other non-indigenous mammals. See J. Sheail, 'The extermination of the musk-rat in inter-war Britain', *Archives of Natural History*, 15 (1988) 155–70; J. Sheail, 'The mink menace: the politics of vertebrate pest control', *Rural History*, 15 (2004) 207–22. Under the 1954 order the penalty for importing, keeping or liberating a non-native rabbit was £20 or £5 per animal if more than four were involved.

Chapter 6. Deliberate Transmission

1. NA MAF 131/113. Minutes of sixth meeting of MAC, 15 March 1954.
2. NA MAF 131/14. Minute of L. R. Sankey, 19 October 1954; Butler and Butler, *British Political Facts*, 24.
3. The LPAC first met in March 1953. Its brief was to consider matters of general interest and advise the ministry about the control of rabbits, grey squirrels, rooks, wood pigeons and other farm pests. The committee remained in existence until 1960 but shed its responsibility for rabbits in 1958. On the origins and early development of the LPAC see NA MAF 131/94.
4. *Report of the Advisory Committee on Myxomatosis*, 6. Lord Listowel, leader of the opposition in the House of Lords, was another advocate: 'I cannot understand why we should be squeamish about the use of this conventional weapon against rabbits when we are prepared to use much more devastating non-conventional weapons against our fellow men.' He thought that the government would have spread the disease deliberately had the country been at war. 5 *Hansard* (Lords) 187 (13 May 1954) 636.
5. 5 *Hansard* 531 (22 October 1954) 1556. See also MAF 131/115. Research report of the MAC's Scientific Sub-Committee, December 1953–December 1955; NA MAF 131/114. Minutes of seventh meeting of MAC, 20 October 1954.
6. 5 *Hansard* (Lords) 189 (22 November 1954) 1756. St Aldwyn and his MAC colleagues accepted that some outbreaks were deliberately induced. See *Second Report of the Advisory Committee on Myxomatosis* (London: HMSO, 1955) 1–2.
7. *PP* 1953–4 xvii, Annual Report of Nature Conservancy, 1953–54, 142.
8. NA MAF 131/12. L. R. Sankey to H. N. White, 16 November 1953.
9. *Farmer & Stock-breeder*, 27–28 April 1954, 76.
10. *Shooting Times*, 14 May 1954, 314. See also 28 May 1954, 338.
11. Lockley, *Private Life of the Rabbit*, 123–4.
12. *Farmers Weekly*, 25 June 1954, 40. See also *Farmer & Stock-breeder*, 22–23 June 1954, 27; *Western Morning News*, 10, 24 June 1954; Tower-Bird, 'Witness this myxomatosis', *Shooting Times*, 23 July 1954, 482, 485; Day, *Poison on the Land*, 55–6.
13. *The Times*, 17 June 1954. The disease reached Devon in June and Somerset in July.
14. *The Times*, 25 June 1954. An RSPCA inspector later told *The Times* of his belief that myxomatosis was 'artificially spread in North Devon in the first instance'. See report of 11 October 1954.

15. 5 *Hansard* 529 (1 July 1954) 1501. See also (8 July 1954) 188.
16. Notwithstanding Munro's comment, official records indicate that Westmorland's first outbreak of myxomatosis did not occur until October 1954. NA MAF 131/115. County-by-county report on the spread of myxomatosis in England and Wales.
17. *Press & Journal*, 14 July 1954. See also *Courier and Advertiser*, 15 July 1954; *Glasgow Herald*, 15 July 1954; *Scotsman*, 19, 21 July 1954; *Scottish Farmer*, 24 July 1954, 1119. Milne later said he was unrepentant about introducing the disease, even after a trapper threatened to sue him for loss of livelihood. *Press & Journal*, 5 August 1954. Bedfordshire was infected in May 1954. When the disease arrived in Ireland, also in July 1954, it was 'generally accepted' that the introduction was 'deliberate, but where the first importation was made, or by whom, is a mystery.' *Courier and Advertiser*, 24, 28 July 1954; *Farmer & Stockbreeder*, 27–28 July 1954, 29; *Shooting Times*, 24 September 1954, 671. See also H. Hudson's statement on Ireland in *La Terre et La Vie*. *Revue d'Histoire Naturelle* 3–4 (1956–7) 263.
18. 5 *Hansard* (Lords) 188 (20 July 1954) 1175–7; 189 (29 July 1954) 410–14. Milne's daughter admitted to selling carcasses. See *Press & Journal*, 23 July, 7 August 1954.
19. 5 *Hansard*, 530 (15 July 1954) 55; (Lords) 189 (29 July 1954) 417; NA MAF 131/114; Minutes of fifth meeting of MAC Scientific Sub-Committee, 22 July 1954.
20. NA MAF 131/22. W. Bakel to G. Sharman, undated (September or October 1954). See also NAS AF70/784. Annual Report of the North of Scotland College of Agriculture, 1953–4. Here it was stated that observations in the Aberdeen area (one of the hardest hit areas of Scotland) 'suggest that most of the spread has been done by man. In only two outbreaks can the human element be eliminated as unlikely.'
21. *Daily Mirror*, 11 August 1954; *Farmer & Stock-breeder*, 17–18 August 1954, 67; *The Times*, 11 August 1954. Legal advice given to the MAC indicated that the deliberate transmission of myxomatosis by moving an infected animal from one place to another (as opposed to inoculating viral matter) constituted a civil rather than criminal offence. The MAC report glossed over the legal implications of deliberate transmission – probably because it was concerned that an accurate exposition of the law might encourage the movement of infected carcasses. NA MAF 131/113. Opinion of Bazil Wingate-Saul, 7 December 1953; *Report of the Advisory Committee on Myxomatosis*, 7.
22. *Farmer & Stock-breeder*, 17–18 August 1954, 67; *The Times*, 12 August 1954.
23. *Shooting Times*, 28 May 1954, 352.
24. Ibid., 16 July 1954, 463; *The Times*, 6 July 1954.
25. *Farmer & Stock-breeder*, 13–14 July 1954, 51; *The Times*, 2 September 1954. See also 6 and 20 September 1954.
26. See *The Times*, 17 September, 14, 18 and 25 October and 8 November 1954.
27. *Daily Mirror*, 3 August 1954; *The Times*, 28 July 1954.
28. *Farmers Weekly*, 9 July 1954, 83. See also 27 August 1954, 71; 29 October 1954, 85.

29. As we now know this request was made because of prime ministerial concern. See NA PREM 11/585. R. Guppy to D. Pitblado, 10 July 1954. Churchill's intervention is discussed below.

30. NA MAF 131/94. Minutes of joint meeting of MAC and LPAC, 26 July 1954. It would not become entirely irrelevant for the likelihood would be that many areas would still have pockets of disease-free rabbits.

31. For further information on Andrewes's views see his article, 'Myxomatosis in Britain', *Nature*, 174 (1954) 529–30.

32. NA MAF 131/94. Minutes of joint meeting of MAC and LPAC, 26 July 1954. C. W. Hume, of UFAW, also thought that a law against deliberate transmission would be unenforceable. See *Field*, 19 August 1954, 348.

33. Anon., 'News and views', *Nature*, 174 (1954) 1130. The MAC's second report states that Thomas took Evans's place on 7 December 1954. However, the minutes of the committee's seventh meeting, in October, record that the chairman 'welcomed Dr Thomas who was taking the place of Dr Evans'. See *Second Report of the Advisory Committee*, ii; NA MAF 131/114. Minutes of seventh meeting of MAC, 20 October 1954.

34. NA MAF 131/22. L. Sankey to D. Westlake, 14 September 1954; MAF 131/114. Minutes of seventh meeting of MAC, 20 October 1954.

35. NA MAF 131/114. Minutes of seventh meeting of MAC, 20 October 1954.

36. 5 *Hansard* (Lords) 184 (10 December 1953) 1172; 185 (26 January 1954) 414–21.

37. Ibid., (26 January 1954) 414–73; (25 February 1954) 1139–92; 186 (1 April 1954) 931–9.

38. P. Clarke, *Hope and Glory: Britain, 1900–1990* (Harmondsworth: Penguin, 1997) 269. Amory's predecessor, Sir Thomas Dugdale, had resigned in July over the Crichel Down affair. Hence Amory 'succeeded to a Ministry that was under a cloud, and one that was liable to be subject in all its actions to the closest scrutiny by Conservatives everywhere'. He was notoriously lacking in ambition. He had never been a farmer but 'forty or more farms were in the possession of his family' and his 'roots went deep into the Devon countryside'. His biographer asserts that 'farmers were well satisfied' with his performance as minister of agriculture. He also had the respect of the opposition in parliament. W. Gore Allen, *The Reluctant Politician: Derick Heathcoat Amory* (London: Christopher Johnson, 1958), 72, 145–50. See also www.oxforddnb.com.

39. 5 *Hansard* 531 (22 October 1954) 1504.

40. Ibid., 1556.

41. Stenton and Lees, *Who's Who of British MPs*, vol. 4, 15–16.

42. 5 *Hansard* 531 (22 October 1954) 1537–8, 1546–9.

43. Ibid., 1526. King entered parliament in 1950 after a long career as a teacher and headmaster. He became Speaker of the House of Commons in 1965. Stenton and Lees, *Who's Who of British Members of Parliament*, 203; www.oxforddnb.com.

44. Day, *Poison on the Land*, 43; *Field*, 9 December 1954, 1186.

45. *The Times*, 29 October 1954.

46. 5 *Hansard* 532 (3 November 1954) 349; *Shooting Times*, 12 November 1954, 781.

47. 5 *Hansard* 532 (10 November 1954) 1308.
48. Ibid., 1313–14.
49. Ibid., 1314–17; *The Times*, 11 and 22 November 1954.
50. *Farmer & Stock-breeder*, 30 November–1 December 1954, 119; 5 *Hansard* 532 (15 November 1954) 168.
51. *Country Life* 118 (1955) 838. For other critical appraisals, see *Scotsman*, 12 October 1955 (letter from A. R. McDougal); *The Times*, 28 November 1955.
52. 5 *Hansard* (Lords) 189 (22 November 1954) 1756–70. The name 'Bunny' was also a humorous allusion to the Jacobite army officer, John Graham, first Viscount Dundee (*circa* 1648–89). His good looks, leadership skills and campaigning brilliance led supporters and 'historians of the romantic school' to dub him 'Bonnie Dundee'. See www.oxforddnb.com
53. MAF 131/14. Dundee to L. Sankey, 11 November 1954.
54. 5 *Hansard* (Lords) 189 (25 November 1954) 1964; 2 & 3 Eliz. 2 c.68.
55. Day, *Poison on the Land*, 59; *Farmer & Stock-breeder*, 23–24 November 1954, 41; *Glasgow Herald*, 18 November 1954; NA MAF 131/14. Dundee to D. Amory, 16 November 1954, H. Woolley to D. Amory, 16 November 1954; *Second Report of the Advisory Committee*, 2; *The Times*, 18, 19, 22 November 1954.
56. *Farmer & Stock-breeder*, 23–24 November 1954, 35.
57. NA PREM 11/585. D. Pitblado to R. Guppy, 7 July 1954, R. Guppy to D. Pitblado, 10 July 1954.
58. NA PREM 11/585. J. Colville to G. Wilde, 12 August 1954; *The Times*, 7 June 1954. In the course of his life Churchill engaged in many field sports including pig-sticking and wild boar hunting. But for all his bulldog reputation, he could be emotional and compassionate. He treated his many pets with great indulgence and often became strongly attached to livestock on his farm. Though not averse to eating animals he had reared, he was reluctant to wield the carving knife himself. N. Rose, *Churchill: An Unruly Life* (London: Simon & Schuster, 1994) 142, 203. The *Daily Mirror* claimed the Queen had 'a personal interest in myxomatosis, partly because she was 'fond of all animals' but also because of Prince Charles's pet rabbit, Harvey, about which 'he has spent hours chattering to her'. She ordered her keepers to make daily patrols in Windsor Forest and Great Park to shoot infected rabbits. *Daily Mirror*, 31 August 1954; *Shooting Times*, 10 September 1954, 621; *Veterinary Record*, 4 September 1954, 516.
59. NA PREM 11/585. G. Wilde to J. Colville, 14 August 1954.
60. NA PREM 11/585. Minute 2, Cabinet Meeting 10 November 1954; *Second Report of the Advisory Committee*, 2. Churchill and Amory were not close but the prime minister held his colleague in high regard: 'He always sat opposite me in Cabinet when I was Prime Minister and he impressed me.' Lord Moran, *Winston Churchill. The Struggle for Survival, 1940–1965* (London: Constable, 1966) 736.
61. 5 *Hansard* 572 (1 July 1957) 71; NA MAF 131/115. Minutes of eleventh meeting of MAC, 3 December 1957; *Farmers Weekly*, 25 April 1958, 53; *Shooting Times*, 3 May 1958, 351; *The Times*, 23 April 1958.

Chapter 7. After the Deluge

1. NA MAF 131/114. Minutes of seventh meeting of MAC, 20 October 1954; Minutes of eighth meeting of MAC, 8 December 1954. Although the MAC issued no further reports, it continued to meet until 3 December 1957 (its eleventh session). It was then subsumed, along with the Rabbit Clearance Committee and Humane Traps Advisory Committee, into the Advisory Council on Rabbit Clearance (from 1961 the Advisory Council on Rabbits and Other Land Pests). See MAF 131/115. Minutes of eleventh meeting of MAC, 3 December 1957; MAF 131/96. J. Hare to R. Verney, 21 March 1958; MAF 131/154. Minutes of first meeting of ACRC, 16 May 1958; MAF 131/142. Note of H. White, 2 June 1960; 5 *Hansard* 587 (8 May 1958) 121–2.

2. *Second Report of the Advisory Committee*, 1–6.

3. Ibid., 3. In December 1954 Robin Lockley predicted that a successful mopping-up campaign would make 1955 'zero hour for the rabbit in Britain' and that by the end of that year numbers would be at their lowest since Norman times. R. M. Lockley, 'Myxomatosis: a factual survey', *Field*, 9 December 1954, 1174–5.

4. Although Harold Macmillan famously declared that 'most of our people have never had it so good' in July 1957, by common consent Britain's 'austerity years' lasted well into the 1950s. Meat was not derationed until July 1954. See P. Addison, *Now the War is Over: A Social History of Britain* (London: Pimlico, 1995) 27; M. Sissons and P. French (eds) *Age of Austerity* (London: Hodder & Stoughton, 1963) 9; Woods, *A Manufactured Plague*, 93; I. Zweiniger-Bargielowska, *Austerity in Britain: Rationing, Controls and Consumption, 1939–1955* (Oxford: Oxford University Press, 2000).

5. NA MAF 131/113. Draft letter of L. Sankey, 22 December 1953; General note by the Earl of Dundee, undated; NA MAF 131/113. MAC (evidence) No. 5; *Report of the Advisory Committee on Myxomatosis*, 8.

6. MAF131/30. H. White to H. Gardner, 18 February 1954; Myxomatosis–mopping-up. Draft notes for a circular to CAECs, undated; note of a meeting held on 25 February; minute of G. V. Smith, 23 March 1954; MAF 131/114. Memorandum to CAECs, myxomatosis in rabbits, 9 April 1954.

7. 2 & 3 Eliz. 2 c.68.

8. 5 *Hansard* 545 (27 October 1955) 42; *Farmer & Stock-breeder*, 30 November–1 December 1954, 91. Subsidized cyanide gas remained available. By October 1956 £33,625 had been distributed in grants, mostly for scrub clearance. NA MAF 131/124. Summary of CAEC progress reports. Position at end of September 1956.

9. 2 & 3 Eliz. 2 c.68.

10. J. C. Wynne-Edwards, 'Common sense about rabbits', *Field*, 5 January 1956, 16.

11. NA MAF 131/136. Minutes of first meeting of Rabbit Policy Group, 6 March 1957.

12. 5 *Hansard* (Lords) 175 (8 April 1952) 34–5; 185 (26 January 1954) 466–7; 531 (22 October 1954) 1546.

13. NA MAF 131/94. Minutes of joint meeting of MAC and LPAC, 26 July 1954.
14. 5 *Hansard* 531 (22 October 1954) 1544.
15. Ibid., 1547.
16. *Farmer & Stock-breeder*, 23–24 November 1954, 89.
17. NA MAF131/30. Myxomatosis: mopping-up. Draft notes for a circular to CAECs, undated; NA MAF 131/114. Memorandum to CAECs, animal and bird pests control campaign, 1954/1955, 24 June 1954; minutes of seventh meeting of MAC, 20 October 1954; MAF 131/115. Minister to chairmen of CAECs, 5 December 1955.
18. NA FT 4/26. Rabbit investigation, note 11.
19. NA MAF 131/30. H. White to H. Gardner, 29 January 1954. See also Minute of H. Gardner, 10 January 1955; MAF 131/101. Note of L. R. Sankey, 12 January 1955.
20. 5 *Hansard* (Lords) 194 (23 November 1955) 762–4, 812–14.
21. NA MAF 131/115. Press notice of 27 January 1955 (MAF 3741); NA MAF 131/30. Minute of H. Gardner, 10 January 1955. See also MAF 131/95. Minutes of sixth meeting of LPAC, 14 December 1954.
22. NA MAF 131/30. Minute by G. V. Smith, 23 March 1954. In July 1954 *Land Worker* carried a condensed version of Harry Thompson's paper, 'Myxomatosis in rabbits', which had previously appeared in MAF's in-house journal, *Agriculture*.
23. MAF 131/30. H. White to H. Gardner, 4 January 1955; Minute by H. White on myxomatosis – follow-up action. Series of articles in *Farmer & Stock-breeder*, 7 January 1955; Publicity Working Party paper 101 & appendix, 24 January 1955; MAF 131/124. Extract from letter from G. Nugent to Sir Robert Gooch, 27 January 1956; Script of Broadcast by J. L. Brighton; Minutes of first meeting of RCC, 18 January 1956; Minutes of second Meeting of RCC, 8 March 1956; Minutes of third meeting of RCC, 19 April 1956; Minutes of sixth meeting of RCC, 5 February 1957; RCC progress report, January 1957; MAF 131/125. RCC progress report, February 1957; *Farmer & Stock-breeder*, 18–19 January 1955, 46–7; *Field* 3 November 1955, 812.
24. BBC Written Archives Centre (WAC) R19/1560/3 A. D. Bird to G. Baseley, 31 August 1955.
25. BBC WAC R19/1560/6. H. C. Hunt to G. Baseley, 30 August 1956. ITV addressed the mopping-up issue in February 1957.
26. NA MAF 131/30. H. White to H. Gardner, 7 January 1955; MAF 131/129. Draft report on rabbit policy, 15 May 1957; Note of meeting of chairmen of CAECs, 28 November 1957; MAF 131/115. Press notice of 13 October 1955; MAF 131/124. Press notice of 13 November 1956.
27. NA MAF 131/129. Draft report on rabbit policy, 15 May 1957; *Farmers Weekly*, 4 December 1959, 57; *Field*, 8 December 1955, 1091.
28. In 1956 a scheme organized by the NFU's Hampshire branch paid 2s (10p) for every pair of rabbit ears. It paid out over £1500 in March and April. Such reward schemes were viewed with ambivalence in official quarters because of the possibility that they would create a vested interest in rabbit survival. NA MAF 131/95. Memorandum on pests act, 1954; MAF 131/96. Summary of

main points and problems discussed at provincial pest conferences, 26 April–
11 May 1956; MAF 131/124. Minutes of third meeting of RCC, 19 April 1956;
Hampshire NFU rabbit scheme, May 1956; *Farmer & Stock-breeder*, 5–6 June
1956, 107.

29. NA MAF 131/115. Minutes of ninth meeting of MAC, 19 May 1955; MAF
    131/95. Minutes of seventh meeting of LPAC, 15 March 1955.

30. In October 1957, with the promulgation of a rabbit clearance order covering
    the West Riding of Yorkshire, the whole of England and Wales became a
    rabbit clearance area. 5 *Hansard* 535 (27 January 1955) 45; 539 (31 March
    1955) 536–7; 540 (2 May 1955) 1324; 542 (16 June 1955) 752; 543 (30 June
    1955) 486; 549 (19 April 1956) 100; NA MAF 131/129. Anglesey rabbit
    clearance order, 22 March 1955; draft press notice, 18 October 1957; MAF
    131/124. Summary of CAEC progress reports. Position at end of
    September 1956; MAF 131/136. Minutes of first meeting of Rabbit Policy
    Group, 6 March 1957; *Farmer & Stock-breeder*, 18–19 October 1955, 41–2;
    25–26 October 1955, 35; 20 November 1956, 34; *Farmers Weekly*, 21
    October 1955, 52; 18 April 1957, 43.

31. 5 *Hansard* 545 (27 October 1955) 42; NA MAF 131/115. Press Notice of 13
    October 1955.

32. NA MAF 131/115. Minutes of ninth meeting of MAC, 19 May 1955.

33. *Farmer & Stock-breeder*, 14–15 June 1955, 49; 5–6 July 1955, 39; 9–10 August
    1955, 33.

34. Ibid., 15–16 May 1956, 99; 26–27 June 1956, 89.

35. *The Times*, 8 September 1956.

36. NA FT 4/26. Rabbit investigation, note 11.

37. *Farmer & Stock-breeder*, 18–19 October 1955, 41; 5 *Hansard* 545 (31 October
    1955) 76. The Agriculture Act, 1947 sought to provide cheap food for
    consumers and stable incomes for farmers by means of guaranteed prices or
    'deficiency payments', in effect subsidies, for a range of basic agricultural
    products. The level of support was determined by annual (and occasionally
    special) price reviews negotiated with great secrecy by the ministry and a
    politically-privileged NFU. See J. Bowers, 'British agricultural policy since the
    Second World War', *Agricultural History Review* 33 (1985) 66–76; B. Holderness,
    British Agriculture since 1945 (Manchester: Manchester University Press, 1985)
    13–21; A. Howkins, *The Death of Rural England: A Social History of the Countryside
    since 1900* (London: Routledge, 2003) 144; Martin, *The Development of Modern
    Agriculture*, 70–1; M. Shoard, *The Theft of the Countryside* (London: Temple Smith,
    1980) 21–2; M. J. Smith, *The Politics of Agricultural Support in Britain* (Aldershot:
    Dartmouth, 1990) 134–5.

38. MAF 131/124. Minutes of first meeting of RCC, 18 January 1956.

39. *Farmer & Stock-breeder*, 20 November 1956, 34; 5 *Hansard* 558 (5 November
    1956) 1929; 561 (28 November 1956) 56; 562 (21 December 1956) 229; NA
    MAF 131/124. Press Notice of 13 November 1956.

40. *Farmers Weekly*, 26 April 1957, 41; NA MAF 131/124. Press notice of 7
    February 1957.

41. NA MAF 131/115. MAC Progress reports, January 1955–May 1957 and

November 1957; MAF 131/125. RCC progress reports, February 1957–December 1957.
42. NA MAF 131/129. Draft Report on rabbit policy, 15 May 1957.
43. 5 *Hansard* 568 (18 April 1957) 2098–9; 572 (1 July 1957) 71; 573 (8 July 1957) 2–3; NA MAF 131/136. B. Engholm to P. Nicholls, 30 August 1957.
44. 5 *Hansard* 573 (15 July 1957) 756–7; 577 (11 November 1957) 9.
45. NA MAF 131/166. Report on rabbit policy, 9 July 1957.
46. *Bulletin of the Ministry of Agriculture, Fisheries and Food*, 5 (1961) 73. See NA MAF 131/124. RCC, summary of progress reports, June 1956; MAF 131/154. Minutes of fourth meeting of ACRC, 14 December 1959. By 1963 there had been two successful prosecutions for failing to deal with rabbits. There were no prosecutions in 1962 and none between 1 October 1964 and 30 September 1967. See MAF 131/166. D. Harty to R. Hornby, 15 March 1963; 5 *Hansard* 674 (27 March 1963) 1291; 755 (29 November 1967) 432.
47. NA MAF 131/136. Rabbit Policy Group. Memorandum on the development of organized rabbit control in England and Wales, 9 January 1957; Minutes of first meeting of Rabbit Policy Group, 6 March 1957; MAF 131/129. M. Keen (NFU) to B. Engholm, 25 November 1957; Submission to Minister, 25 November 1957; *Farmers Weekly*, 25 April 1958, 65.
48. New Zealand had had a serious problem with European wild rabbits since their introduction in the nineteenth century. Government attempts to introduce myxomatosis in the early 1950s failed because of the absence of a suitable insect vector. Since 1947 rabbit control had mainly involved the establishment of mandatory rabbit boards in areas where a majority of landholders were in favour. All occupiers in an area covered by a board were required to contribute to its running costs. Boards received matching funds from the government and employed staff to kill rabbits on all land in their district, mostly by poisoning. From 1948 taxes on skin sales progressively curtailed the value of carcasses. In 1956 the sale and export of rabbit products was made illegal. Anon., 'Editorial note', *Country Life*, 122 (1957) 912; R. Hudson, 'The rabbit problem: lessons from New Zealand', *Country Life*, 122 (1957) 288; Livestock Division, NZ Department of Agriculture Bulletin no. 284, 'The rabbit pest and its control' (Oxford University, Department of Zoology, BAP reprint, 1947); NA MAF 131/166. New Zealand Rabbit Policy, April 1958; H. V. Thompson, 'Rabbit control in Australia and New Zealand', *Agriculture*, 65 (1958) 388–92, 440–4.
49. NA MAF 131/129. Draft report on rabbit policy, 15 May 1957; Minutes of meeting to discuss formation of Rabbit Clearance Societies, 11 November 1957; Submission to minister, 25 November 1957; MAF 131/136. B. Engholm to P. Nicholls, 30 August 1957; MAF 131/96. Press notice of 7 February 1958; J. Hare to R. Verney, 21 March 1958; MAF 131/154. Minutes of first meeting of ACRC, 16 May 1958; Minutes of second meeting of ACROLP, 31 October 1961; 5 *Hansard* 579 (12 December 1957) 153–4; 581 (7 February 1958) 215.
50. *Farmer*, 26 September 1959, 32.
51. NA MAF 131/129. Note of meeting of chairmen of CAECs, 28 November 1957; B. Engholm to Sir R. Manktelow, 10 December 1957; MAF 131/154. Minutes of first meeting of ACRC, 16 May 1958; 5 *Hansard* 587 (8 May 1958) 121.

52. *Farmers Weekly*, 10 January 1958, 34; *Scottish Farmer*, 15 October 1955, 1578; 5 October 1957, 1480.
53. MAF 131/154. Minutes of first meeting of ACRC, 16 May 1958; *Farmers Weekly*, 25 April 1958, 53, 65; *The Times*, 5 May 1958. Subscription rates varied. One of the largest societies, in Wales, charged only 3d (1.25p) per acre. In difficult areas the charge could be as high as 2s 6d (12.5p) per acre. See *The Times*, 20 June 1960.
54. *Farmers Weekly*, 6 February 1959, 49; *Veterinary Record*, 14 February 1959, 132.
55. *Farmers Weekly*, 21 March 1958, 94.
56. Ibid., 25 July 1958, 82.
57. *Country Life*, 18 December 1958, 1458.
58. *The Times*, 5 May 1958.
59. *Country Life*, 12 February 1959, 290; *Farmer & Stock-breeder*, 27 January 1959, 87; 10 February 1959, 61; *Farmers Weekly*, 6 February 1959, 49.
60. *The Times*, 13 January 1960.
61. MAF 131/245. Review of Rabbit Clearance Societies in England and Wales, 1964–5, August 1965; MAF 131/243. Minister's Message to Rabbit Clearance Societies, 22 March 1967.
62. *The Times*, 20 June 1960; NA MAF 131/154. Minutes of second meeting of ACROLP, 31 October 1961.
63. *The Times*, 30 October 1961.
64. NA MAF 131/155. Minutes of fifth meeting of ACROLP, 22 May 1963.
65. NA MAF 131/166. J. Austin to R. Maynard, 4 March 1964; R. Maynard to J. Austin, 9 April 1964. The motion passed was for a pilot scheme in Cornwall.
66. NA MAF 131/245. Review of Rabbit Clearance Societies in England and Wales, 1964–65, August 1965.
67. Ibid; MAF 131/167. Submission to Minister, 16 December 1965.
68. NA MAF 131/80. Land Pests Research Report No. 34. West Wales rabbit survey, 1961–65 (March 1966) 1.
69. Minutes of twelfth meeting of ACROLP, 9 April 1968; MAF 131/243. Minister's Message to Rabbit Clearance Societies, 22 March 1967; 5 *Hansard* 743 (21 March 1967) 242.
70. *The Times*, 21 August 1978. The coypu, a large amphibious rodent native to South America, was farmed in Britain for its fur. Escapees established themselves in parts of East Anglia, particularly in the Norfolk Broads, where they damaged crops and undermined river banks.
71. NA MAF 131/113. MAC Scientific Sub-Committee. Summary of evidence available … for consideration at meeting of sub-committee on 3 December 1953; Minutes of second meeting of MAC Scientific Sub-Committee, 3 December 1953.
72. NA MAF 131/115. Minutes of ninth meeting of MAC, 19 May 1955.
73. NA MAF 131/115. MAC progress report, January 1955–May 1957.
74. *Farmer & Stock-breeder*, 31 January–1 February 1956, 33; 5 *Hansard* 542 (16 June 1955) 751–2; MAF 131/115. Research report of MAC Scientific Sub-Committee, December 1953–December1955, Minutes of tenth meeting of MAC, 18 June 1956, MAC progress report, January 1955–May 1957; *Manchester*

Guardian, 15 February 1956; NA MAF 131/96. Minutes of joint meeting of MAC and LPAC, 12 October 1955; *Veterinary Record*, 24 September 1955, 746–7.

75. NA MAF 131/122. Rabbits in the Dukeries. Undated and unsigned memorandum.

76. NA MAF 131/122. Notes of meeting of 10 October 1955; H. N. White to A. C. Sparks, 21 October 1955; A. K. H. Atkinson to I. Thomas, 5 January 1956.

77. *Daily Express*, 15 February 1956; NA MAF 131/122. Rabbits in the Dukeries. Undated and unsigned memorandum; W. Davies to D. Williams, 23 December 1955.

78. NA MAF 131/122. W. Davies to D. Williams, 23 December 1955; A. K. H. Atkinson to I. Thomas, 5 January 1956; MAF 131/24. Minutes of first meeting of RCC, 18 January 1956.

79. *Daily Express, Manchester Guardian, Newark Advertiser, Nottingham Evening News*, all 15 February 1956; *Retford Times*, 17 February 1956.

80. *Manchester Guardian*, 15 February 1956.

81. NA MAF 131/115. MAC progress report, January 1955–May 1957; 5 *Hansard* 552 (30 April 1956) 2.

82. NA MAF 131/122. Press Notice of 22 March 1956; P. F. Williams's Report on Operation Dukeries, 24 March 1956; W. Pringle to Lord St Aldwyn, 26 March 1956; undated report on rabbit clearing operations in The Dukeries; MAF 131/124. Minutes of second meeting of RCC, 8 March 1956.

83. *Farmers Weekly*, 10 January 1958, 34; NA MAF 131/115. MAC progress report, January 1955–May 1957; MAC progress report, November 1957; Minutes of eleventh meeting of MAC Scientific Sub-Committee, 11 June 1956. The Micheldever outbreak was 'dealt with successfully with the cooperation of the occupiers'.

84. *Farmers Weekly*, 27 December 1957, 21; 5 *Hansard* 552 (30 April 1956) 1; 580 (19 December 1957) 606.

85. NA MAF 131/122. Myxomatosis and rabbit control. Note by L. R. Sankey, 19 October 1958.

86. 5 *Hansard* 596 (4 December 1958) 1339; 607 (23 July 1959) 160.

87. NA MAF 168/14. Investigation of strains of virus, 14 September 1962; Pests newsletter no. 6, July 1964; MAF 131/155. Minutes of eighth meeting of ACROLP, 2 June 1965; ninth meeting of ACROLP, 3 November 1965.

88. *Farmer & Stock-breeder*, 25–26 October 1955, 35. See also *Farmers Weekly*, 19 August 1955, 39, 23 November 1956, 82, 15 March 1957, 59, 21 June 1957, 36 and 19 July 1957, 67; *Gamekeeper & Countryside*, October 1956, 3; *Shooting Times*, 30 December 1955, 843.

89. *Veterinary Record*, 29 January 1955, 105.

90. *Farmers Weekly*, 4 February 1955, 52.

91. NA MAF 131/31. Summary of replies to rabbit questionnaire, July 1955; MAF 131/95. Proposals for 1955–56 land pests destruction campaign; *Field*, 23 June 1955, 1107 and 19 August 1955, 39; *Scottish Farmer*, 18 June 1955, 1042.

92. *Farmers Weekly*, 20 May 1955; 5 *Hansard* 540 (2 May 1955) 1324; NA MAF 131/95. Proposals for 1955–56 land pests destruction campaign.

93. NA MAF 131/95. Minutes of third meeting of LPAC for Wales, 3 May 1955; Minutes of eighth meeting of LPAC, 19 May 1955; MAF 131/96. Minutes of joint meeting of the MAC and LPAC, 12 October 1955; MAF 255/597. D. Heathcoat Amory to H. F. C. Crookshank, 8 December 1955; Press notice of 22 December 1955; *Farmer & Stock-breeder*, 20–21 December 1955; *Field* thought 'all reasonable opinion' would welcome the bill. See *Field*, 2 February 1956, 165, 7 June 1956, 1008 and 19 July 1956, 101; 5 *Hansard* (Lords) 194 (8 December 1955) 1302; 557 (2 August 1956) 191; *Shooting Times*, 20 January 1956, 46, 10 February 1956, 81 and 8 June 1956, 563.

94. *Farmers Weekly*, 23 November 1956, 82 and 19 July 1957, 67; MAF 131/115. Minutes of tenth meeting of MAC, 18 June 1956; MAF 131/124. Minutes of sixth meeting of RCC, 5 February 1957; C. W. Hume's comment on Lord Merthyr's bill, *La Terre et La Vie. Revue d'Histoire Naturelle* 3–4 (1956–7) 263.

95. *Veterinary Record*, 9 July 1955, 534–5.

96. *Farmer & Stock-breeder*, 1–2 May 1956, 77; *Farmers Weekly*, 27 April 1956, 51; 5 *Hansard* 547 (12 December 1955) 794–5; *The Times*, May 28 1956.

97. *Glasgow Herald*, 23 July 1955. See also 10 August, 14 November 1955.

98. NA MAF 131/115. Minutes of eleventh meeting of MAC Scientific Sub-Committee, 11 June 1956; MAC Paper no. 20, use of myxomatosis for rabbit control, 12 June 1956.

99. NA MAF 131/115. Minutes of eleventh meeting of MAC Scientific Sub-Committee, 11 June 1956; Note of L. R. Sankey on use of myxomatosis for rabbit control, 12 June 1956; Minutes of tenth meeting of MAC, 18 June 1956; NA MAF 131/115. MAC progress report, January 1955–May 1957.

100. NA MAF 131/136. Minutes of first meeting of Rabbit Policy Group, 6 March 1957.

101. NA MAF 131/136. Analysis of rabbit situation in 12 counties, 17 April 1957.

102. NA MAF 131/136. B. Engholm to P. Nicholls, 30 August 1957.

103. NA MAF 131/115. Minutes of eleventh meeting of MAC, 3 December 1957.

104. NA MAF 131/154. Minutes of first meeting of ACRC, 16 May 1958.

105. NA MAF 131/154. Minutes of first meeting of ACROLP, 25 April 1961; Minutes of second meeting of ACROLP, 31 October 1961.

106. NA MAF 131/115. Press notice of 13 October 1955; see Anon., 'It's war now to the last rabbit', *Farmers Weekly*, 21 October 1955, 52–3.

107. 5 *Hansard* 548 (16 February 1956) 2505. See *Field*, 5 January 1956, 16; *Southern Weekly News*, 30 December 1955.

108. See for example *Field*, 27 October 1955, 752.

109. Barrett-Hamilton, *A History of British Mammals*, vol. 2, 211–12; *Land Worker*, 34 (December 1953) 9; Livestock Division, 'The rabbit pest and its control', 1. Dugald Macintyre estimated that a pair of rabbits, taking into account losses caused by vermin, was capable of producing 1000 descendants in three years. See Macintyre, *Nature Notes*, 160.

110. *The Times*, 28 November 1955.

111. A. G. Street, *Feather Bedding* (London: Faber & Faber, 1954) 127. See also *Farmers Weekly*, 6 August 1954, 67.

112. C. S. Jarvis, 'A countryman's notes', *Country Life*, 114 (1953) 1031.

113. Lockley, *Private Life of the Rabbit*, 16.
114. 5 *Hansard* (Lords) 194 (23 November 1955) 778.
115. *Farmers Weekly*, 27 August 1954, 71, 3 September 1954, 53, 12 August 1955, 61, 29 March 1957, 65, 3 May 1957, 75, 12 July 1957, 47, 13 September 1957, 82, 14 February 1958, 47, 25 July 1958, 82, 9 January 1959, 47, 23 January 1959, 51, 13 February 1959, 52, 60 and 20 February 1959, 50; 5 *Hansard* 570 (14 May 1957) 13.
116. MAF 131/167. Submission to minister, 16 December 1965; V. H. Bath, 'The rabbit clearance society movement: a new look', *Agriculture* (July 1967) 307–8.
117. *Farmers Weekly*, 3 September 1954, 53.
118. See for example P. W. J. Bartrip and P. T. Fenn, 'The evolution of regulatory style in the nineteenth century British factory inspectorate', *Journal of Law and Society*, 10 (1983) 201–27; W. G. Carson, 'White collar crime and the enforcement of factory legislation', *British Journal of Criminology*, 10 (1970) 383–98; K. O. Hawkins, *Environment and Enforcement* (Oxford: Clarendon Press, 1984); B. Hutter, *Compliance, Regulation and Environment* (Oxford: Clarendon Press, 1997).
119. NA MAF 131/125. Minutes of seventh meeting of RCC, 8 May 1957.
120. NA MAF 131/166. Report on rabbit policy, 9 July 1957.
121. NA MAF 131/129. Note of meeting of chairmen of CAECs, 28 November 1957. For further discussion of these issues, see MAF 131/154. Minutes of second meeting of ACROLP, 31 October 1961; MAF 131/155. Minutes of fifth meeting of ACROLP, 22 May 1963.
122. M. Winter, *Rural Politics* (London: Routledge, 1996) 110.
123. See for example D. Vogel, *National Styles of Regulation: Environmental Policy in Great Britain and the United States* (Ithaca: Cornell University Press, 1986).

Chapter 8. Agriculture and Environment

1. NA FT 1/2. Lord Rothschild to E. M. Nicholson, 8 June 1953. Note by E. M. Nicholson on rabbits and the balance of payments, 14 July 1948.
2. Middleton, *The Control*, 3.
3. NA FT 1/2. Lord Rothschild to E. M. Nicholson, 8 June 1953.
4. *Field*, 22 July 1954, 171 and 3 March 1955, 353; 5 *Hansard* (Lords) 184 (11 November 1953) 211; 185 (26 January 1954) 447–8, 471; NA MAF 131/113. MAC Paper No. 11, undated.
5. *Report of the Advisory Committee on Myxomatosis*, 5. See Report of the Committee on Cruelty, 520–1; 5 *Hansard* 531 (22 October 1954) 1515. Surveys of rabbit damage to crops in Britain before the arrival of myxomatosis included B. M. Church et al., 'Surveys of rabbit damage to wheat in England and Wales, 1950–2', *Plant Pathology*, 2 (1953) 107–12; B. M. Church et al., 'Survey of rabbit damage to winter cereals, 1953–4', *Plant Pathology*, 5 (1956) 66–9; H. C. Gough and F. W. Dunnett, 'Rabbit damage to winter corn', *Agriculture*, 57 (1950) 374–8; H. V. Thompson, 'The grazing behaviour of the wild rabbit, *oryctolagus cuniculus* (l.)', *British Journal of Animal Behaviour*, 1 (1953) 1–4.
6. Thompson and Worden, *The Rabbit*, 161–2, 171–2.

7. Day, *Poison on the Land*, 62–3; *Field*, 3 March 1955, 353; 24 March 1955, 487; 2 June 1955, 986 and 17 December 1955, 904; *Shooting Times*, 18 March 1955, 174, 6 May 1955, 281, 18 November 1955, 742 and 2 December 1955, 775–6.

8. Marchington, *Pugs and Drummers*, 119.

9. Thompson, 'The rabbit in Britain', 93.

10. Anon., 'Value of myxomatosis', extract from *Rural Research in CSIRO*, 8 (1954) Oxford University Zoology Library, BAP Reprint Collection; P. A. Reid, 'Some economic results of myxomatosis', *Quarterly Review of Agricultural Economics*, 6 (1953) 93–4.

11. *Farmer & Stock-breeder*, 29–30 March 1955, 42–3.

12. NA MAF 131/115. Minutes of ninth meeting of MAC, 19 May 1955.

13. *Field*, 4 August 1955, 223. See *Farmer & Stock-breeder*, 19–20 July 1955, 38–9.

14. *Field*, 27 October 1955, 752.

15. *Farmers Weekly*, 5 August 1955, 67, 16 September 1955, 48. See also A. G. Armitage and R. E. Rogers, 'Crops not rabbits', *Agriculture*, 62 (1955) 313–15; *Land Worker*, 36 (1955) 3; *Lancet*, 7 January 1956, 32; *Scottish Farmer*, 22 October 1955, 1603; H. V. Thompson, 'Myxomatosis: a survey', *Agriculture*, 63 (1956) 52–3.

16. 5 *Hansard* (Lords) 194 (23 November 1955) 757. See 5 *Hansard*, 195 (20 December 1955) 376–77.

17. 5 *Hansard* (Lords) 194 (23 November 1955) 767.

18. *Southern Weekly News*, 30 December 1955. See *Shooting Times*, 19 August 1955, 522.

19. *Farmer & Stock-breeder*, 25–26 October 1955, 35; *Farmers Weekly*, 4 November 1955, 37; *Glasgow Herald*, 3 December 1955; 5 *Hansard* (Lords) 194 (23 November 1955) 773–4.

20. *Field*, 29 July 1954, 218, 3 March 1955, 353, 24 March 1955, 487, 28 April 1955, 727 and 2 June 1955, 986. See also 29 September 1955, 559.

21. NA MAF 131/115. Minutes of ninth meeting of MAC, 19 May 1955.

22. NA MAF 131/115. Press notice of 13 October 1955. See 5 *Hansard* 545 (27 October 1955) 42–3.

23. 5 *Hansard* 545 (31 October 1955) 76. See 547 (5 December 1955) 14. On the APR see Chapter 7.

24. *Farmer & Stock-breeder*, 29–30 November 1955, 119.

25. *Field*, 8 December 1955, 1091 and 2 February 1956, 165. Though some places experienced the 'worst drought in living memory', the 'brilliant summer of 1955 was accompanied by bumper harvests of many crops'. See also *Farmer & Stock-breeder*, 25–26 October 1955, 35, 39; Thompson, 'Myxomatosis: a survey', 52. See 5 *Hansard* (Lords) 194 (23 November 1955) 767.

26. *Land Worker*, 36 (November 1955) 3. See also *Farmer & Stock-breeder*, 8–9 November 1955, 41, 101 and 103, 15–16 November 1955, 40, 29–30 November 1955, 37, 46, 119; *Farmers Weekly*, 28 October 1955, 49.

27. 5 *Hansard* 547 (5 December 1955) 547; 548 (16 February 1956) 2505. See (2 February 1956) 1055–6, (13 February 1956) 225–6; 549 (20 February 1956) 23–4.

28. *Farmer & Stock-breeder*, 10 February 1959, 53.

29. *Farmers Weekly*, 6 February 1959, 39.
30. *Farmer & Stock-breeder*, 19–20 June 1956, 29, 4–5 September 1956, 44–5. See I. S. Macadam (ed.) *Annual Register of World Events, 1957* (London: Longmans, Green & Co., 1958) 49; I. S. Macadam (ed.) *Annual Register of World Events, 1958* (London: Longmans, Green & Co., 1959) 31, 50.
31. Martin, *The Development of Modern Agriculture*, 98. See also Holderness, *British Agriculture since 1945*; Howkins, *The Death of Rural England*, 150.
32. Martin, *The Development of Modern Agriculture*, 76–7.
33. Thompson, 'The rabbit in Britain', 91.
34. J. Ross, 'Myxomatosis: the natural evolution of the disease', *Symposia of the Zoological Society of London*, 50 (1982) 89.
35. B. Boag, 'Reduction in numbers of the wild rabbit (*oryctolagus cuniculus*) due to agricultural practices and land use', *Crop Protection*, 6 (1987) 347–51; M. J. Crawley, 'Rabbits as pests of winter wheat', in R. J. Putnam (ed.) *Mammals as Pests* (London: Chapman Hall, 1989) 168–77; S. Mills, 'Rabbits breed a growing controversy', *New Scientist*, 109 (1986) 50–4; W. A. Rees et al., 'Humane control of rabbits', in D. P. Britt (ed.) *Humane Control of Land Animals and Birds* (Potters Bar: UFAW, 1985) 96; J. Ross and A. M. Tittensor, 'Influence of myxomatosis in regulating rabbit numbers', *Mammal Review*, 16 (1986) 163–8; Thompson, 'The rabbit in Britain', 93; R. C. Trout et al., 'Recent trends in the rabbit population in Britain', *Mammal Review*, 16 (1986) 117–23; www.mammal.org. uk/rabbit.
36. www.abdn.ac.uk/mammal/estimates2004.
37. A. S. Thomas, 'Changes in vegetation since the advent of myxomatosis', *Journal of Ecology*, 48 (1960) 287–30.
38. A. Wallis, 'The flora of the Cambridge district', in J. E. Marr and A. E. Shipley (eds) *Handbook to the Natural History of Cambridgeshire* (Cambridge: Cambridge University Press, 1904) 224.
39. E. P. Farrow, 'On the ecology of the vegetation of Breckland. III. General effects of rabbits on the vegetation', *Journal of Ecology*, 5 (1917) 1–18; Tansley, *The British Islands*, 136.
40. Tansley, *The British Islands*, 136; A. S. Watt, 'Studies in the ecology of Breckland. I. Climate, soil and vegetation', *Journal of Ecology*, 24 (1936) 117; A. S. Watt, 'Studies in the ecology of Breckland. II. The origin and development of blow-outs', *Journal of Ecology*, 25 (1937) 91.
41. E. P. Farrow, *Plant Life on East Anglian Heaths: Being Observational and Experimental Studies of the Vegetation of Breckland* (Cambridge: Cambridge University Press, 1925) 25. See also C. Elton, *Animal Ecology* (London: Sidgwick & Jackson, 1927) 51–2; E. W. Fenton, 'The influence of rabbits on the vegetation of certain hill-grazing districts of Scotland', *Journal of Ecology*, 28 (1940) 438–49.
42. A. G. Tansley, *Britain's Green Mantle: Past, Present and Future* (London: George Allen & Unwin, 1949) 50.
43. Tansley, *The British Islands*, 138.
44. A. S. Watt, 'The effect of excluding rabbits from grassland A (*xerobrometum*) in Breckland, 1936–60', *Journal of Ecology*, 50 (1962) 197.

45. A. S. Thomas, 'Further changes in vegetation since the advent of myxomatosis', *Journal of Ecology*, 51 (1963) 179.

46. See H. N. Southern, 'If rabbits should disappear', *Country Life*, 115 (8 April 1954) 1024–26; Tansley, *Britain's Green Mantle*, 51–2; Wallis, 'The flora', 227.

47. W. Davies, 'The grasslands of Wales', in R. G. Stapledon (ed.) *A Survey of the Agricultural and Wastelands of Wales* (London: Faber & Faber, 1936) 51; F. W. Oliver, 'Some remarks on Blakeney Point, Norfolk', *Journal of Ecology*, 1 (1913) 14; H. N. Southern, 'Ecologists are excited by England's "rabbit disease"', *Animal Kingdom*, 59 (1956) 117; Tansley, *The British Islands*, 138–9; Tansley, *Britain's Green Mantle*, 50–2.

48. Barrett-Hamilton, *A History of British Mammals*, vol. 2, 212–13; Simpson, *The Wild Rabbit*, chapter 3; Wallis, 'The flora', 227–8.

49. E. P. Farrow, 'On the ecology of the vegetation of Breckland. II Factors relating to the relative distributions of *calluna*-heath and grass-heath in Breckland', 4 (1916) 64; R. G. Stapledon, 'Permanent grass', in W. G. R. Paterson (ed.) *Farm Crops. III. Pastures and Hay* (London: Gresham, 1925) 88–9.

50. Tansley, *Britain's Green Mantle*, 52.

51. J. F. Hope-Simpson, 'The utilization and improvement of chalk down pastures', *Journal of the Royal Agricultural Society of England*, 100 (1940) 44–9. See NA FT 1/1. J. F. Hope–Simpson to H. V. Thompson, 9 March 1949; Stapledon, 'Permanent grass', 75.

52. Smith, *Ecology of the English Chalk*, 262.

53. British Ecological Society, 'Nature conservation and nature reserves', *Journal of Ecology*, 32 (1944) 62; Smith, *Ecology of the English Chalk*, 262.

54. Elton, *Animal Ecology*, 51–2.

55. Moore, *Bird of Time*, 125, 135.

56. H. N. Southern and J. S. Watson, 'Summer food of the red fox (*vulpes vulpes*) in Great Britain: a preliminary report', *Journal of Animal Ecology*, 10 (1941) 1–11.

57. C. M. Morrison, 'Second thoughts on rabbits', *Field*, 31 December 1953, 1181. See G. Cobnut, 'Foxes and myxomatosis in Kent', *Oryx: British Mammals*, 3 (1955) 156–7; R. Henriques, 'Farmers' ordinary', *Field*, 21 January 1954, 109.

58. NA FT 1/2. Note by E. M. Nicholson on rabbits and the balance of payments, 14 July 1948. Nicholson was then secretary of the Lord President of the Council's office.

59. Moore, *Bird of Time*, 124.

60. NA FT 1/2. E. M. Nicholson to R. Franklin, 23 October 1953. The Nature Conservancy (later Nature Conservancy Council and, later still, English Nature) was established under the terms of the national parks and access to the countryside act, 1949 (12 & 13 Geo. 6 c.97).

61. An NC officer, Norman Moore, attended MAC meetings as an observer and served as a member of its scientific subcommittee. See Moore, *Bird of Time*, 124.

62. NA MAF 131/113. Minutes of second meeting of MAC Scientific Sub-Committee, 3 December 1953.

63. NA FT 1/2. J. D. Ovington to E. M. Nicholson, 10 November 1953; FT 1/3. N. W. Moore to E. M. Nicholson, 14 December 1953.

64. NA FT 4/26. Minutes of Grants Sub-Committee, 19 November 1953; *PP* 1953–4 xvii, Annual Report of Nature Conservancy, 1953–54, appendix vi, 142–3, 184; *The Times*, 18 January 1956. Lockley later wrote that 'my experience in studying rabbit control methods at Skokholm led to an invitation from the Nature Conservancy to investigate on their behalf the progress of myxomatosis, when it broke out in England in 1953.' However, his rabbit research project was under consideration months before myxomatosis reached Britain. See FT 4/26. R. M. Lockley to E. M. Nicholson, 22 July 1953.

65. NA FT 4/26. R. Lockley to M. Nicholson, 22 July 1953; M. Southern to M. Nicholson, 18 August 1953; C. Elton to M. Nicholson, 26 August 1953; Minutes of Grants Sub-Committee, 19 November 1953. Lockley, born 1903, was an author, naturalist and farmer. He published his first book in 1932. Many others, on birds, farming, natural history and travel, followed. In 1977 the University of Wales awarded him an honorary M.Sc. Lockley emigrated to New Zealand in the 1970s. *The Times*, 28 November 1977; *Who's Who 1991* (London: A & C Black, 1991) 1120.

66. NA CAB 124/2884. Memorandum by GMN [Nicholson], 18 November 1954.

67. In his book Lockley 'particularly' acknowledged Nicholson's 'interest and help'. In 1974 Adams wrote an introduction to a reissue in which he described *The Private Life of the Rabbit* as 'an exceptional work of observation and natural history'. *Watership Down* includes several references to myxomatosis, sometimes called the 'white blindness'. See Lockley, *Private Life of the Rabbit*, 5–6, 16; *Times Literary Supplement*, 28 January 1965 and 8 October 1976.

68. NA FT 4/26. Extract from Comments from C. Elton, 10 November 1953.

69. NA FT1/2. Lockley's typescript on 'The effect which a substantial reduction in the wild rabbit population would have on the fauna and flora of Great Britain', 25 November 1953.

70. NA FT 4/26. Rabbit investigation, note 6.

71. Ibid.

72. NA FT 4/26. Rabbit investigation, note 9; Rabbit investigation, note 10. See R. M. Lockley, 'The observed effects of myxomatosis on rabbit populations and behaviour and on wild life generally', *La Terre et La Vie. Revue d'Histoire Naturelle* 3 (4) 1956–57, 211–19.

73. NA FT 4/26. R. Lockley's draft paper, 'Survival of the wild rabbit', 5 December 1959.

74. Lockley, *Private Life of the Rabbit*, 128.

75. K. J. Sumption and J. R. Flowerdew, 'The ecological effects of the decline in rabbits (*oryctolagus cuniculus* L.) due to myxomatosis', *Mammal Review*, 15 (1985) 151–86.

76. Fenner and Fantini, *Biological Control*; Thompson, 'The rabbit in Britain', 64–107.

77. Rackham, *History of the Countryside*, 303.

78. K. M. Backhouse and H. V. Thompson, 'Myxomatosis', *Nature*, 176 (1955) 155–6; *Country Life*, 15 August 1957, 288; Fenner and Fantini, *Biological Control*, 281; A. S. Thomas, 'Biological effects of the spread of myxomatosis among rabbits', *La Terre et La Vie. Revue d'Histoire Naturelle*, 103 (1956) 239–42.

79. Rackham, *The History of the Countryside*, 48.

80. Rees et al., 'Humane control', 96.

81. Thomas, 'Biological effects of the spread of myxomatosis', 239–42.

82. J. A. Thomas, 'Why did the Large Blue become extinct in Britain', *Oryx*, 15 (1980) 243–7. The Large Blue was successfully reintroduced to certain areas in the 1980s. In 2006 the British population was estimated at 7000. The adonis blue has also recovered. *The Times*, 15 May 2006.

83. Moore, *Bird of Time*, 135.

84. On foxes, see for example Cobnut, 'Foxes and myxomatosis', 156–7; J. S. Fairley, 'An indication of the food of the fox in Northern Ireland after myxomatosis', *Irish Naturalists' Journal*, 15 (1966) 149–51; 5 *Hansard*, 535 (17 February 1955) 533; R. Hewson and H. H. Kolb, 'Changes in the number and distribution of foxes (*Vulpes vulpes*) killed in Scotland from 1949 to 1970', *Journal of Zoology*, 171 (1973) 345–65; J. A. Ingleby, 'Sheep, foxes and rabbits', *Scottish Agriculture*, 36 (1956) 69–70; R. A. Lever, 'The diet of the fox since myxomatosis', *Journal of Animal Ecology*, 28 (1959) 359–75; R. A. Lever et al., 'Myxomatosis and the fox', *Agriculture*, 64 (1957) 105–11; J. D. Lockie, 'After myxomatosis: notes on the food of some predatory animals in Scotland', *Scottish Agriculture*, 36 (1956) 65–9; H. N. Southern, 'A second year of myxomatosis', *Country Life*, 118 (17 November 1955) 1134–5; H. N. Southern, 'Myxomatosis and the balance of nature', *Agriculture*, 63 (1956) 10–13; H. V. Thompson, 'Myxomatosis in the United Kingdom', Oxford University Zoology Library. BAP Reprint Collection.

85. C. King, *The Natural History of Weasels and Stoats* (London: Christopher Helm, 1989) 208–9; Southern, 'Myxomatosis and the balance', 10–13.

86. N. W. Moore, 'Rabbits, buzzards and hares: two studies on the indirect effects of myxomatosis', *La Terre et La Vie. Revue d'Histoire Naturelle*, 103 (1956) 220–5 and 266–7; N. W. Moore, 'The past and present status of the buzzard in the British Isles', *British Birds*, 50 (1957) 173–97; Moore, *Bird of Time*, 126–32; J. Sheail, 'The management of an animal population: changing attitudes towards the wild rabbit in Britain', *Journal of Environmental Management*, 33 (1991) 200; C. R. Tubbs, *The Buzzard* (Newton Abbot: David & Charles, 1974) 20, 73–6.

87. Southern, 'A second year', 1134–5; Southern, 'Ecologists are excited', 116–23; Southern, 'Myxomatosis and the balance', 10–13; Southern, 'The natural control of a population of tawny owls, *strix aluco*', *Journal of Zoology*, 162 (1970) 197–285.

88. Southern, 'Myxomatosis and the balance', 13; Thomas, 'Biological effects of the spread of myxomatosis', 239–42; H. V. Thompson, 'The origin and spread of myxomatosis with particular reference to Great Britain', *La Terre et La Vie. Revue d'Histoire Naturelle*, 103 (1956) 149. See also P. Bourlière, 'Biological consequences due to the presence of myxomatosis', *La Terre et La Vie. Revue d'Histoire Naturelle*, 103 (1956) 131–6.

89. Thomas, 'Further changes in vegetation', 181–3.

90. Rackham, *The History of the Countryside*, 48.

91. L. Durrell, *State of the Ark* (London: Bodley Head, 1986) 113.

92. Moore, *Bird of Time*, 135.

93. 5 *Hansard* 557 (26 July 1956) 612.
94. *The Times*, 18 January 1956.
95. Moore, *Bird of Time*, 135; Ross, 'Myxomatosis: the natural evolution', 89.
96. Thompson, 'The rabbit in Britain', 81–2. See Thompson, 'Myxomatosis: a survey', 54.

Chapter 9. Attitude and Opinion

1. Quoted in Day, *Poison on the Land*, 44–5. I have been unable to locate a copy of the sermon except in Day's book. No trace of it could be found in Winchester Cathedral archives. The date of its delivery is uncertain but internal evidence points to August 1954 or soon after.
2. *Daily Mirror*, 31 August 1954; *Glasgow Herald*, 31 August 1954; *Kent & Sussex Courier*, 3 September 1954; *Press & Journal*, 23 September 1954; RSPCA, Annual Report, 1954, 19–20; *Shooting Times*, 10 September 1954, 621; *The Times*, 31 August 1954; *Veterinary Record*, 4 September 1954, 516.
3. *Kent & Sussex Courier*, 10 September 1954.
4. British Library. National Sound Archive. BBC Home Service broadcast on myxomatosis, *War on the Warren*, 14 September 1954.
5. A. Briggs, *The History of Broadcasting in the United Kingdom*, vol 4, *Sound and Vision, 1945–55* (Oxford: Oxford University Press, 1995) 522.
6. *Listener*, 12 August 1954.
7. *Southern Weekly News* appeared between 1876 and 1965. It continued for a few more years as the *Brighton and Hove Gazette and Southern Weekly News*.
8. *Southern Weekly News*, 30 October 1953.
9. Ibid., 6 November 1953.
10. Ibid., 11 June 1954.
11. Ibid., 2 July 1954.
12. Ibid., 6 August 1954.
13. Ibid., 30 December 1955; *Shooting Times*, 25 November 1955, 753.
14. *Southern Weekly News*, 6 January 1956. See also 13 and 20 January and 3 February 1956.
15. *Essex Chronicle*, 4 November 1955; *Shooting Times*, 9 December 1955, 798.
16. *Essex Chronicle*, 11, 18 and 25 November 1955.
17. *Louth and North Lincolnshire Advertiser*, 5 June 1954.
18. *Kent and Sussex Courier*, 3 September 1954; *West Sussex Gazette*, 22 July, 12 August 1954. See also *Western Morning News*, 8 May, 10 June, 1, 3, 6 and 14 July 1954.
19. *The Times*, 2, 4, 7 and 10 November 1953, 18 June, 31 July and 2 August 1954, and 18 January 1956.
20. Ibid., 11, 13 and 17 November 1953, 25 and 28 June, and 30 July 1954. See also 18 January 1956.
21. Ibid., 5 November 1953.
22. Ibid., 16 November 1953; see 2 December 1955.
23. *Manchester Guardian*, 27 July 1954.
24. Ibid., 14, 25, 30 August 1954. The *Guardian* also printed C. W. Hume's letter appealing for people to help with the mercy killing of infected animals.

25. *News Chronicle*, 13 November 1953.
26. *Daily Mail*, 28 January 1955.
27. *Daily Mirror*, 20 July 1954.
28. Ibid., 3 August 1954.
29. Ibid., 24 August 1954.
30. *People*, 4 and 7 July 1954.
31. *Daily Dispatch*, 17 July 1954.
32. *News of the World*, 1 November 1953.
33. Ibid., 11 July 1954. See also 26 December 1954. Wightman (1901–1971), a Durham graduate, became a freelance journalist and broadcaster in 1948 following a 25-year career as an agricultural lecturer and adviser in Devon, Wiltshire and Dorset. Between 1948 and 1970 he wrote many books on farming and the countryside. See www.knowuk.co.uk (*Who Was Who*).
34. *Glasgow Herald*, 1 and 2 February 1954.
35. Ibid., 19 June 1954.
36. Ibid., 2 August 1954.
37. See for example ibid., 19 July 1954.
38. Ibid., 24, 26, 27, 28, 30, 31 July, 2 August 1954.
39. *Scotsman*, 24 July 1954.
40. *Press & Journal*, 15, 22, 31 July 1954.
41. See for example ibid., 29 July, 4, 11 August , 8 September
42. Ibid., 5 August 1954.
43. *Gamekeeper & Countryside*, December 1953, 33, 40–1.
44. Ibid., May 1954, 135. See August 1954, 197, September 1954, 216, November 1954, 26–7 and April 1955, 134.
45. Ibid., August 1956, 187, October 1956, 3 and November 1956, 35.
46. Ibid., September 1954, 227.
47. Ibid., October 1954, 15. See also November 1954, 35 and September 1955, 235.
48. Ibid., December 1954, 54.
49. Ibid., September 1955, 235.
50. *Gamekeepers' Gazette*, August 1955, 4335.
51. *Shooting Times*, 17 October 1953, 660. See also 14 November 1953, 727.
52. Ibid., 12 February 1954, 100, 23 April 1954, 272, 17 September 1954, 647, 658, 6 May 1955, 281–2, 2 December 1955, 775–6, 20 April 1956, 266, 3 May 1957, 343 and 11 December 1959, 927.
53. Ibid., 28 May 1954, 338, 352, 9 July 1954, 442. See also 4 June 1954, 354, 23 July 1954, 482, 485, 20 August 1954, 562, 24 September 1954, 662, 17 December 1954, 874, 11 February 1955, 82, 19 August 1955, 522, 11 May 1956, 294, 8 June 1956, 368, 20 March 1959, 228.
54. Ibid., 20 March 1959, 228.
55. Ibid., 7 November 1953, 705, 19 December 1953, 809, 9 July 1954, 455, 16 July 1954, 463.
56. Ibid., 11 June 1954, 374, 18 June 1954, 390, 25 June 1954, 415, 2 July 1954, 435, 9 July 1954, 455, 30 July 1954, 514–15, 6 August 1954, 534–5, 20 August 1954, 574–5, 27 August 1954, 595; 3 September 1954, 615, 10 September 1954,

634, 8 October 1954, 711; 29 October 1954, 758, 5 November 1954, 774, 12 November 1954, 790, 18 November 1955, 742, 31 December 1954, 942, 7 January 1955, 10, 4 March 1955, 143, 25 November 1955, 765.

57. Ibid., 8 October 1954, 711.

58. Ibid., 17 September 1954, 654–55, 1 October 1954, 694–55, 697, 15 October 1954, 726–27, 29 October 1954, 758, 5 November 1954, 774, 19 November 1954, 810, and 27 May 1955, 335.

59. See for example ibid., 24 September 1954, 662.

60. See R. N. Rose, *The Field 1853–1953: A Centenary History* (London: Michael Joseph, 1953).

61. *Field*, 12 November 1953, 834.

62. Ibid., 31 December 1953, 1181.

63. Ibid., 15 July 1954, 111. See also 12 August 1954, 289.

64. Ibid., 1 July 1954, 31. See also 19 August 1954, 357.

65. Ibid., 5 August 1954, 243.

66. Ibid., 4 November 1954, 872, 17 February 1955, 255, 19 July 1956, 101, 4 July 1957, 13, 18 July 1957, 118, and 15 August 1957, 265.

67. Ibid., 10 June 1954, 1981, 29 July 1954, 218, 19 August 1954, 348, 26 August 1954, 387, 23 September 1954, 577, 7 October 1954, 671, 21 October 1954, 791, 28 October 1954, 840, 4 November 1954, 884, 2 December 1954, 1132, 6 January 1955, 27, 13 January 1955, 67, 27 January 1955, 147, 3 February 1955, 187; 6 October 1955, 601, 22 December 1955, 1196, 8 March 1956, 377, 1 August 1957, 199, 22 August 1957, 315, 8 January 1959, 69.

68. Ibid., 2 September 1954, 429, 13 January 1955, 67, 20 January 1955, 107, 27 January 1955, 147, 16 February 1956, 247, 19 April, 1956, 677, 13 May 1954, 858, 15 July 1954, 125, 18 July 1957, 118.

69. *Scottish Field*, September 1954, 8. See also October 1956, 16.

70. Ibid., August 1955, 2.

71. *Country Life*, 29 October 1953, 1403.

72. Ibid., 29 October 1953, 1402. See also 1 December 1955, 1242.

73. Ibid., 24 February 1955, 552.

74. Ibid., 26 August 1954, 655, 10 May 1956, 995.

75. Ibid., 9 September 1954, 815–16. See also 16 September 1954, 903–4, 30 September 1954, 1080.

76. *Countryman*, 49 (1954) 169–70, 391–2, and 52 (1955) 386.

77. *Farmers Weekly*, 5 September 1952, 60–1.

78. Ibid., 17 April 1953, 36.

79. Ibid., 23 October 1953, 38.

80. Ibid., 25 June 1954, 40, 6 August 1954, 36, and 3 September 1954, 52.

81. Ibid., 26 April, 1957, 41

82. Ibid., 6 February 1959, 39

83. Ibid., 8 October 1954, 711.

84. www.oxforddnb.com.

85. *Farmers Weekly*, 27 November 1953, 63.

86. Ibid., 9 July 1954, 83, 6 August 1954, 67, 27 August 1954, 29 March 1957, 65, 3 May 1957, 75, 19 June 1957, 67, 13 September 1957, 82, 17 January 1958, 75, 25 July 1958, 82.

87. Ibid., 25 September 1953, 37.

88. Ibid., 6 November 1953, 36, 20 November 1953, 36, 27 November 1953, 38.

89. Ibid., 16 July 1954, 35.

90. Ibid., 6 August 1954, 37.

91. Ibid., 3 September 1954, 54. See 10 September 1954, 48.

92. Ibid., 23 July 1954, 33.

93. Ibid., 10 September 1954, 48.

94. *Farmer & Stock-breeder*, 7–8 September 1954, 115, 117, 5–6 October 1954, 115, 16–17 November 1954, 51, 23–24 November 1954, 101, 30 November–1 December 1954, 109, 29–30 March 1955, 99, 101, 8–9 November 1955, 103.

95. Ibid., 27–28 October 1953, 35. See 27–28 April 1954, 35, 22–23 June 1954, 27, and 17–18 August 1954, 37.

96. Ibid., 10–11 November 1953, 87, and 17–18 August 1954, 116.

97. *Scottish Farmer*, 24 July 1954, 1115. See also 7 August 1954.

98. Ibid., 31 July 1954, 1141. See also 28 August 1954, 1245.

99. Ibid., 11 September 1954, 1307. See also 4 September 1954, 1275.

100. Ibid., 12 March 1955, 593.

101. Ibid., 20 August 1955, 1323.

102. *Shooting Times*, 20 August 1954, 574.

103. See, for example, *Quarterly Journal of Forestry*, 44 (1950) 181–2.

104. *Quarterly Journal of Forestry*, 47 (1953) 123–5.

105. *Quarterly Journal of Forestry*, 48 (1954) 3.

106. P. L. Shanks et al., 'Experiments with myxomatosis in the Hebrides', *British Veterinary Journal*, 111 (1955) 25–30.

107. Editorial, 'Man's concern for his animals', *British Veterinary Journal*, 110 (1954) 445–6.

108. *Veterinary Record*, 29 January 1955, 105. See also 12 March 1955, 211.

109. Ibid., 26 February 1955, 173–4.

110. Ibid., 5 March 1955, 191.

111. *Farmers Weekly*, 4 February 1955, 52.

112. The issue of cruelty is discussed in the Conclusion.

113. *Field*, 14 January 1954, 69.

114. *Illustrated London News*, 28 August 1954.

115. See for example Tower-Bird, 'Witness this myxomatosis', *Shooting Times*, 23 July 1954, 485.

116. See for example Moore, *Bird of Time*, 137; Page, *Decline of an English Village*, 117; *The Times*, 6 July 1957 and 6 February 1959.

117. Report of the Committee on Cruelty, 437.

118. http://www.wikipedia.org.

119. *Field*, 14 January 1954, 69.

120. See NA MH 56/324. Newspaper and periodical cuttings plus letters from and to various individuals, 1954–5; MAF 131/125. RCC progress report, June 1957.

121. *The Times*, 6 February 1959.
122. *Field*, 14 January 1954, 69.

Chapter 10. Conclusion

1. Moore, *Bird of Time*, 122. The virus actually arrived in 1953.
2. Ibid., 141.
3. Evans, *History of Nature Conservation in Britain*, xxiii.
4. P. D. Lowe, 'Values and institutions in the history of British nature conservation', in A. Warren and F. B. Goldsmith (eds) *Conservation in Perspective* (Chichester: John Wiley, 1983) 329.
5. Ibid.
6. B. W. Clapp, *An Environmental History of Britain since the Industrial Revolution* (London: Longman, 1984) 1.
7. K. Thomas, *Man and the Natural World* (Harmondsworth: Allen Lane, 1983).
8. P. Brimblecombe, *The Big Smoke: A History of Air Pollution in London since Medieval Times* (London: Routledge, 1987); A. Wheeler, *The History of a River and its Fishes* (London: Routledge, 1979).
9. J. Sheail, *Conservation: The British Experience, 1950–1975* (Oxford: Clarendon Press, 1985) 1–2; J. Sheail, *An Environmental History of Twentieth-Century Britain* (Basingstoke: Palgrave, 2002) 235, 271–82.
10. Until the end of the decade, when a major recruitment drive commenced, membership of the Royal Society for the Protection of Birds, which can be regarded as an index for public concern about conservation and the natural environment, remained stagnant at the 1945 level of about 8000. Lowe, 'Values and institutions', 346.
11. Brimblecombe, *The Big Smoke*, 169–73; Clapp, *An Environmental History of Britain*, 50–5; Sheail, *An Environmental History*, 248–50.
12. Sheail, *An Environmental History*, 235–45; Shoard, *The Theft of the Countryside*, 18–19.
13. Moore, *Bird of Time*, 164.
14. J. Sheail, *Pesticides and Nature Conservation: The British Experience* (Oxford: Clarendon Press, 1985) 120–2.
15. J. Burchardt, *Paradise Lost: Rural Idyll and Social Change since 1800* (London: I.B.Tauris, 2002) 169.
16. *Oxford Times*, 21 October 2005.
17. Day, *Poison on the Land*, ix. Day (1899–1983) has been called a 'high Tory patriot of extreme right wing views' and 'a caricature of a reactionary English country gentleman of the old school'. Highly irascible and personally difficult, he briefly occupied many journalistic positions, including with the *Daily Express*, *Field*, and *Country Life*. *Poison on the Land*, which predates *Silent Spring* by five years, deserves recognition as a pioneering contribution to the popular literature on conservation and environmental protection. See www.oxforddnb.com; www.knowuk.co.uk (*Who Was Who*); *The Times*, 6 January 1983.
18. *Field*, 19 August 1954, 348; Hume, *Man and Beast*, 44–5; NA MAF 131/113. MAC (evidence) No. 5. Hume's pronouncements on myxomatosis were not

entirely consistent. On other occasions he described it as 'unpleasant' but also a 'blessing in disguise' in that it led to bumper harvests that convinced enlightened farmers that rabbits did not pay and therefore that trapping could be abandoned. See BBC Written Archives Centre (WAC). WE1/56. Features. 'Myxomatosis'. C. W. Hume to J. H. B. Irving, 11 October 1954.

19. See for example www.dictionary.oed.com.

20. Report of the Committee on Cruelty, 442–3. On the legal position see M. Cooper, *An Introduction to Animal Law* (London: Academic Press, 1987); M. Radford, *Animal Welfare Law in Britain* (Oxford: Oxford University Press, 2001) 13–36; P. Todd, 'The protection of animals acts, 1911–64', in D. Blackman et al. (eds) *Animal Welfare and the Law* (Cambridge: Cambridge University Press, 1989) 13–36.

21. 5 *Hansard* (Lords) 184 (11 November 1953) 285; NA FT1/2. R. Lockley to M. Nicholson, 17 October 1953.

22. NA MAF 131/113. Minutes of fourth meeting of MAC, 20 January 1954. See *Field*, 5 April 1956, 579; E. J. Moynahan, 'Myxomatosis', *Practitioner*, 174 (1955) 709–14.

23. 5 *Hansard* (Lords) 189 (22 November 1954) 1759–62; NA MAF 131/113. Minutes of fifth meeting of MAC, 23 February 1954. See MAF 131/194. Minutes of a Joint Meeting of the MAC and LPAC, 26 July 1954; *Second Report of the Advisory Committee*, 1; R. B. Verney, 'Thoughts on myxomatosis', *Country Landowner*, 5 (1954) 266–7.

24. Report of the Committee on Cruelty, 432. Tower-Bird had no objection to poisoning rats and mice but objected to spreading myxomatosis on the grounds that rabbits had 'a higher level of sensitivity' and could be killed by more humane means, *Shooting Times*, 28 May 1954, 338; *Gamekeeper & Countryside*, October 1954, 4 agreed that otherwise 'humane people seem to approve the use of almost anything against rats'; see also *Field*, 20 January 1955.

25. 5 *Hansard* (Lords) 184 (11 November 1953) 257.

26. *The Times*, 6 and 12 July 1957.

27. *Report of the Advisory Committee on Myxomatosis*, 7–8.

28. C. H. Andrewes, 'Myxomatosis in Britain', *Nature*, 174 (1954) 529.

29. NA MAF 131/113. Paper MAC (evidence) No. 7.

30. 5 *Hansard* (Lords) 189 (29 July 1954) 412.

31. Day, *Poison on the Land*, 61; *Farmers Weekly*, 6 August 1954, 67; *Field*, 19 August 1954, 357; Report of the Committee on Cruelty, 436, 458, 462–3, 472–3, 523–44.

32. T. Gould, *A Summer Plague: Polio and its Survivors* (New Haven: Yale University Press, 1955) 161–2; A. Hardy, *Health and Medicine in Britain since 1860* (Basingstoke: Palgrave, 2001) 155.

33. B. H. Liddell Hart, *History of the First World War* (London: Cassell, 1970 edn) 195–6.

34. R. Garner, *Animals, Politics and Morality* (Manchester: Manchester University Press, 2004 edn) 45–51.

35. Ibid., 71, 80–1.

36. Report of the Committee on Cruelty, 425–545.

37. Woods, *A Manufactured Plague*, 140.
38. www.defra.gov.uk/animalh/bse
39. Woods, *A Manufactured Plague*. See D. Campbell and R. Lee, '"Carnage by computer": the blackboard economics of the 2001 foot and mouth epidemic', *Social and Legal Studies*, 12 (2003) 425–58; D. Campbell and R. Lee, 'How MAF caused the 2002 foot-and-mouth outbreak', in B. Hill (ed.) *The New Rural Economy: Change, Dynamism and Government Policy* (London: Institute of Economic Affairs, 2005) 185–94.
40. *Sunday Times*, 9 April 2006; *The Times*, 6 April 2006.
41. *The Times*, 5, 6 February 2007.
42. In 1956 Kangol Ltd reported that the fur felt hat section of one of its subsidiaries had incurred 'substantial losses' owing to a recession in the men's hat trade related to 'the high price of rabbit fur caused by myxomatosis'. *The Times*, 21 July 1956. See also 31 August 1957.
43. *The Times*, 30 November, 1, 17 December 1966, and 12, 17 and 19 January 1967.
44. www.news.bbc.co.uk (23 and 28 April 2001).
45. www.food.gov.uk/bse; www.alzheimers.org.uk; www.cjd.ed.ac.uk/figures.
46. *Guardian*, 28 February 2007; *Sunday Times*, 9 April 2006; *The Times*, 6 May 2006.
47. *Guardian*, *Sunday Times* and *The Times*, 7 February 2007.
48. C. J. Martin, 'Observations and experiments with *myxomatosis cuniculi* (Sanarelli) to ascertain the suitability of the virus to control the rabbit population', *Fourth Report of the University of Cambridge Institute* (1934–5) 32–3.
49. Fenner and Fantini, *Biological Control*, 141–2.
50. NA MAF 255/216. Third report of C. P. Quick, 13 October 1953.
51. Anon., 'Myxomatosis', *Practitioner*, 173 (1954) 629; *Report of the Advisory Committee on Myxomatosis*, 2; J. N. Ritchie et al., 'Myxomatosis', *Veterinary Record*, 66 (1954) 796–802; *Second Report of the Advisory Committee*, 4.
52. *Daily Telegraph*, 13 November 1953. See also NA MH56/324. Newspaper and periodical cuttings plus letters from and to various individuals, 1954–5. Cass achieved fleeting fame by virtue of an appearance on a television panel game. E. J. Moynahan, 'Myxomatosis: a note', *Guy's Hospital Gazette*, 68 (1954) 391.
53. *Gamekeeper & Countryside*, December 1953, 40–1, September 1954, 216, and October 1954, 5.
54. *Daily Dispatch*, 17 July 1954.
55. *Farmer & Stock-breeder*, 7–8 September 1954, 115, 117.
56. *The Times* (6 and 7 September 1954) ran a story about a dog in Buckinghamshire 'feared to be suffering from myxomatosis'.
57. Moynahan, 'Myxomatosis: a note', 391.
58. See, for example, *The Times*, 17 March 1955.
59. www.news.bbc.co.uk (23 April 2001).
60. *Municipal Journal*, 6 May 1955; NA MH 56/324. See for example S. A. Heald's note, 1 October 1954; N. R. Beattie's minute, 12 January 1955; *The Times*, 9 September 1954.

Bibliography

Archive Sources
BBC Research Central
BBC Written Archives Centre (Caversham, Reading). Files: R19/1560/3, R19/1560/6, WE1/56
British Library. National Sound Archive
BBC Written Archives Centre (Caversham, Reading). Files: R19/1560/3, R19/1560/6, WE1/56
British Library. National Sound Archive
National Archives (Kew). Files: CAB 124/2884. FT 1/1, 1/2, 4/26. HO 45/21811. MAF 105/311, 112/181, 113/367, 131/2, 131/5, 131/10, 131/12, 131/13, 131/14, 131/19, 131/22, 131/23, 131/30, 131/31, 131/37, 131/80, 131/94, 131/95, 131/96, 131/100, 131/101, 131/113, 131/114, 131/115, 131/122, 131/124, 131/125, 131/129, 131/132, 131/136, 131/142, 131/152, 131/154, 131/155, 131/166, 131/167, 131/243, 131/245, 147/73, 168/14, 170/11, 191/143, 191/145, 255/216, 255/597. PREM 11/585. MH 56/324
National Archives of Scotland (Edinburgh). Files: AF 43/200, AF 70/128, AF70/722, AF70/784, AF74/24, AF 74/177, GD 325/1/182

Recorded Interviews
Lord Carrington
Georgina Coleby (née Ottaway)
Cyril Skinner
Stuart Wicks

Official Publications
Annual Reports of Nature Conservancy
Hansard
PP xii 1921 (Cmd. 1401) Game and Heather-Burning (Scotland) Committee (Edinburgh: HMSO, 1921)
PP 1950–1 viii (Cmd. 8266) Report of the Committee on Cruelty to Wild Animals
PP 1846 ix (2) Select Committee on Game Laws
PP 1872 x Select Committee on Game Laws
PP 1873 xii Select Committee on Game Laws

Report of the Select Committee of the House of Lords on Agriculture (Damage by Rabbits) together with the proceedings of the committee and minutes of evidence (London: HMSO, 1937)

Report of the Advisory Committee on Myxomatosis (London: HMSO, 1954)

Second Report of the Advisory Committee on Myxomatosis (London: HMSO, 1955)

Select Committee appointed to consider the Rabbits and Rook Bill [H.L.] (London: HMSO, 1927)

Statutes of the Realm

Statutory Instruments

Statutory Rules and Orders (SR & O)

Secondary Sources

Abbott, W. E. *The Rabbit Pest and the Balance of Nature* (n.p.: Wingen, NSW, 1913)

Adams, R. *Watership Down* (Harmondsworth: Penguin, 1974 edn)

Addison, P. *Now the War is Over: A Social History of Britain* (London: Pimlico, 1995)

Allan, R. M. 'A study of the populations of the rabbit flea *spilopsyllus C cuniculi* (Dale) on the wild rabbit *oryctolagus cuniculus* in the north-east of Scotland', *Proceedings of the Royal Entomological Society of London. Series A. General Entomology*, 31 (1956) 145–52

Allen, W. Gore, *The Reluctant Politician: Derick Heathcoat Amory* (London: Christopher Johnson, 1958)

Ambrosioni, P. 'Giuseppe Sanarelli', in C. C. Gillispie (ed. in chief) *Dictionary of Scientific Biography* (New York: Charles Scribner's Sons, 1980 edn) vol 12, 96–7

Andrewes, C. H. 'Myxomatosis in Britain', *Nature*, 174 (1954) 529–30
    The Natural History of Viruses (London: Weidenfeld & Nicholson, 1967)

Anon., 'Control of rabbit infestation by the use of a virus', *Nature*, 138 (1936) 396–7
    'Rabbit control by virus infestation', *Nature*, 144 (1939) 145
    'Information for the press, for release to morning papers published on Thursday 1 March 1951', Oxford University Zoology (Elton) Library. BAP Reprint Collection (1951)
    'Myxomatosis,' *Practitioner*, 173 (1954) 629
    'News and views,' *Nature*, 174 (1954) 1130
    'Value of myxomatosis', extract from *Rural Research in CSIRO*, 8 (1954) Oxford University Zoology Library, BAP Reprint Collection
    'It's war now to the last rabbit', *Farmers Weekly*, 21 October 1955, 52–3
    'Editorial Note', *Country Life*, 122 (1957) 912

Armitage, A. G. and R. E. Rogers, 'Crops not rabbits', *Agriculture*, 62 (1955) 313–15

Armour, C. J. and H. V. Thompson, 'Spread of myxomatosis in the first outbreak in Great Britain', *Annals of Applied Biology*, 43 (1955) 511–18

Arscott, C. 'Sentimentality in Victorian paintings', in G. Waterfield (ed.) *Art for the People* (Dulwich: Dulwich Picture Gallery, 1994) 65–81

Ayrton, E. *The Cookery of England* (London: Penguin, 1974)

Backhouse, K. M. and H. V. Thompson, 'Myxomatosis,' *Nature*, 176 (1955) 155–6

Barrett-Hamilton, G. E. H. *A History of British Mammals*, 2 vols (London: Gurney & Jackson, 1913)

Bartrip P. W. J. and Fenn, P. T. 'The evolution of regulatory style in the nineteenth century British factory inspectorate', *Journal of Law and Society*, 10 (1983) 201–27

Bath, V. H. 'The rabbit clearance society movement: a new look', *Agriculture* (July 1967) 307–8

Beeton, I. *Mrs Beeton's Book of Household Management* (London: Ward Lock, 1888 edn)
Mrs Beeton's All-About Cookery: With over 2000 Practical Recipes (London: Ward Lock, 1923)
Mrs Beeton's Book of Household Management: A Complete Cookery Book (London: Ward Lock, 1950)

Boag, B. 'Reduction in numbers of the wild rabbit (*oryctolagus cuniculus*) due to agricultural practices and land use', *Crop Protection*, 6 (1987) 347–51

Boden, E. (ed.) *Black's Veterinary Dictionary*, 20th edn (London: A&C Black, 2001)

Bourlière, P. 'Biological consequences due to the presence of myxomatosis', *La Terre at La Vie. Revue d'Histoire Naturelle*, 103 (1956) 131–6

Bowers, J. 'British agricultural policy since the Second World War', *Agricultural History Review*, 33 (1985) 66–76

Briggs, A. *The History of Broadcasting in the United Kingdom*, vol 4, *Sound and Vision, 1945–55* (Oxford: Oxford University Press, 1995)

Brimblecombe, P. *The Big Smoke: A History of Air Pollution in London since Medieval Times* (London: Routledge, 1987)

British Ecological Society, 'Nature conservation and nature reserves', *Journal of Ecology*, 32 (1944) 45–82

British Imperial Calendar and Civil Service List (London: HMSO, various dates)

Brown, P. W. et al. 'Rabbits and myxomatosis in the north east of Scotland', *Scottish Agriculture*, 35 (1956) 204–7

Buckley, W. H. 'Report on a solution of the rabbit problem: cyanide gassing', *Veterinary Journal*, 91 (1935) 210–15
'One man's war against the rabbit', *Field*, 24 October 1957, 724–5

Bull, L. B. and C. G. Dickinson, 'The specificity of the virus of rabbit myxomatosis', *Journal of the Council for Scientific and Industrial Research*, 10 (1937) 291–4

Bull, L. B. and M. W. Mules, 'An investigation of *myxomatosis cuniculi* with special reference to the possible use of the disease to control rabbit populations in Australia', *Journal of the Council for Scientific and Industrial Research*, 17 (1944) 1–15

Burchardt, J. *Paradise Lost: Rural Idyll and Social Change since 1800* (London: I.B.Tauris, 2002)

Burnet, F. M. 'Myxomatosis as a method of biological control against the Australian rabbit', *American Journal of Public Health*, 42 (1952) 1522–26

Burnet, F. M. *Mosquito-Borne Myxomatosis* (Melbourne: CSIRO, 1951)
Viruses and Man (London: Penguin, 1953)

Burnett, J. *Plenty and Want: A Social History of Diet in England, 1815 to the Present Day* (London: Scolar, 1979 edn)

Butler, D. and G. Butler, *British Political Facts 1900–1994* (Basingstoke: Macmillan, 1994 edn)

Button, J. A. 'The insect vector in relation to myxomatosis in Australia', *Journal of Agriculture. West Australia*, 3rd ser. 1 (1952) 819–21, 823, 825, 827–9

Campbell, D. and R. Lee, '"Carnage by computer": the blackboard economics of the 2001 foot and mouth epidemic', *Social and Legal Studies*, 12 (2003) 425–59

'How MAF caused the 2002 foot-and-mouth outbreak', in B. Hill (ed.) *The New Rural Economy: Change, Dynamism and Government Policy* (London: Institute of Economic Affairs, 2005) pp.185–94

Cannadine, D. *The Decline and Fall of the British Aristocracy* (New Haven: Yale University Press, 1990)

Carrington, P. *Reflect on Things Past: The Memoirs of Lord Carrington* (London: Collins, 1988)

Carson, W. G. 'White collar crime and the enforcement of factory legislation', *British Journal of Criminology*, 10 (1970) 383–98

Cartwright, T. J. *Royal Commissions and Departmental Committees in Britain* (London: Hodder & Stoughton, 1975)

Church, B. M. et al. 'Surveys of rabbit damage to wheat in England and Wales, 1950–2', *Plant Pathology*, 2 (1953) 107–12

'Survey of rabbit damage to winter cereals, 1953–4', *Plant Pathology*, 5 (1956) 66–9

Clapp, B. W. *An Environmental History of Britain since the Industrial Revolution* (London: Longman, 1984)

Clarke, P. *Hope and Glory: Britain, 1900–1990* (Harmondsworth: Penguin, 1997)

Cobnut, G. 'Foxes and myxomatosis in Kent', *Oryx: British Mammals*, 3 (1955) 156–7

Cooper, M. *An Introduction to Animal Law* (London: Academic Press, 1987)

Crawley, M. J. 'Rabbits as pests of winter wheat', in R. J. Putnam (ed.) *Mammals as Pests* (London: Chapman Hall, 1989) 168–77

Crowcroft, P. *Elton's Ecologists: A History of the Bureau of Animal Population* (Chicago: University of Chicago Press, 1991)

Davies, W. 'The grasslands of Wales', in R. G. Stapledon (ed.) *A Survey of the Agricultural and Wastelands of Wales* (London: Faber & Faber, 1936) 13–107

Day, J. Wentworth, *Poison on the Land: The War on Wildlife and some Remedies* (London: Eyre & Spottiswood, 1957)

Drakeford, J. *Rabbit Control* (Wykey, Shrewsbury: Swan Hill Press, 2002)

Drummond J. C. and A. Wilbraham, *The Englishman's Food: A History of Five Centuries of English Diet* (London: Cape, 1957 edn)

Durrell, L. *State of the Ark* (London: Bodley Head, 1986)

Editorial, 'Man's concern for his animals', *British Veterinary Journal*, 110 (1954) 445–6

Elton, C. *Animal Ecology* (London: Sidgwick & Jackson, 1927)
  'Research on rodent control by the Bureau of Animal Population', in D. Chitty
  and H. N. Southern (eds) *Control of Rats and Mice* (Oxford: Clarendon Press,
  1954) vol. 1, pp.1–24
Evans, D. *A History of Nature Conservation in Britain* (London: Routledge, 1992)
Fairley, J. S. 'An indication of the food of the fox in Northern Ireland after
  myxomatosis', *Irish Naturalists' Journal*, 15 (1966) 149–51
Farrow, E. P. 'On the ecology of the vegetation of Breckland. II. Factors relating
  to the relative distributions of *calluna*-heath and grass-heath in Breckland', 4
  (1916) 57–64
  'On the ecology of the vegetation of Breckland. III. General effects of rabbits on
  the vegetation', *Journal of Ecology*, 5 (1917) 1–18
  *Plant Life on East Anglian Heaths: Being Observational and Experimental Studies of the
  Vegetation of Breckland* (Cambridge: Cambridge University Press, 1925)
Fenner, F. and B. Fantini, *Biological Control of Vertebrate Pests: The History of Myxoma-
  tosis in Australia* (Wallingford: CABI, 1999)
Fenner, F. and F. N. Ratcliffe, *Myxomatosis* (Cambridge: Cambridge University
  Press, 1965)
Fenner, F. and J. Ross, 'Myxomatosis', in H. V. Thompson and C. King (eds) *The
  European Rabbit: The History and Biology of a Successful Colonizer* (Oxford: Oxford
  University Press, 1994) 205–39
Fenton, E. W. 'The influence of rabbits on the vegetation of certain hill-grazing
  districts of Scotland', *Journal of Ecology*, 28 (1940) 438–49
Findlay, G. M. 'Notes on infectious myxomatosis of rabbits', *British Journal of
  Experimental Pathology*, 10 (1929) 214–19
Fletcher, N. *500 Sixpenny Recipes* (London: Harrap, 1934)
Garner, R. *Animals, Politics and Morality* (Manchester: Manchester University Press,
  2004 edn)
Gathorne-Hardy, A. E. *Autumns in Argyleshire with Rod and Gun* (London: Longmans
  Green, 1900)
Glasse, H. *'First Catch Your Hare': The Art of Cookery Made Plain and Easy* (Totnes:
  Prospect Books, 1995 edn)
Gough H. C. and Dunnett, F. W. 'Rabbit damage to winter corn', *Agriculture*, 57
  (1950) 374–8
Gould, T. *A Summer Plague: Polio and its Survivors* (New Haven: Yale University
  Press, 1955)
Grigson, J. *English Food* (London: Penguin, 1993 edn)
Hardy, A. *Health and Medicine in Britain since 1860* (Basingstoke: Palgrave, 2001)
Harrison Matthews, L. *Man and Wildlife* (London: Croom Helm, 1975)
  Mammals in the British Isles (London: Collins, 1982)
Harting, J .E. *The Rabbit* (London: Longmans, Green & Co., 1898)
Hartley, D. *Food in England* (London: Macdonald, 1954)

Hawkins, K. O. *Environment and Enforcement* (Oxford: Clarendon Press, 1984)

Henriques, R. 'Farmers' ordinary', *Field*, 21 January 1954, 109

Hewson, R. and H. H. Kolb, 'Changes in the number and distribution of foxes (*vulpes vulpes*) killed in Scotland from 1948 to 1970', *Journal of Zoology*, 171 (1973) 345–65

Hobbs, J. R. 'Studies on nature of infectious myoma virus of rabbits', *American Journal of Hygiene*, 8 (1928) 800–39

Holderness, B. *British Agriculture since 1945* (Manchester: Manchester University Press, 1985)

Hope-Simpson, J. F. 'The utilization and improvement of chalk down pastures', *Journal of the Royal Agricultural Society of England*, 100 (1940) 44–9

Howkins, A. *The Death of Rural England: A Social History of the Countryside since 1900* (London: Routledge, 2003)

Hudson, R. 'The rabbit problem: lessons from New Zealand', *Country Life*, 122 (1957) 293

Hume, C. W. *Instructions for Dealing with Rabbits* (London: Universities Federation for Animal Welfare, 1936)
Man and Beast (London: Universities Federation for Animal Welfare, 1962)

Hutter, B. *Compliance, Regulation and Environment* (Oxford: Clarendon Press, 1997)

Ingleby, J. A. 'Sheep, foxes and rabbits', *Scottish Agriculture*, 36 (1956) 69–70

Jarvis, C. S. 'A countryman's notes', *Country Life*, 114 (1953) 1031

Kean, H. *Animal Rights: Political and Social Change in Britain since 1800* (London: Reaktion Books, 1998)

Kessel, J. F. et al. 'Occurrence of infectious myxomatosis in southern California', *Proceedings of the Society for Experimental Biology and Medicine*, 28 (1930–31) 413–14

King, C. *The Natural History of Weasels and Stoats* (London: Christopher Helm, 1989)

Kirkman, A. H. B. *Man versus Rabbit* (London: ULAWS, 1934)

Lever, R. A. 'The diet of the fox since myxomatosis', *Journal of Animal Ecology*, 28 (1959) 359–75

Lever, R. A. et al., 'Myxomatosis and the fox,' *Agriculture*, 64 (1957) 105–11

Lewis, P. *The People's War* (London: Thames Methuen, 1986)

Liddell Hart, B. H. *History of the First World War* (London: Cassell, 1970 edn)

Livestock Division, NZ Department of Agriculture Bulletin no. 284, 'The rabbit pest and its control' (Oxford University, Department of Zoology, BAP reprint, 1947)

Lockie, J. D. 'After myxomatosis: notes on the food of some predatory animals in Scotland', *Scottish Agriculture*, 36 (1956) 65–9

Lockley, R. M. 'My island and our life there. 19. An experiment in the extermination of rabbits – our boat beaten back', *Countryman* (July 1939) 557–71
'Some experiments in rabbit control', *Nature*, 145 (1940) 767–9
'Myxomatosis: a factual survey', *Field*, 9 December 1954, 1174–5
'Has the rabbit a future?' *Countryman*, 53 (1956) 658–60

'The observed effects of myxomatosis on rabbit populations and behaviour and on wild life generally', *La Terre et La Vie. Revue d'Histoire Naturelle*, 3 (4) 1956–57, 211–19

The Island (London: Andre Deutsch, 1969)

The Private Life of the Rabbit (London: Andre Deutsch, 1978 edn)

Lorwin, M. *Dining with William Shakespeare* (New York: Atheneum, 1976)

Lowe, P. D. 'Values and institutions in the history of British nature conservation', in A. Warren and F. B. Goldsmith (eds) *Conservation in Perspective* (Chichester: John Wiley, 1983) 329–52

Lush, D. 'The virus of infectious myxomatosis of rabbits on the chorioallantoic membrane of the developing egg', *Australian Journal of Experimental Biology and Medical Science*, 15 (1937) 131–9

Macadam, I. S. (ed.) *Annual Register of World Events* (London: Longmans, Green & Co., various dates)

Macintyre, D. *Nature Notes of a Highland Gamekeeper* (London: Seeley, Service & Co. Ltd, 1960)

McKendry, M. *The Seven Centuries Cookbook* (New York: McGraw-Hill, 1973)

Marchington, J. *Pugs and Drummers: Ferrets and Rabbits in Britain* (London: Faber & Faber, 1978)

Marks, H. F. and D. K. Britton, *A Hundred Years of British Food and Farming: A Statistical Survey* (London: Taylor & Francis, 1989)

Martin, C. J. 'Observations and experiments with *myxomatosis cuniculi* (Sanarelli) to ascertain the suitability of the virus to control the rabbit population', *Fourth Report of the University of Cambridge Institute* (1934–35) 16–38

'Observations on *myxomatosis cuniculi* (Sanarelli) made with a view to the use of the virus in the control of rabbit plague', *Commonwealth of Australia Council for Scientific and Industrial Research, Bulletin no. 96* (Melbourne, 1936) 28pp

Martin, J. *The Development of Modern Agriculture: British Farming since 1931* (Basingstoke: Macmillan, 1931)

Middleton, A. D. *The Control and Extermination of Wild Rabbits* (Oxford: Bureau of Animal Population, 1940)

Mills, S. 'Rabbits breed a growing controversy', *New Scientist*, 109 (1986) 50–4

Minett, F. C. 'Diseases of animals: prevention and treatment', *Journal of the Royal Agricultural Society of England*, 98 (1937) 246–72

Ministry of Information, *Land at War: The Official Story of British Farming, 1939–1944* (London: HMSO, 1945)

Moore, N. W. 'Rabbits, buzzards and hares: two studies on the indirect effects of myxomatosis', *La Terre et La Vie. Revue d'Histoire Naturelle*, 103 (1956) 220–5

'The past and present status of the buzzard in the British Isles', *British Birds*, 50 (1957) 173–97

The Bird of Time: The Science and Politics of Nature Conservation (Cambridge: Cambridge University Press, 1987)

Moran, Lord, *Winston Churchill: The Struggle for Survival, 1940–1965* (London: Constable, 1966)

Morrison, C. M. 'Second thoughts on rabbits', *Field*, 31 December 1953, 1181

Morton, J. M. (ed.) *Morton's Medical Bibliography* (Aldershot: Scolar, 1991 edn)

Moynahan, E. J. 'Myxomatosis: a note', *Guy's Hospital Gazette*, 68 (1954) 391
'Myxomatosis', *Practitioner*, 174 (1955) 709–14

Muirhead-Thompson, R. C. 'Field studies of the role of *anopheles atroparvus* in the transmission of myxomatosis in England', *Journal of Hygiene*, 54 (1956) 472–7
'The part played by woodland mosquitoes of the genus *aëdes* in the transmission of myxomatosis in England', *Journal of Hygiene*, 54 (1956) 461–71

Munsche, P. *Gentlemen and Poachers: The English Game Laws, 1671–1831* (Cambridge: Cambridge University Press, 1981)

Myers, K. 'Studies in the epidemiology of infectious myxomatosis of rabbits II: field experiments, August–November 1950, and the first epizootic of myxomatosis in the riverine plain of south-eastern Australia', *Journal of Hygiene*, 52 (1954) 47–59

Newby, H. *Country Life: A Social History of Rural England* (London: Weidenfeld & Nicholson, 1987)

Nichols, J. E. 'Rabbit control in Australia: problems and possibilities', *Nature*, 168 (1951) 932–4

Oddy, D. J. *From Plain Fare to Fusion Food: British Diet from the 1890s to the 1990s* (Woodbridge: Boydell, 2003)

Oliver, F. W. 'Some remarks on Blakeney Point, Norfolk', *Journal of Ecology*, 1 (1913) 4–15

Page, R. *The Decline of an English Village* (London: Denis-Poynter, 1974)

Rackham, O. *The History of the Countryside* (London: J&M Dent, 1986)

Radford, M. *Animal Welfare Law in Britain* (Oxford: Oxford University Press, 2001)

Ratcliffe, F. N. *The Rabbit Problem: A Survey of Research Needs and Possibilities* (Melbourne: CSIRO, 1951)

Ratcliffe, F. N. et al. 'Myxomatosis in Australia: a step towards the biological control of the rabbit', *Nature*, 170 (1952) 7–11

Rees, W. A. et al., 'Humane control of rabbits', in D. P. Britt (ed.) *Humane Control of Land Animals and Birds* (Potters Bar: Universities Federation for Animal Welfare, 1985) 96–104

Reid, P. A. 'Some economic results of myxomatosis', *Quarterly Review of Agricultural Economics*, 6 (1953) 93–4

Rhodes, G. *Committees of Inquiry* (London: Allen & Unwin, 1975)

Ritchie, J. N. et al. 'Myxomatosis', *Veterinary Record*, 66 (1954) 796–802

Rivers, T. M. 'Changes observed in epidermal cells covering myxomatous masses induced by virus myxomatosum (Sanarelli)', *Proceedings of the Society for Experimental Biology and Medicine*, 24 (1926–27) 435–7

'Some general aspects of pathological conditions caused by filterable viruses', *American Journal of Pathology*, 4 (1928) 91–124

'Infectious myxomatosis of rabbits: observations on the pathological changes induced by virus myxomatosum (Sanarelli)', *Journal of Experimental Medicine*, 51 (1930) 965–76

Rolls, E. C. *They All Ran Wild* (Sydney: Angus & Robertson, 1969)

Rose, N. *Churchill: An Unruly Life* (London: Simon & Schuster, 1994)

Rose, R. N. *The Field 1853–1953: A Centenary History* (London: Michael Joseph, 1953)

Ross, J. 'Myxomatosis: the natural evolution of the disease', *Symposia of the Zoological Society of London*, 50 (1982) 77–95

Ross, J. and A. M. Tittensor, 'Influence of myxomatosis in regulating rabbit numbers', *Mammal Review*, 16 (1986) 163–8

RSPCA, Annual Report, 1954

Sellers, R. F. 'Possible windborne spread of myxomatosis to England in 1953', *Epidemiology and Infection*, 98 (1987) 119–25

Service, M. W. 'A reappraisal of the role of mosquitoes in the transmission of myxomatosis in Britain', *Journal of Hygiene*, 69 (1971) 105–11

Shanks, P. L. et al. 'Experiments with myxomatosis in the Hebrides', *British Veterinary Journal*, 111 (1955) 25–30

'Myxomatosis in rabbits with special reference to the north of Scotland', *Transactions of the Royal Highland and Agricultural Society of Scotland*, 68 (1957) 1–16

Sheail, J. *Rabbits and their History* (Newton Abbot: David & Charles, 1971)

Conservation: The British Experience, 1950–1975 (Oxford: Clarendon Press, 1985)

Pesticides and Nature Conservation: The British Experience (Oxford: Clarendon Press, 1985)

'The extermination of the muskrat in inter-war Britain', *Archives of Natural History*, 15 (1988) 155–70

'The management of an animal population: changing attitudes towards the wild rabbit in Britain', *Journal of Environmental Management*, 33 (1991) 189–203

An Environmental History of Twentieth-Century Britain (Basingstoke: Palgrave, 2002)

'The mink menace: the politics of vertebrate pest control', *Rural History*, 15 (2004) 207–22

Shoard, M. *The Theft of the Countryside* (London: Temple Smith, 1980)

Simpson, J. *The Wild Rabbit in a New Aspect* (Edinburgh: Blackwood & Sons, 1893)

Sissons, M. and P. French (eds) *Age of Austerity* (London: Hodder & Stoughton, 1963)

Smith, C. J. *Ecology of the English Chalk* (London: Academic Press, 1980)

Smith, M. J. *The Politics of Agricultural Support in Britain* (Aldershot: Dartmouth, 1990)

Southern, H. N. 'If rabbits should disappear', *Country Life*, 115 (8 April 1954) 1024–26

'A second year of myxomatosis', *Country Life*, 118 (1955) 1134–5

'Ecologists are excited by England's "rabbit disease"', *Animal Kingdom*, 59 (1956) 116–23

'Myxomatosis and the balance of nature', *Agriculture*, 63 (1956) 10–13

'The natural control of a population of tawny owls, *Strix Aluco*' *Journal of Zoology*, 162 (1970) 197–285

Southern, H. N. and J. S. Watson, 'Summer food of the red fox (*vulpes vulpes*) in Great Britain: a preliminary report', *Journal of Animal Ecology*, 10 (1941) 1–11

Spry C. and R. Hume, *The Constance Spry Cookery Book* (London: J&M Dent, 1956)

Stamp, L. D. *Man and the Land* (London: Collins, 1973 edn)

Stapledon, R. G. 'Permanent grass', in W. G. R. Paterson (ed.) *Farm Crops. III. Pastures and Hay* (London: Gresham, 1925) pp.74–136

    The Plough-up Policy and Ley Farming (London: Faber & Faber, 1939)

Stead, D .G. *The Rabbit Menace in Australia in 1933 and the Way Out* (Sydney: F. E. Moore, 1932)

Stenton, M. and S. Lees, *Who's Who of British MPs* (Hassocks: Harvester, 1976–81)

Stewart, F. W. 'The fundamental pathology of infectious myxomatosis', *American Journal of Cancer*, 15 (1931) 2013–28

Street, A. G. *Feather Bedding* (London: Faber & Faber, 1954)

Sumption, K. J. and J. R. Flowerdew, 'The ecological effects of the decline in rabbits (*oryctolagus cuniculus* L.) due to myxomatosis', *Mammal Review*, 15 (1985) 151–86

Tansley, A. G. *Britain's Green Mantle: Past, Present and Future* (London: George Allen & Unwin, 1949)

    The British Islands and their Vegetation (Cambridge: Cambridge University Press, 1949)

Tansley, A. G. and R. S. Adamson, 'Studies of the vegetation of the English chalk. III. The chalk grasslands of the Hampshire–Sussex border', *Journal of Ecology*, 13 (1925) 177–223

Thomas, A. S. 'Biological effects of the spread of myxomatosis among rabbits', *La Terre et La Vie. Revue d'Histoire Naturelle*, 103 (1956) 239–42

    'Changes in vegetation since the advent of myxomatosis', *Journal of Ecology*, 48 (1960) 287–306

    'Further changes in vegetation since the advent of myxomatosis', *Journal of Ecology*, 51 (1963) 151–83

Thomas, J. A. 'Why did the Large Blue become extinct in Britain?' *Oryx*, 15 (1980) 243–7

Thomas, K. *Man and the Natural World* (London: Allen Lane, 1983)

Thompson, H. V. 'Myxomatosis in the United Kingdom', Oxford University Zoology Library. BAP Reprint Collection

    'Myxomatosis for rabbit destruction', *Quarterly Review of the Royal Agricultural Society of England* (1953) 15–16

'The grazing behaviour of the wild rabbit, *oryctolagus cuniculus* (l.)', *British Journal of Animal Behaviour*, 1 (1953) 1–4

'Myxomatosis of rabbits', *Agriculture*, 60 (1954) 503–8

'The rabbit disease: myxomatosis', *Annals of Applied Biology*, 41 (1954) 358–66

'Myxomatosis: a survey', *Agriculture*, 63 (1956) 52–3

'The origin and spread of myxomatosis with particular reference to Great Britain', *La Terre et La Vie. Revue D'Histoire Naturelle*, 3–4 (1956–7) 137–52

'Rabbit control in Australia and New Zealand', *Agriculture*, 65 (1958) 388–92

'The rabbit in Britain', in H. V. Thompson and C. King (eds) *The European Rabbit: The History and Biology of a Successful Colonizer* (Oxford: Oxford University Press, 1994) pp.64–107

Thompson H. V. and A. N. Worden, *The Rabbit* (London: Collins, 1956)

Todd, P. 'The protection of animals acts, 1911–64', in D. Blackman et al. (eds) *Animal Welfare and the Law* (Cambridge: Cambridge University Press, 1989) 13–36

Tower-Bird, 'Witness this myxomatosis', *Shooting Times* (23 July 1954) 482, 485

Trout, R. C. et al., 'Recent trends in the rabbit population in Britain', *Mammal Review*, 16 (1986) 117–23

Tubbs, C. R. *The Buzzard* (Newton Abbot: David & Charles, 1974)

Turner, E. S. *All Heaven in a Rage* (London: Michael Joseph, 1964)

Veale, E. 'The rabbit in England,' *Agricultural History Review*, 5 (1957) 85–90

Verney, R. B. 'Thoughts on myxomatosis', *Country Landowner*, 5 (1954) 266–7

Vogel, D. *National Styles of Regulation: Environmental Policy in Great Britain and the United States* (Ithaca: Cornell University Press, 1986)

Wallis, A. 'The flora of the Cambridge district', in J. E. Marr and A. E. Shipley (eds) *Handbook to the Natural History of Cambridgeshire* (Cambridge: Cambridge University Press, 1904)

Watt, A. S. 'Studies in the ecology of Breckland. I. Climate, soil and vegetation', *Journal of Ecology*, 24 (1936) 117–38

'Studies in the ecology of Breckland. II. The origin and development of blow-outs', *Journal of Ecology*, 25 (1937) 91–112

'The effect of excluding rabbits from grassland A (*xerobrometum*) in Breckland, 1936–60', *Journal of Ecology*, 50 (1962) 181–98

Wheeler, A. *The History of a River and its Fishes* (London: Routledge, 1979)

Whetham, E. H. *The Agrarian History of England and Wales vol viii 1914–1918* (Cambridge: Cambridge University Press, 1978)

Who's Who 1991 (London: A & C Black, 1991)

Winter, D. *Death's Men: Soldiers of the Great War* (London: Penguin, 1979)

Winter, M. *Rural Politics* (London: Routledge, 1996)

Woods, A. *A Manufactured Plague: The History of Foot and Mouth Disease in Britain* (London: Earthscan, 2004)

Wynne-Edwards, J. C. 'Common sense about rabbits', *Field*, 5 January 1956, 16

Zweiniger-Bargielowska, I. *Austerity in Britain: Rationing, Controls and Consumption, 1939–1955* (Oxford: Oxford University Press, 2000)

Newspapers and Periodicals

Agriculture

Animal World

Bulletin of the MAFF

Country Life

Countryman

Courier and Advertiser

Daily Dispatch

Daily Express

Daily Mail

Daily Mirror

Daily Telegraph

Essex Chronicle

Farmer

Farmer & Stock-breeder

Farmers Weekly

Field

Gamekeeper & Countryside

Gamekeepers' Gazette

Glasgow Herald

Guardian

Illustrated London News

Kent & Sussex Courier

La Terre et La Vie

Land Worker

Listener

Louth and North Lincolnshire Advertiser

Manchester Guardian

Municipal Journal

Newark Advertiser

News Chronicle

News of the World

Nottingham Evening News

Oxford Times

People

Press & Journal

Quarterly Journal of Forestry

Retford Times

Scottish Farmer

Scottish Field

Scotsman

Shooting Times

Southern Weekly News

Sunday Times

The Times

Times Literary Supplement

Veterinary Record

Western Morning News

West Sussex Gazette

DVD, Audio-Tape and Internet

Rabbits Wanted: Dead or Alive, BBC Television (30 January 1977)

War on the Warren, BBC Home Service broadcast on myxomatosis (14 September 1954)

www.abdn.ac.uk/mammal/estimates2004

www.cjd.ed.ac.uk/figures

www.dictionary.oed.com

www.knowuk.co.uk

www.oxforddnb.com

www.alzheimers.org.uk

www.defra.gov.uk/animalh/bse

www.food.gov.uk/bse

www.news.bbc.co.uk

www.wikipedia.org

Index